ESSENTIALS IN DENTISTRY

ESSENTIALS IN DENTISTRY

(A Student's Manual)

Author

Priyanka Jain BDS MDS MSc
Senior Ex-Lecturer
Department of Conservative Dentistry
and Endodontics
DAV College, Yamuna Nagar, Haryana, India

Ex-Officer
Department of Restorative Dentistry
St George's Hospital, UK

Co-author

Balaram Naik BDS MDS BSc
Professor and Head
Department of Conservative Dentistry
and Endodontics
SDM College of Dental Sciences and Hospital
Sattur, Dharwad, Karnataka, India

Foreword

Ronald S Brown

JAYPEE *The Health Sciences Publishers*

New Delhi | London | Philadelphia | Panama

Jaypee Brothers Medical Publishers (P) Ltd.

Headquarters
Jaypee Brothers Medical Publishers (P) Ltd.
4838/24, Ansari Road, Daryaganj
New Delhi 110 002, India
Phone: +91-11-43574357
Fax: +91-11-43574314
Email: jaypee@jaypeebrothers.com

Overseas Offices

J.P. Medical Ltd.
83, Victoria Street, London
SW1H 0HW (UK)
Phone: +44 20 3170 8910
Fax: +44 (0)20 3008 6180
Email: info@jpmedpub.com

Jaypee-Highlights Medical Publishers Inc.
City of Knowledge, Bld. 237, Clayton
Panama City, Panama
Phone: +1 507-301-0496
Fax: +1 507-301-0499
Email: cservice@jphmedical.com

Jaypee Medical Inc.
The Bourse
111, South Independence Mall East
Suite 835, Philadelphia, PA 19106, USA
Phone: +1 267-519-9789
Email: joe.rusko@jaypeebrothers.com

Jaypee Brothers Medical Publishers (P) Ltd.
17/1-B, Babar Road, Block-B, Shaymali
Mohammadpur, Dhaka-1207
Bangladesh
Mobile: +08801912003485
Email: jaypeedhaka@gmail.com

Jaypee Brothers Medical Publishers (P) Ltd.
Bhotahity, Kathmandu, Nepal
Phone: +977-9741283608
Email: kathmandu@jaypeebrothers.com

Website: www.jaypeebrothers.com
Website: www.jaypeedigital.com

Inquiries for bulk sales may be solicited at: jaypee@jaypeebrothers.com

Essentials in Dentistry (A Student's Manual)

First Edition: **2015**

ISBN: 978-93-5152-539-4

Printed at Sanat Printers, Kundli

Dedicated to

My parents for making me
who I am today

Foreword

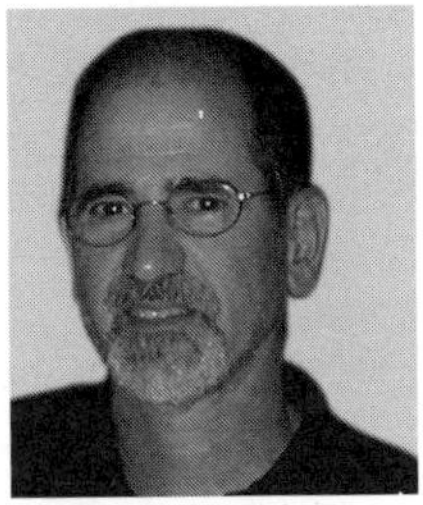

Dr Priyanka Jain has recently completed her text on *Essentials in Dentistry (A Student's Manual)* and it is a must for dentists to add to their libraries. The text is your basic "Dentistry from Soup to Nuts, in a Nutshell". The concept is to provide detailed relevant clinical information in a comprehensive text as a general dental resource for clinical dentistry. For most of us practicing dentists, this text will provide up-to-date information, to answer the most likely clinical questions that come up within our ongoing dental practices.

The text is arranged in thirteen chapters which include: Analgesia and Sedation, Preventive Dentistry, Isolation and Soft Tissue Protection in Dentistry, Dental Radiography, Radiographic Diagnosis of Caries, Radiographic Diagnosis of Periodontitis, Dental Materials, Noncarious Tooth Surface Loss, Treatment of Discolored Teeth, Drug Prescribing and Therapeutics, Drug Interactions, Dental Considerations in Medically Compromised Patients, and Medical Emergencies.

The overall layout of the text, allows the reader to reference many important clinical areas of interest and concern. Furthermore, each area is involved in quickly elucidating these areas of concern in a comprehensive manner. It is my pleasure to recommend this text as a great reference for us all to complete our dental resource libraries.

Dr Jain's background is as a restorative and endodontic dentist with clinical hospital dentistry experience and previous academic experience as a Senior Lecturer at DAV Dental College in Yamuna Nagar, Haryana, India. She received her BDS from Jawaharlal Nehru Medical College, Karnataka University, Dharwad, Karnataka, India, an MDS in Conservative Dentistry and Endodontics from Shri Dharmasthala Manjunatheshwara College, Rajiv Gandhi University, Dharwad, Karnataka, India, and an MSc in Health Care Management from the University of Surrey, Guildford, Surrey (UK).

Ronald S Brown DDS MS Dipl ABOM FACD FICD
Director
Continuing Education at the Howard University
College of Dentistry, Washington DC, USA

Preface

The dental literature already contains a great number of books which, for the most part deal with exclusively, in some depth, with a particular branch or aspect of dentistry. The aim of this book is not to replace these specialist dental texts, but rather to complement them by putting together theory and practical information into a more accessible format. The sole purpose of this book is to enable you, the reader, to gain easy access to the sometimes confusing facts, ideas, opinions, and truth that constitutes clinical dentistry in today's world. This book will provide a consolidated and easily referenceable source of information when it is most needed. The information has been provided with an effort to keep a balance between the amount of detailed information and the depth of knowledge required for the young professional.

Diagnosing and dealing with critical subjects in oral health and management is very important. With reference to information provided in certain chapters, diagnosis can be made more easily as the author has explained subjects (such as caries and periodontitis and their radiological diagnosis) with classifications and diagrams thus simplifying it wherever possible. Advisory notes and cautions are provided to help the practitioner take a more informed decision.

Specific chapters within the book, such as, *Dental Considerations in Medically Compromised Patients,* will, also be of benefit to postgraduates and specialist dental practitioners. Complications may arise during dental treatment of a patient who has a disease of an organ system. The first issue in such cases is that it is often difficult to detect such patients. Subsequently, after determining the disease and the drug treatment available, it is imperative to determine the implications of them on the dental treatment. And as such, it is necessary to determine how to best deal with such complications. The structure and formatting of these chapters provide sufficient information about the drug use and their implications in dentistry. The importance of these diseases and drugs is also outlined and their treatment accordingly in dentistry. All this will prove beneficial for dental practitioners in the primary care sector, and applies to all patients, including the elderly, children and those with special needs.

Common drug interactions that could have serious consequences are identified within the book. It is important that dentists are aware of potential drug interactions. Treating the elderly, pregnant and nursing mothers might differ from treatment for the general adult population. Also, dentists need to be aware of whether any patient is taking other medications as modification to the management of the patient's dental condition might be required in such cases.

We believe that this book will allow the reader to organize and apply knowledge in a practical way and sincerely hope that the readers find this book a useful addition.

Priyanka Jain
Balaram Naik

Acknowledgments

It has taken hundreds of hours and many months in preparing this book which could not have been achieved without the help, support and encouragement of many people. First, our appreciation to the publishers in giving us the opportunity in writing and publishing the book.

We would like to start by thanking Mrs Maryanna Annibale who helped to format and edit the entire book. Maryanna has been a beacon of support and spent many hours including over weekends to work on the book. Thanks also to her husband, Marcus, for his patience with us.

And many thanks to Dr Ronald S Brown for his kind words of introduction in the foreword.

Also whilst there have been many people who have been supportive during this venture, a special mention to Ms Kyleen Bushroe, a friend who has been an immense source of encouragement throughout the process.

Our special thanks to Dr C Bhasker Rao, founder principal and former director, SDM College of Dental Sciences and Hospital, Sattur, Dharwad, Karnataka, India for his continuous encouragement in this endeavor.

Last but not least, I would like to thank Dr Brij Sabharwal, my mentor and Dr Balaram Naik for always being supportive and encouraging throughout the journey.

Contents

Chapter 1 ❖ Analgesia and Sedation **1**
Priyanka Jain

• Local anesthetics *1* • Local anesthetic solution *2* • Drugs used in dental anesthesia *8* • Dental anesthetic techniques *10* • Other anesthetic techniques *12* • Use of local anesthetics *14*

Chapter 2 ❖ Preventive Dentistry **15**
Priyanka Jain

• Purpose *15* • Precautions *15* • Dental caries *16* • Types of caries *21* • Early childhood caries *24* • Caries risk assessment *24* • Preventive dentistry *27* • Caries prevention *27* • Fluoride therapy *29* • Methods of fluoride delivery *31* • Safety and toxicity of fluoride *34* • Prevention *35* • Dental health education *38* • Oral hygiene instructions *41* • Indices *41*

Chapter 3 ❖ Isolation and Soft Tissue Protection in Dentistry **44**
Priyanka Jain

• Methods of isolation *46* • Control of the operating field in different quadrants *52* • Gingival retraction *54* • Surgical methods of gingival retraction *59* • Some clinical applications *62*

Chapter 4 ❖ Dental Radiography **66**
Priyanka Jain

• Biological effects of radiation *68* • Radiation protection and safety *69* • Radiological interpretation and diagnosis *73* • Interpretation and diagnosis *75* • Image analysis *75* • Films used in taking radiographs *78* • Various radiographic techniques *80* • Recent advances in radiographic techniques *83* • Other radiographic techniques in the head and neck *85* • Radiographic errors and artefacts *86*

Chapter 5 ❖ Radiographic Diagnosis of Caries **90**
Balaram Naik, Priyanka Jain

• Radiographic diagnosis and techniques *91* • Caries classification *93* • Interproximal caries *93* • Occlusal caries *97* • Buccal and lingual caries (cervical caries) *98* • Root surface caries (cemental caries) *98* • Recurrent caries/secondary caries *99* • Rampant caries *99* • Radiation caries/drug related caries *99* • Arrested caries *99* • Conditions resembling caries on radiographs *100* • Mach band effect *104*

Chapter 6 ❖ Radiographic Diagnosis of Periodontitis **105**
Priyanka Jain

• Limitations of radiographs *105* • Radiographic techniques for periodontal disease *106* • Normal radiographic anatomy *111* • Radiographic changes seen in periodontal disease *113* • Gingival diseases *114*

Chapter 7 ❖ Dental Materials **119**
Priyanka Jain

• Physical properties of materials *120* • Metallurgical terms *122* • Amalgam *122* • Liners and bases *126* • Dental adhesives *135* • Resins *137* • Pit and fissure sealants *139* • Cavity lining varnish *139* • Intermediate restorative material *139* • Direct filling gold *139* • Indirect restorative materials *140* • Cast metal restorations *142* • Dental porcelain (ceramics) *145* • Porcelain fused to metal *146* • Machined restorations *147* • Dental cements *147* • Miscellaneous *147* • Safety and efficacy *150*

Chapter 8 ❖ Noncarious Tooth Surface Loss **152**
Balaram Naik, Priyanka Jain

• Factors precipitating tooth wear *152* • Types of wear *153* • Tooth wear *155* • Abrasion *156* • Abfraction *158* • Demastication *159* • Resorption *159* • Erosion *159* • Diagnosis *164* • Measurements of wear *165* • Treatment *167* • Prevention *170* • Dentin hypersensitivity *171* • Evaluation strategies *176* • Management of dentine hypersensitivity *178* • Other procedures *182*

Chapter 9 ❖ Treatment of Discolored Teeth **185**
Balaram Naik, Priyanka Jain

• Discolorations *185* • Management of discolorations *190* • Treatment options for discolored teeth *191* • Microabrasion and macroabrasion *191* • Stain removal and prevention by the use of dentifrice *192* • Bleaching *193* • Composite resin restorations *201* • Porcelain veneers *201* • Crowns *201*

Chapter 10 ❖ Drug Prescribing and Therapeutics **203**
Balaram Naik, Priyanka Jain

• Drugs used to control pain *203* • Nonsteroidal anti-inflammatory drugs *205* • Opioid analgesics (narcotics) *210* • Drugs used to treat dental infections *215* • Therapeutic antibiotics *216* • Prophylactic antibiotics *219* • Topical antibiotics *220* • Antifungal agents *222* • Antiviral agents *223* • Agents used to control anxiety *224* • Other drugs used in dentistry *226* • Pregnant patient *227* • Newer drugs of use in dentistry (approved by FDA in 1996) *231*

Chapter 11 ❖ Drug Interactions **234**
Balaram Naik, Priyanka Jain

• Types of drug interactions *237* • Adverse oral and dental effects of drugs *239* • Dental drug reactions *243* • Local anesthesia interactions *247* • Sedative and anxiolytic drugs *250*

Chapter 12 ❖ Dental Considerations in Medically Compromised Patients **255**
Priyanka Jain

• Medical history and assessment *258* • Significant investigations in dentistry *259* • Blood tests for renal function *262* • Blood test for diabetes *262* • Liver function tests and hepatic serology *263* • HIV/AIDS assessment tests *263* • Infective endocarditis, surgically corrected heart disease and antibiotic coverage *265* • Endocarditis prophylaxis recommended *265* • Endocarditis prophylaxis not recommended *265* • Dental procedures for which prophylaxis is recommended *266* • Antibiotic prophylaxis for dental patients with total joint replacements (ADA) *267* • Dental management in specific illnesses *268* • Bleeding disorders *270* • Cardiac problems *271* • Endocrine conditions *276* • Hyper/hypothyroidism *278* • Patient on corticosteroids *278* • Epilepsy *279* • Renal disease *279* • Pulmonary diseases *280* • Chronic obstructive pulmonary disease and tuberculosis *281* • Liver disorders *281* • Infectious diseases *282* • HIV/AIDS *284*

Chapter 13 ❖ Medical Emergencies **286**
Priyanka Jain

• Preparation for emergencies/medical risk assessment *286* • Emergency training *288* • Drugs *291* • Proposed office emergency plan *292* • Handling specific medical emergencies *295* • Airway obstruction *295* • Asthma/bronchospasm/chronic obstructive pulmonary disease *296* • Allergy *298* • Anaphylaxis *299* • Accidental anesthetic overdose *300* • Acute adrenal insufficiency *302* • Cardiac emergencies angina pectoris (chest pain) *303* • Myocardial infarction (heart attack) *304* • Heart failure/sudden cardiac arrest *306* • Diabetes *306* • Hypoglycemia *307* • Hyperglycemia/diabetic ketoacidosis *308* • Syncope (fainting) *309* • Seizures *311* • Transient ischemic attack/cerebrovascular accidents (stroke) *313* • Hyperventilation *315* • Respiratory arrest *315*

Index *317*

Symbols and Abbreviations

>	greater than
<	less than
1/4	one-fourth
AAC	antibiotic associated colitis
ACP	amorphous calcium phosphate
ADH	antidiuretic hormone
AED	automatic external defibrillator
Ag	antigen
AIDS	acquired immuno-deficiency syndrome
APF	acidulated phosphate fluoride
ARF	acute renal failure
ASA	American Society of Anesthesiology
AST	aspartate transaminase
bd	twice daily
BDA	British Dental Association
Bis-GMA	bisphenol A glycidylmethacrylate
BP	blood pressure
CAT	caries risk assessment tool
CDC	center for disease control
CEJ	cemento-enamel junction
CNS	central nervous system
CO_2	carbon dioxide
COPD	chronic obstructive pulmonary disease
CPP	casein phosphopeptide
CPR	cardiopulmonary resuscitation
CRF	chronic renal failure
CT	computed tomography
CTZ	chemoreceptor trigger zone
DEJ	dentino enamel junction
DH	dentinal hypersensitivity
DPT	dental panoramic tomogram (politically correct: OPT/OPG)
DSR	digital subtraction radiography
DVT	digital volume tomography
ECC	early childhood caries
EDTA	ethylene diamine tetra-acetic acid
e.g.	for example
EH	enamel hypoplasia
EMLA	eutectic mixture of prilocaine and lidocaine
FDA	Food and Drug Administration
Fe	iron
FOTI	fiber optic transillumination
g	gram
GABA	gamma aminobutyric acid
GI	gastrointestinal
GTN	glyceryl trinitrate
H_2O_2	hydrogen peroxide
Hb	hemoglobin
HBeAg	hepatitis B e antigen (high-risk marker)
HBsAg	hepatitis B surface antigen
HCl	hydrochloric acid
Hep B/C	hepatitis B/C
Hg	mercury
HIV	human immunodeficiency virus
HSV	herpes simplex virus
IDB	inferior dental block
i.e.	that is
IE	infective endocarditis
Ig	immunoglobulin (e.g. IgA, IgG, etc.)

i.m./IM	intramuscular
INR	international normalized ratio
IOPA	intraoral periapical
i.v.	intravenous
Kg	kilogram
L	liter
LA	local anesthetic
LB	*lactobacillus*
LFT	left ventricular failure
mg	milligram
MI	myocardial infarction
MIH	molar incisor hypo-mineralization
MNB	mandibular nerve block
MRI	magnetic resonance imaging
MRSA	methicillin resistant *Staphylococcus aureus*
MS	*Streptococcus mutans*
N_2O	nitrous oxide
Na	sodium
NaF	sodium fluoride
NGF	nerve growth factor
NIH	National Institute of Health
NICE	National Institute of Clinical Excellence
NSAID	nonsteroidal anti-inflammatory drug
od	once daily
OH	oral hygiene
OHI	oral hygiene instruction
OVD	occlusal vertical dimension
PDL	periodontal ligament
PMMA	polymethylmethacrylate
PO	per oral
PSA	posterior superior alveolar nerve block
PT	prothrombin time
PTT	partial thromboplastin time
qds	four times daily
QLF	quantitative light induced fluorescence
Rx	treatment
RVF	right ventricular failure
SARS	severe acute respiratory syndrome
TB	tuberculosis
TCA	tricyclic antidepressants
tds	thrice daily
TIA	transient ischemic attack
μm	micrometer
yrs	years
ZOE	zinc oxide eugenol

CHAPTER 1

ANALGESIA AND SEDATION

Priyanka Jain

LOCAL ANESTHETICS

Introduction

Local anesthetics are chemical agents that produce loss of sensation to pain in a specific area of the body without the loss of consciousness by the depression or excitation in the nerve endings. In clinical dental practice, a localized loss of pain is desired. Although dental analgesia and dental anesthesia are used synonymously in dentistry, local analgesia is more accurate. Local anesthesia can be achieved by a number of different mechanisms including the use of neurolytic agents in addition to the traditional agents. However, in clinical dental practice, only reversible local anesthetic agents are used. These agents block the nerve conduction impulses reversibly and can be administered via a spray, drops or an injection. The most common route of administration is by injection to the area requiring numbing. This works as the anesthetic selectively targets nerves to block them transmitting pain signals and sending them to the brain.

The use of reversible local anesthetic chemical agents is the most preferred method of achieving pain control in dental practice. Some ideal properties of a local anesthetic agent are:

- Reversible action
- Nonirritant
- Should not produce any secondary local reactions like allergies
- Should have rapid onset
- Potent in nature
- Should have sufficient penetrating properties
- Should be stable in its form
- Should not interfere with the healing of local tissues
- Nonaddictive
- Suitable duration of action
- No systemic toxicity
- Sterilizable without the loss of properties.

Classification

Local anesthetics can be classified according to their (Table 1.1):

Chemical Structure

- Amides
- Esters.

Duration of Action

- Short acting
- Intermediate acting
- Long acting.

Mechanism of Action of Local Anesthetics

All local anesthetics agents used in dentistry work by obstructing the exchange in Na^+ permeability which is essential for the initial phases of a neuronal action potential. In general terms, these agents prevent nerve conduction by obstructing the depolarization which is effected by the influx of sodium ions. In the axon wall there are numerous pores which allow the ionic changes (influx of sodium ions). Local anesthetics (LA) cations block these channels. As a result, the nerve loses the capacity to create the impulse and the patient loses the sensation in the area supplied by the nerve.

LOCAL ANESTHETIC SOLUTION

Constituents

- *Vasoconstrictor:* This is added to delay the removal of the anesthetic by decreasing the blood flow. A vasoconstrictor has the following

Table 1.1 Various types of local anesthetics used in dentistry

Local anesthetic	*Type*	*Duration of action*
Lidocaine	Amide	Intermediate
Prilocaine	Amide	Intermediate
Mepivacaine	Amide	Intermediate
Bupivacaine	Amide	Long acting
Etidocaine	Amide	Long acting
Articaine	Amide with an ester side chain	Intermediate
Procaine	Ester	Short acting

advantages—(a) longer duration of action of the local anesthetic agent (b) reduces bleeding at the injection site and (c) has reduced systemic effects. The most commonly used vasoconstrictors in dental anesthetic agents are epinephrine (adrenaline) and octapressin (felypressin). Certain chemicals are included in local anesthetic to protect the vasoconstrictor drug from being broken down. Contraindications of local anesthesia with vasoconstrictor include diabetics (as they increase the blood glucose level by counteracting the action of Insulin), hypertensive patients, cardiac patients (as they produce tachycardia and increased heart rate), pregnancy (as they can cause uterine contractions and may sometimes cause abortion), extraction of teeth with chronic peri apical sepsis (as they decrease the blood flow to the tissues which may lead to dry socket), and hyperthyroidism.

- *Reducing agent:* This prevents the oxidation of the vasoconstrictor and acts by competing with the vasoconstrictor for the oxygen available in the solution. Sodium metabisulphite (0.5 mg/mL) is most commonly used.
- *Fungicide:* Thymol is used as a fungicide. Sodium hydroxide is included to enhance the numbing effect of the drug.
- *Preservative:* This helps to prolong the shelf life of the solution. They are bacteriostatic in nature. The typical shelf life of an anesthetic agent without preservative is approximately 18 months to 2 years. Methylparaben (1 mg/mL) is added as a preservative to articaine.

Structure

The injectable local anesthetics used in dentistry have a common core structure consisting of:

- Hydrophilic amino terminal
- Intermediate chain
- Lipophilic aromatic terminal.

The combination of hydrophilic and lipophilic properties is essential in one molecule for the local anesthetic to be effective (Fig. 1.1). The hydrophilic portion of the anesthetic consists of a substituted secondary or tertiary amine. This hydrophilic property (solubility in water) is essential to allow for the dissolution in a solvent to permit injection and to allow sufficient penetration through the interstitial fluid after injection. The lipophilic part of the anesthetic molecule is an aromatic residue that is essential for its ability to penetrate fatty tissue such as lipid sheaths of nerves to reach its site of action.

The intermediate chain consists of either an amide or ester linkage. This allows the spatial separation of the hydrophilic and the lipophilic components of the molecule.

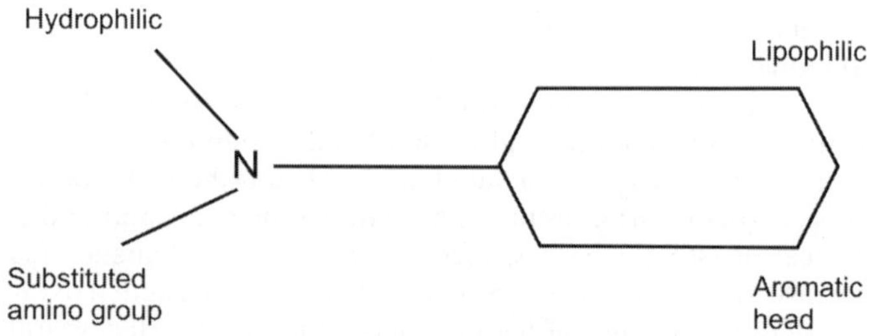

Fig. 1.1 Structure of a local anesthetic molecule

Differences of Esters and Amides

All local anesthetics are weak bases. Chemical structure of the local anesthetic molecule have an amine group on one end connected to an aromatic ring on the other and an amine group on the right side (Fig. 1.2). The amine end is hydrophilic (soluble in water) and the aromatic head is lipophilic (soluble in lipids). Therefore, a local anesthetic molecule can either have an amide group (Fig. 1.3) or an ester group (Fig. 1.4).

The older agents like procaine and cocaine were ester based but are no longer used due to their unwanted side effects of allergic reactions.

Different drugs have different proportions of hydrophilic and lipophilic components. These differences modify the characteristics and/or the properties of the anesthetic agents (Table 1.2).

Factors Affecting the Reaction of Local Anesthetics

Lipid Solubility: All local anesthetics are weak bases. Increasing the lipid solubility leads to faster nerve penetration and increases the onset of action. Onset of action is also dependent upon the proximity of the site of injection to the nerve to be anesthetized and the diameter of the nerve fibers. Thin fibers are anesthetized more rapidly as compared to thick fibers possibly because the nodes of Ranvier are closer together.

pH Influence: pH of the local anesthetics ranges from 7.6 to 8.9. Decrease in the pH shifts the equilibrium towards the ionized form of the local anesthetics thus delaying the onset of action.

Duration of Action: This is dependent on the rate of diffusion along a concentration gradient away from the site of injection. Lower vasodilator activity of a local anesthetic leads to slower absorption and longer duration of action (Table 1.3). Other factors affecting the duration and depth of the local anesthesia can be:

- *Patient factors:* Children with problems of pediatric anesthesia, individuals with learning difficulties may be uncooperative and communication may be challenging, or patients who are highly

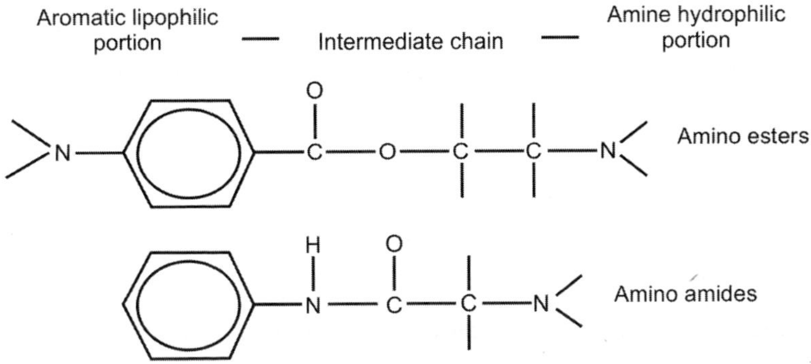

Fig. 1.2 Chemical structure of local anesthetics

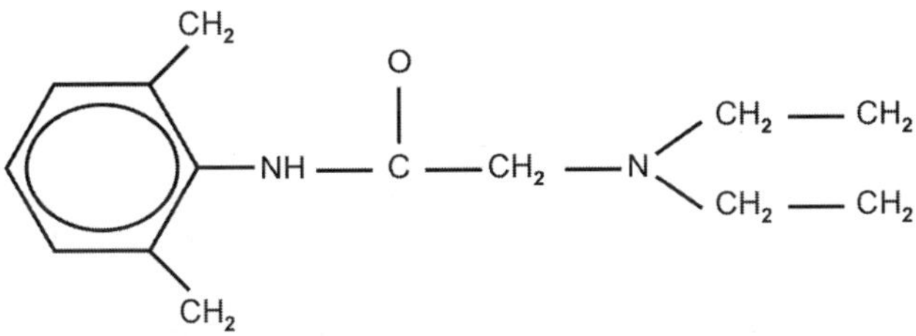

Fig. 1.3 Local anesthetic molecule with the amide link

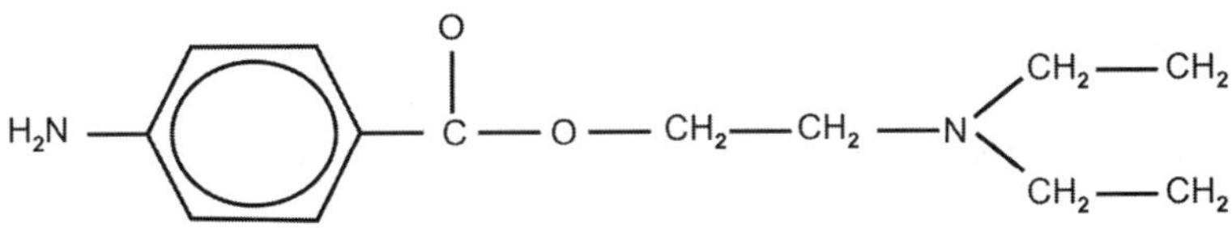

Fig. 1.4 Local anesthetic molecule with the ester link

Table 1.2 Differences between amide and ester groups of local anesthetics

Amide	*Ester*
• Amide link between intermediate chain and aromatic ring	• Ester link between intermediate chain and aromatic ring
• Metabolized in the liver by amidase enzymes	• Metabolized in the plasma through pseudocholinesterases and in the liver by lipase enzyme
• Soluble in the solution	• Stable in the solution
	• Causes allergic reactions

Table 1.3 Some commonly used local anesthetics in dentistry

Anesthetic	*Onset*	*Duration (with epinephrine) in minutes*
Procaine	Slow	45–90
Lidocaine	Rapid	120–240
Bupivacaine	Slow	4–8 hours

Table 1.4 Maximum recommended doses

Drug	*Maximum dose*	*Equivalent cartridges*
Lidocaine (lignocaine)	4.4 mg/kg	6–7 cartridges of 2.2 mL
Prilocaine	6 mg/kg	For 3% prilocaine about 5–6 cartridges of 2.2 mL For 4% prilocaine about 4 cartridges of 2.2 mL
Articaine	7 mg/kg	4 cartridges of 2.2 mL

anxious and needle phobic. In such patients there may be high levels of autonomic activity with increased propensity to arrhythmias and vasovagal responses.

- *Factors related to the type of technique:* Type of technique (infiltration or a nerve block), volume of solution and the accuracy of technique.

Effects on Other Tissues Including Toxicity: The functions of lipid containing organs and tissues such as the brain and heart may be affected by high levels of local anesthetics. Toxicity is the peak circulation levels of local anesthetics. Levels of local anesthetics administered to patients are varied according to age, weight and health. Some common toxic effects are light headedness, shivering or twitching, seizures, hypotension and numbness (Table 1.4).

Rate of Degradation: Amide local anesthetics are broken down by hepatic dealkylation and hydrolysis and excreted in the urine. Esters are metabolized by esterases.

Failure of Anesthesia

Failure to achieve profound analgesia during treatment procedure may be related to a variety of factors, like:

- Inaccurate anatomic placement of the anesthetic solution
- Injecting too little solution
- Allowing insufficient time for the solution to diffuse and take effect

- Injecting into infected or inflamed tissues
- Using an outdated or improperly stored anesthetic solution.

A local anesthetic should not be injected in inflamed tissues because of the risk of spreading the infection and the increased probability of achieving less than effective anesthesia due to the low pH within the infected tissue which maintains the ionized and the nonlipid soluble state of the anesthetic.

Complications of Local Anesthetics

These include both local and systemic effects.

Local Complications

Spread of Infection: Infection may spread into the tissues due to the needle passing through a contaminated tissue or the needle being contaminated before use.

Hematoma: Damage of a blood vessel by the tip of the needle may cause bleeding into the tissues. Small hematomas (in sulcus) are of little significance but significant bleeding may produce swelling and cause pain and trismus.

Needle Fracture: The chances are less likely due to the disposable use of needles these days.

Needle Stick Injury: The risk can be minimized by needle sheathing or the use of safe syringes.

Trismus: This occurs after inferior dental (ID) block and is attributed to damage in the medial pterygoid muscle. Either injection given too low or faster rate of deposition are the common factors. Management usually involves reassurance and encouragement to open the mouth slowly. If needed, antibiotics can be prescribed.

Blockage of the Facial Nerve: If the injection is given in close proximity to the facial nerve, a motor blockage causing temporary paralysis of the facial muscles may occur. The effect can last for 1–2 hours. In these cases, the desired branch of the trigeminal nerve will not be anesthetized.

Nerve Damage: Very rarely, the tip of the needle may pierce or hit a nerve bundle during injection causing an immediate electric shock like sensation to the patient. A complete return to normal sensation occurs soon.

Systemic Complications

Syncope: This is the most common systemic complication. It can be minimized by administering LA with patient in a supine position.

Allergy: Some drugs may react with the anesthetic solution that causes allergies to the patient. For this, dentists should be careful keeping the medical history of the patient in mind.

Regional Infection: Infection can spread within the perioral tissues through planes of the head and neck by the passage of the needle through an infected area.

Cardiovascular Risk/Collapse: This may be related to stress in a susceptible patient (patients with angina pectoris, previous myocardial infarction or who have had previous cardiac surgery or circulatory dysfunction like cardiac failure. Excessive amounts of LA, faster delivery of the anesthetic solution and lack of aspiration can be contributing factors. The maximum safe dose of the lidocaine should be halved in such patients.

Liver Disease: Patients with reduced hepatic function may exhibit an increased rate of metabolism of the amide type of local anesthetics. Dosage levels should therefore be adjusted for these patients.

Methemoglobinemia: This is caused by a metabolite of prilocaine which reduces their oxygen delivering capacity and results in hypoxia. This is a rare complication.

DRUGS USED IN DENTAL ANESTHESIA

The drugs used for anesthesia in dentistry are (Table 1.5).

Lidocaine

In 1940, the first modern local anesthetic agent was lidocaine, trade name xylocaine. Used for blocks and infiltrations; however, effectiveness of analgesia is limited and of brief duration. This belongs to the amide class

Table 1.5 Dilutions of the local anesthetic molecule

Dilution of local anesthetics
The dilution of an LA agent as 2% means that there is 2 grams (2000 mg) of LA agent in 100 mL of solution. 0.2% means 2 g/100 mL and 0.2% means 2000 mg/100 mL.
Dilution of vasoconstrictor
1:1000 means that there is 1 g (1000 mg) of vasoconstrictor in 1000 mL (1 L) of the solution or 1.0 mg/mL of the solution.

and causes little allergic reaction. The addition of 1:80,000 epinephrine prolongs effectiveness to over 90 minutes.

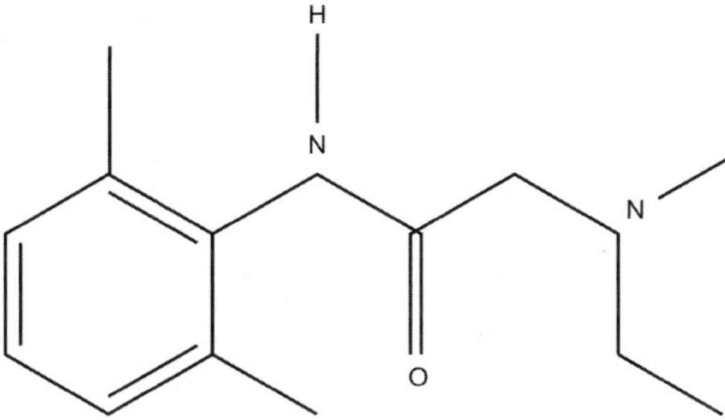

2 – (diethylamide) – N – (2, 6 – dimethylphenyl) acetamide monohydrochloride "Lidocaine"

Prilocaine (Citanest)

This is less toxic in higher doses than lidocaine because of the small vasodilatory activity. Used for blocks and infiltrations, effective analgesia over 90 minutes, but predisposes to methemoglobinemia. It should be avoided in pregnancy.

Articaine (Septocaine)

This is the newest local anesthetic drug approved by the FDA in 2000. Its half-life is less than about one-fourth of lidocaine. This is used with a vasoconstrictor and enters the blood barrier smoothly. It is currently recommended for infiltration use only as it has rapid onset (<2 minutes) with exceptional ability to penetrate dense mandibular cortical bone. It is therefore ideal where blocks are contraindicated.

Bupivacaine (Marcaine)

This drug produces long anesthetic affect and is used for blocks and infiltrations where up to 8 h of anesthesia is required. This is available as 0.5% solution with a vasoconstrictor (Table 1.6).

Table 1.6 Local anesthetic solutions

Duration	*Solution*	*Infiltration (pulpal)*	*Nerve block (pulpal)*	*Soft tissue duration*
Short duration – plain	• 2% lidocaine HCl	5 m	Not indicated	2 h
	• Mepivacaine HCl 3%	20–30 m	45–65 m	2–3 h
	• Prilocaine HCl 4%	10–15 m	45–65 m	3–4 h
Normal duration with vasoconstrictor	• Articaine HCl 4% with epi 1:100,000	60–75 m	Up to 120 m	3–5 h
	• Articaine HCl 4% with epi 1:200,000	60–75 m	Up to 120 m	3–5 h
	• Lidocaine HCl 2% with epi 1:50,000	55–65 m	80–90 m	3–5 h
	• Lidocaine HCl 2% with epi 1:100,000	55–65 m	80–90 m	3–5 h
	• Prilocaine HCl 4% with epi 1:200,000	35–45 m	50–70 m	3–6 h
Long duration	• Bupivacaine HCl 0.5% with epi 1:200,000	Up to 7 h	Up to 7 h	Up to 12 h

Abbreviations: epi, epinephrine; m, minutes; h, hours

DENTAL ANESTHETIC TECHNIQUES

There are various types of dental anesthetic techniques used. These are mentioned in brief below:

Infiltration

The anesthetic solution is deposited at/near the apex of the tooth and diffuses through the bone to affect the peripheral nerves and those nerves serving the periodontal ligament, adjacent bone and soft tissues. This may be used for minor procedures such as fillings.

Regional/Nerve Block

This is a common form of local dental anesthesia which blocks the reception of pain for one quadrant of the mouth at a time. This type of block is typically given in the buccal surface cheek. The anesthetic solution is deposited around a nerve trunk and causes anesthesia to tissues within the distribution of the nerve peripheral to the point of administration (Table 1.7). The different types of nerve blocks used in dentistry are:

- Nasopalatine
- Greater palatine

Table 1.7 Types of nerve blocks

Type of anesthesia	*Tissues anesthetized*	*Comments*
Inferior dental nerve block	• Mandibular teeth (including their pulp and periodontium), buccal gingivae from premolars to midline • Lower lip • Anterior two-thirds of the tongue • Floor of the mouth • Lingual gingivae	The buccal gingivae and the sulcus in the molar region are not anesthetized fully and require separate infiltration of the long buccal nerve. The needle is introduced from premolars of the opposite side and inserted slightly above the occlusal plane lateral to the pterygomandibular raphae
Mental nerve block	• Mandibular first premolar to central incisor (including the pulp and the periodontium) • Lip, chin and adjacent sulcus and cheek of the above mentioned teeth	Provides effective soft tissue analgesia. A lingual infiltration may be given for extractions
Posterior superior alveolar	• Upper molars	Rarely indicated technique. The anesthetic solution is deposited distal to the maxillary second molar
Infraorbital	• Upper lip, cheek, side of the nose and lower eyelid • Buccal gingivae and sulcus from midline to premolar region • Incisors, canine and premolars	The needle is aligned parallel to the long axis of the premolars while injecting
Greater palatine	• Palatal mucoperiosteum of the canine and posterior to it	This injection is painful. Only a few drops need to be introduced very slowly for anesthesia. The anesthetic solution is deposited in the compressible area of the hard palate between the midline and the gingival margin of the teeth
Nasopalatine	• Palatal mucoperiosteum of the anterior hard palate related to canines and incisors	This injection is also painful. A very small amount of anesthetic solution is required. Immediate blanching of the area is noted

- Inferior alveolar
- Posterior superior
- Mental nerve block
- Infraorbital.

Intraosseous

An injection of local anesthetic is given directly into the osseous (bone) structure of the tooth. This provides profound single tooth analgesia.

Intraligamentary

The anesthetic solution is deposited along the periodontal membrane of individual teeth (to be anesthetized). This technique has the advantage of rapid onset and specific analgesia to isolated teeth and is a useful adjunct to conventional local anesthesia. The disadvantages include post injection discomfort due to temporary extrusion.

OTHER ANESTHETIC TECHNIQUES

Topical Anesthetics

Benzocaine (10–20%), eugenol, and forms of xylocaine (5–10%) are used topically to numb various areas before injections or other minor procedures. They produce their effect by acting on the free nerve endings (spray, gel or ointment). Ice bags can also be used for this purpose and act by means of refrigerant action on the surface of the mucous membrane. Another example is ethyl chloride.

General Anesthesia

Drugs such as midazolam, ketamine, propofol and fentanyl are used to put the patient in a twilight sleep or render them completely unconscious and unaware of pain.

Conscious Sedation

Conscious sedation is defined as a technique in which the use of a drug or drugs produces a state of depression of the central nervous system enabling treatment to be carried out, but during which verbal contact with the patient is maintained. The patient is able to retain their protective airway reflexes, and is able to respond to and understand verbal communication. It is a means to control an unmanageable child where all other means of restraint have failed. Patients should be carefully selected and medically pre-assessed and written consent must be obtained. The principal methods currently in use are inhalation, intravenous and oral although other methods are occasionally used.

Inhalation Sedation

A titrated mixture of up to 70% nitrous oxide may be administered. Clinical monitoring of patient color, respiration and pulse is required. It can be combined with an oral anxiolytic drug. Adult patients need not be accompanied home afterwards. This is the technique of choice in children felt to be candidates for sedation with mild and moderate anxiety and anxiety related gagging reflex. Works best in children aged 5 and above. Nitrous oxide (N_2O), also known as "laughing gas", easily crosses the alveoli of the lung and is dissolved into the passing blood, where it travels to the brain, leaving a dissociated and euphoric feeling for most patients. Nitrous oxide is used in combination with oxygen. Often (especially with children) a sweet-smelling fruity scent similar to an auto scent is used with the gas to inspire deep inhalation. The most common delivery system for this is the Quantiflex system. Written and informed consent is required for inhalational sedation. Advantages of conscious sedation include safe to use with minimal side effects, extremely useful in fearful, uncontrollable patients and provide comfortable and efficient dental treatment without compromising on quality.

Contraindications to Inhalational Sedation Include: These could be local or systemic. This technique cannot be used in patients with nasal obstruction, intolerance to mask, cold. Systemic contraindications include severe respiratory disease or mental/physical handicap.

Intravenous Sedation

Various intravenous sedatives have been used in the past. Titrated benzodiazepine is used to achieve anesthesia. Pulse oximetry and blood pressure monitoring is a must. Facilities must be available to administer oxygen or ventilation if needed.

It is relatively simple in comparison to general anesthesia. The technique is fast with few adverse effects and patient remains conscious throughout the procedure. Patients must be recovered appropriately and be accompanied by a responsible adult. Other intravenous agents used include a mixture of pentobarbitone, pethidine, hyoscine, and methohexitone. Advantages of intravenous sedation include sedation without loss of consciousness, verbal contact maintained with the patient during the procedure, and anterograde amnesia of 20–30 minutes duration.

USE OF LOCAL ANESTHETICS

During Pregnancy

Any adverse drug interactions during pregnancy may affect either the mother or the fetus. Doses of dental local anesthetics are relatively small and are unlikely to cause any complications during pregnancy. All local anesthetics cross the placenta to some degree. Prilocaine has been found in highest concentration in the fetal circulation following its injection with bupivacaine as the lowest and lidocaine in between. Felypressin can cause uterine contractions; therefore it is best avoided in pregnancy although the dosage used in dental local anesthetics is very low to cause any unlikely effects. Lidocaine with epinephrine is most commonly used for pregnant patients. The anesthetics should have minimum epinephrine concentrations. Acetaminophen is the best analgesic used in pregnancy for dental patients. Penicillin, cephalosporin and erythromycin are the antibiotics of choice if needed. In the first trimester of pregnancy, radiographs should be limited to a minimum and performed only if deemed absolutely necessary.

In Children

Maximum recommended doses of local anesthetics are based on the weight of the child (expressed as mg/kg of the body weight). For obese children, maximum doses are calculated on the basis of ideal body weight and not the true body weight.

CONCLUSION

The level of anesthesia can be controlled to regulate how long the pain block lasts for as well as the level of numbness. This is meticulously controlled by concentration, amount administered as well as the actual solutions used in the anesthetic.

BIBLIOGRAPHY

1. Aitkenhead Ar, Rowbotham DJ, Smith G. Textbook of Anesthesia, 4th edn. Churchill Livingstone, Edinburgh, 2001.
2. Cantlay K, Wiilaimson S, Hawkings J. Anesthesia for Dentistry. Continuing Education in Anesthesia, Critical Care and Pain. 2005;5:3.
3. Meechan JG, Robb ND, Seymour RA. Pain and Anxiety Control for the Conscious Dental patient. Oxford University Press, Oxford, 1998.
4. Poswillo D. General anesthesia, sedation and resuscitation in dentistry. Report of an Expert Working Party for the Standing Dental Advisory Committee. London: Department of Health, 1990.
5. Robinson PD, Pitt Ford TR, Mc Donald F. Local anesthesia in dentistry. Wright, Oxford, 2000.
6. The Royal College of Anesthetists. Standards and Guidelines for General Anesthesia for Dentistry. London: The Royal College of Anesthetists, 1999.

CHAPTER **2**

PREVENTIVE DENTISTRY

Priyanka Jain

INTRODUCTION

The word prevention has a Latin origin meaning "to anticipate". Preventive dentistry is that area of dentistry that focuses on the procedures and practices that help people to prevent the beginning or progression of oral disease like caries. It includes at-home dental care performed by patients, as well as dental care and education by professional dental staff in the office or clinic.

Operative dentistry can most certainly be improved by anticipating the problems that may reduce the effectiveness of restorative therapy. Like most other health sciences, modern day dentistry has also assumed a role of prevention rather than intervention. We promote periodic oral examination as a means of prevention.

PURPOSE

Preventive dentistry includes two aspects of dental care which are both performed to help patients to avoid any new dental disease or to catch it in its early, more treatable stages. Firstly, it is the *oral hygiene* care performed by the patient at home. Also what is done by the dental staff in their offices to help patients maintain healthy teeth and gums is also considered a part of preventive dentistry. In either case, the objective is to stop the development or progression of oral disease or to find it at an early stage. Dental health professionals most often look for early signs of periodontal disease, dental decay, and other changes in the soft tissue of the mouth.

PRECAUTIONS

Preventive dentistry should always be prescribed and not harm patients when done correctly. At times, dentists do need to take precautions when someone has a medical condition that would be affected by some of the procedures. Dentists need to be aware of certain medical conditions, such as heart diseases, which may need to be treated with prophylactic antibiotics.

Allergies to any of the medications or materials used in preventive dentistry are rare. The most important part in the treatment of any disease is its prevention. The loss of tooth in most instances is the result of the cumulative effect of a series of preventable disorders that in effect were not prevented. In the final analysis, all dental treatment can be considered preventive in nature. The ultimate goal of preventive dentistry is to have a healthy mouth throughout one's lifetime. In order to achieve this, any new or recurring diseases must be prevented and treated.

DENTAL CARIES

Dental caries is an infectious microbiologic disease of the teeth that results in localized dissolution and destruction of the calcified tissues (*Sturdevant*). *Dental caries* is an infectious communicable disease resulting in the destruction of the tooth structure by acid forming bacteria found in dental plaque, in the presence of sugar (*National Institute of Health*, USA 2002). Dental caries, better known as "tooth decay", is the disease process that leads to the loss of tooth mineral and eventually, cavitation of the tooth surface ("cavity"). It is a diet-bacterial, infectious, transmissible, oral disease. Caries is a dynamic process, where there is an imbalance between mineral loss and gain. Overtime, if there is a net mineral loss, it leads to cavitation. Studies of incipient lesions have shown that in the same lesion, some areas can be demineralizing while some remineralizing (surface layer—remineralizing; subsurface—demineralizing).

Dependency Factors Necessary for Dental Caries

Dental caries is a sugar-dependent infectious disease (Fig. 2.1). The primary components of dental plaque are bacteria (Table 2.1). Acid produced by these bacterial species (*Streptococcus mutans*) is considered to be most important in the production of tooth decay. Acid is produced during the metabolism of dietary carbohydrate by these bacteria present in the plaque, which results in a drop in pH at the tooth surface. Due to this, to counteract this action, calcium and phosphate ions diffuse out of enamel, resulting in demineralization process. But this process is reversed, when the pH rises again. Caries is therefore, a dynamic process characterized by episodic demineralization and remineralization occurring overtime. If this demineralization/destruction continues over a period of time, disintegration of the mineral component of the enamel will occur, leading to cavitation.

Host (Tooth)

- Age
- Fluoride
- Nutrition
- Pit and fissures

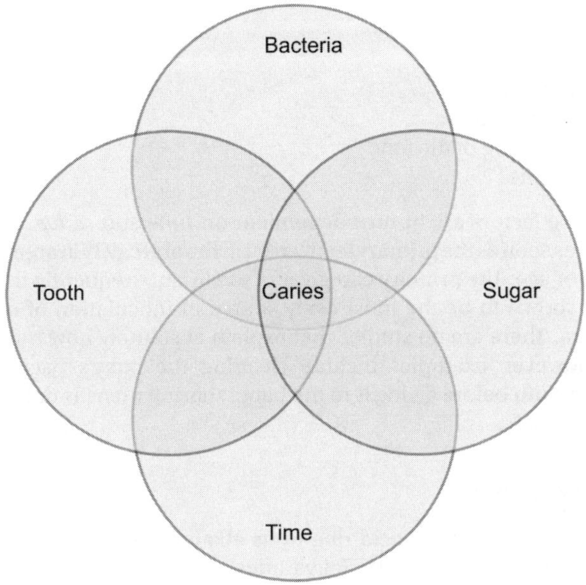

Fig. 2.1 Keyes diagram to show the factors involved in the development of caries

Table 2.1 Microorganisms in dental caries

Streptococcus	*Lactobacillus (Lb)*	*Actinomyces*
• *Mutans (MS)* • *Sorbinus* • *Gordonii* • *Oralis* • *Salivarius*	• *Casei* • *Fermentum* • *Oris*	• *Israelii* • *Naeslundii*

Source: DCNA and Caries Research, 2001

- Morphology of teeth.

Oral Flora

- *Streptococcus mutans*
- Oral hygiene of the individual
- Presence of fluoride in plaque
- Virulence factors.

Substrate Environment

- Saliva
- Carbohydrates
- Frequency of eating
- Physical nature of the food
- Oral hygiene.

All these factors are in turn dependent on *time* and *saliva*. Infants are colonized as soon as the primary teeth erupt in the oral cavity at approximately 6 months of age. The primary caregiver of the infant, frequently the mother, has been shown to be the most likely source of inoculation of an infant's dental flora. There are no studies that explain absolutely how transmission occurs; however, examples include cleaning the baby's pacifier in the mother's mouth before giving it to the baby, sharing utensils or prechewing the baby's food.

Saliva and Caries

Saliva acts as an intraoral acid due to its alkali pH at high flow rates and buffering capacity (Table 2.2). Saliva affects all the three components of Keyes classic Venn diagram of caries etiology (Dodd et al., 2005) namely tooth, substrate and oral flora.

Salivary factors to be taken into consideration are:

- pH of saliva
- Flow rate
- Composition
- Buffering capacity
- Bicarbonate levels.

Importance of saliva can be gained by examining a patient with a dry mouth. The main functions of saliva are:

- To decrease plaque accumulation and aids clearance of foodstuffs
- To act as a reservoir of calcium, phosphate, and fluoride ions
- Has an antibacterial action because of its IgA, lysozyme, lactoferritin, and lactoperoxidase content.

Table 2.2 Salivary flow rate

Xerostomia (dry mouth)	*Hypo salivation*
• Genetic • Drugs • Therapy • Miscellaneous	• Objective salivary rate that is under or 0.16 mL/min

Source: Tanathipanont and Korwanich, 2008

Sugar and Caries

Exposure to sugar is an important factor in the development of caries. Frequency and the quantity of sugar intake have been shown to affect the caries incidence in a population (Fig. 2.2). Individuals should be recommended to reduce the frequency with which they consume foods containing free sugar to four times a day to limit the amount of free sugar consumed.

European Workshop on Oral Care and General Health, 2003

Sugar refers to the mono and disaccharides group of the carbohydrates. Monosaccharides include glucose, fructose, galactose and mannose. Disaccharides include lactose, maltose, and sucrose (Table 2.3).

Dietary sugars are classified as *intrinsic sugars* (when they are part of the cells in a food like vegetables and fruits) or *extrinsic sugars* (milk, table sugar). Both these types are known to cause decay. Various epidemiological studies have shown the role of sugar as one of the causative factors in dental caries. Cross sectional studies relate the caries experience of a population to their sugar intake. Clinical studies like Vipeholm study, Turku sugar study (xylitol), plaque pH studies and animal experiments, all show the evidence of sugar in causing dental caries.

This shows the pH drop that occurs after a sugary drink is consumed. The dashed line indicates the critical pH. Below the critical pH, demineralization will occur. The shape of this curve is affected by a variety of factors like:

- Buffering potential of saliva
- Type of the sugary food ingested
- Food or drinks taken after the sugar consumption.

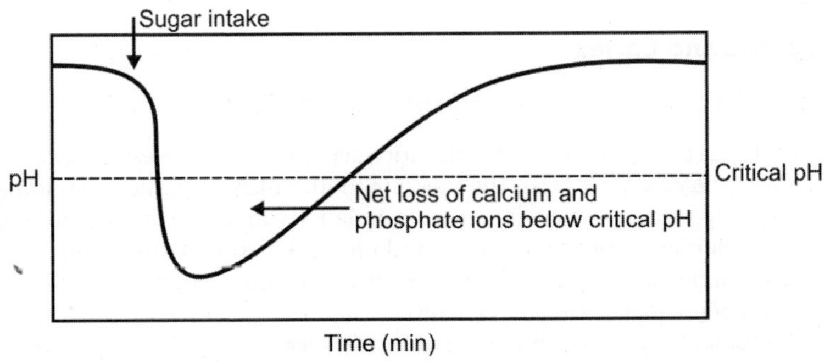

Fig. 2.2 Stephan's Curve—to show the drop in pH after the consumption of a sugary drink

Table 2.3 Classification of sugars

Intrinsic sugars: Sugars forming an integral part of certain unprocessed foodstuffs called intrinsic because they are enclosed within a cell. Found in whole fruits and vegetables; mainly fructose, glucose, sucrose.
Extrinsic sugars: In food without cellular structure. Further classified as: • Milk sugars: In milk and milk-containing products, mainly lactose.
Non-milk extrinsic sugars: In confectionery, soft drinks, biscuits and cakes. Include sucrose, fructose and glucose. Constitute two-thirds of all sugar in the diet and have the greatest cariogenic potential.

Sucrose is considered to be the main sugar in causing dental caries due to its ability to facilitate production of extracellular polysaccharide in plaque. But this is dependent on a variety of factors like:

- Frequency of sugar intake
- Interval between sugar intakes
- Total amount of sugar eaten in the diet
- Concentration of the sugar consumed
- Stickiness of a particular food.

The acidigenicity of a sugar containing food can be modified by other foodstuffs in the diet. Food that stimulates the salivary flow can speed the return of plaque pH to normal like cheese, salted peanuts.

Suggestions for caries prevention by reducing the availability of the microbial substrate

- Remove sugar from food
- Substitute with nonsweetened sweeteners
- Modify the diet so that it is less cariogenic

Bacteria and Caries

Properties of Cariogenic Bacteria (Plaque and Tooth Decay)

Three things are required for dental caries activity to become established:

1. *Susceptible tooth surfaces:* The sites on a tooth which are particularly prone to decay are those where plaque accumulation can occur like the proximal tooth surfaces, cervical margins, and pits and fissures. Other factors like the volume and composition of the saliva, can also affect susceptibility.
2. Cariogenic (decay causing) bacteria.
3. Fermentable carbohydrates (particularly sucrose).

MS and LB remain active and viable at low pH and grow and metabolize acids. They also have the ability to produce extra and intracellular polysaccharides. They can rapidly transport fermentable sugars into acids (acidogenic) and also have the ability to maintain sugar metabolism under extreme conditions (aciduric). However, caries can develop in the absence of *Streptococcus mutans* and its presence do not inevitably lead to decay; e.g. root caries has been associated with *Streptococcus salivarius* and actinomyces species. Lactobacilli are also acidophilic and have been implicated in fissure caries.

TYPES OF CARIES

Enamel Caries

The initial lesion occurs as a white spot. Fissure caries often starts as two white spot lesions on opposing walls, which coalesce later.

Enamel Caries Process

Decay causing bacteria like *Streptococcus mutans* and *Lactobacillus* ingest sugar and other fermentable carbohydrates from the diet and produce acid as a by product, causing a drop in the plaque pH and increasing the H^+ ion concentration. The acid attacks the outer surface of the tooth (enamel) resulting in mineral loss (demineralization). Perhaps the single strongest predictor of disease acquisition and progression is frequency (rather that quantity or source) of fermentable carbohydrates. With this acid attack, the surface changes from being smooth to rough, and may become stained. As the lesion progresses, pitting and eventually cavitation occur.

Clinical Manifestations of Enamel Caries

The early changes in enamel which occur directly after the demineralization process cannot be detected clinically.

White Spot Lesion: This is a reversible stage of the carious process and is the first clinically and visually detectable sign. It is an area of demineralization characterized by a chalky, white appearance. There is a loss of translucency due to the enamel subsurface loss. This lesion can present itself as arrested which clinically will manifest as white or brown in colour and remain like that. This is an incipient lesion and this stage is reversible.

Cavities

When demineralization exceeds remineralization as a result of frequent acid attacks, the result is a breakdown of the enamel, and the formation of a "cavity " in the tooth surface. This is a late-stage sign of tooth decay. This is not reversible, but can be arrested with intense diet control, oral hygiene measures and topical application of fluoride.

It is very important to be able to differentiate a white spot lesion from enamel hypoplasia.

Enamel hypoplasia is defined as a deficiency in enamel formation that manifests clinically as grooves or pits, or a lack of surface enamel. These surface irregularities act as "plaque traps" allow for an increased colonization of harmful bacteria and increase the risk for developing cavities (Table 2.4).

Dentine Caries

This comprises demineralization followed by bacterial invasion, but differs from enamel caries by producing secondary dentine which is protective in nature. Once bacteria reach the ADJ, lateral spread occurs, undermining the overlying enamel.

Rate of Progression of Caries through Enamel and Dentine

The mean time that the lesions remain confined radiographically to the enamel is normally 3–4 years, but there are variations and sometimes the lesions may even regress. The rate of progression through dentine is unknown; however, it is likely to be faster than through enamel. Progression of fissure caries is usually rapid due to the morphology of the area.

Smooth Surface Caries

Noncavitated: These lesions do not exhibit any signs of cavitation after visual or tactile examination. It occurs where dental plaque accumulates (gingival margin) and is not glossy in appearance when a tooth is dried. Areas of demineralization are not in close proximity to the gingival margin, and are not covered by plaque.

Cavitated Carious Lesion: Where there is visual breakdown of a tooth surface, it is classified as cavitated carious lesion.

Caries in Pit or Fissure Surfaces

All discolored areas should be explored using gentle pressure. If a discolored and noncavitated area is soft when explored, it is classified as noncavitated carious pit or fissure. A cavity is detected when there is an actual hole in

Table 2.4 Differences between enamel hypoplasia and white carious spot

	Enamel hypoplasia	*White carious spot*
On drying	Appears opaque	Appears opaque
On wetting	Appears opaque	Appears translucent
Surface characteristics	Hard in consistency	Softer than normal enamel

the tooth in which an explorer could easily enter the space and there is a justifiable catch. An active cavity has soft walls or floors (detected using gentle exploring). If there is visual enamel opacity under a sound or stained pit or fissure, then the enamel is undermined because of the carious process and the tooth surface is classified as a noncavitated carious lesion in dentin. If a discolored area is hard when gently explored, then it should be marked as questionable cavitated carious lesion.

Root Caries

Root surface caries comprises of a series of changes ranging from small discolored areas to cavitation that may extend into the pulp. For diagnostic purpose; they may be either be active root surface lesion characterized by well-defined area showing yellowish or light brown discoloration covered by visible plaque, with the presence of softening/leathery consistency on probing with moderate pressure or inactive root surface lesion (arrested) characterized by well-defined dark brown/black discoloration smooth and shiny in appearance and hard on probing with moderate pressure.

Arrested Caries

Arrested (remineralized) lesions can be seen clinically as brown or black spots of discoloration. The change in color is presumably due to trapped organic debris and metallic ions within the enamel. These discolored, remineralized lesions are intact and are highly resistant to subsequent caries. The arrested caries need not be removed. Under favorable conditions, a lesion may become inactive and even regress.

Arrested dentine caries has a hard or leathery consistency and is darker in color. Arrested enamel caries can be stained dark-brown.

Recurrent Caries

This instead of IT is diagnosed, whenever there is softness of the tooth surface due to caries at a defective margin, and the tip of a probe can enter the defect without any resistance. A restoration with a discolored margin or a small marginal ditch (<0.5 mm or the head of the probe) is recorded as an early recurrent carious area. A larger defect may be classified as advanced recurrent carious area.

Rampant Caries

This is an acute, widespread caries with early pulpal involvement of teeth that are usually immune to decay affecting both the dentitions with rapid appearance of new lesions. Mandibular incisors are also affected in this.

Nursing Bottle Caries

This is a specific form of rampant caries (Table 2.5) in which only the primary dentition is affected. It has a specific clinical pattern of involving the maxillary molars and incisors. Mandibular incisors are not affected.

EARLY CHILDHOOD CARIES

Early childhood decay, also known as "nursing bottle caries" or "baby-bottle tooth decay", is a particular form of tooth decay that affects the teeth of infants and preschool going children. It results from an overgrowth of specific organisms that are a part of dental plaque (sticky white or yellow film found on the tooth surface). Although numerous types of bacteria live in the mouth, tooth decay results from the overgrowth of cariogenic (decay causing) organisms like *Streptococcus mutans* (*S. mutans*), counts that exceed 30% of the cultivable plaque flora. Thus, *S. mutans* have been implicated as the most likely infectious etiologic agents of tooth decay.

CARIES RISK ASSESSMENT

This helps us to determine the probability of caries incidence during a given period of time. This science is the use of knowledge associated with the disease to determine which patients are more or less likely to prevent/control their disease. Our primary goal should be to reduce the risk factors associated with the disease and promote factors that help maintain a healthy life. Caries risk assessment advances in the understanding of dietary influences and fluoride on dental disease has become instrumental in supporting early intervention. Every child should have an examination and oral health risk assessment by 12 months of age by a dentist or qualified pediatric health care professional.

The *caries risk assessment tool (CAT) (Table 2.6)*, provided by the American Academy of Pediatric Dentistry, was designed to assist both dental and health professionals in assessing the risk of tooth decay in infants, children and adolescents. The CAT can be used to determine the relative risk

Table 2.5 Differences between nursing bottle and rampant caries

Nursing bottle caries	*Rampant caries*
Specific form of rampant caries	Acute widespread caries with early involvement of teeth
Primary dentition affected	Both dentitions affected
Specifically affects maxillary incisors and molars	Mandibular incisors are affected

Table 2.6 Caries risk assessment

Risk assessment for infants and toddlers		
	Assessment	*Treatment*
Low-risk	• No active carious lesions at examination • Good oral hygiene habits • Shallow, coalesced grooves • No white spot lesions • Does not sleep with a bottle	• Oral hygiene instruction • Fluoride toothpaste and • Assess for systemic supplements 6–12 month recall
High-risk	• Any cavitated or white spot lesions • High *Streptococcus mutans* level • Bottle fed beyond 12–14 months • Diet high in refined sugars • Family caries history • Inadequate exposure to fluoride • Inadequate saliva flow	• Oral hygiene instruction • Fluoride toothpaste • Assess for systemic supplements • Sealants (behavior permitting) • Fluoride varnish treatments • Restore any carious lesions • Dietary counseling • Discourage bottle use at bedtime 3–6 month recall

of caries of the patient. Questions are directed at dietary practices, fluoride exposure, oral hygiene, utilization of dental services, socioeconomic status and general level of health. All this can help determine if a child is at low, moderate or high-risk for dental disease.

Benefits of Caries Risk Assessment

- Helps us to identify percentage of population that will benefit from preventive measures
- Better and more thorough examination and diagnosis
- Can help us to predict who will get the disease and who will not.

This assessment can be further sub classified into:
- Different age groups—key risk age groups are from 1 to 3 and 5–7 years of age and young adults
- Individuals at risk—by combining various factors like etiology, incidence and prevalence, diet, individuals at risk may be predicted
- Teeth
- Tooth surfaces.

Assessment can also be done according to:
- Behavioral factors like age, breastfeeding, nocturnal bottle usage, drinking sweet beverage, on pacifier during sleep

- Based on past caries experience
  The most consistent predictor of caries risk in children is the past caries experience (*National Institute of Health, USA, 2001)*
  Previous caries experience was an important predictor in most models tested for primary, permanent and root surface caries (*Zero et al.*, 2001)
- Based on salivary factors and microbial colonization
- Based on socioeconomic status, oral hygiene and dietary factors (sugar exposures).

High-risk Group

- Low income
- Special health care needs
- Parents/siblings have decay
- Existing decay/fillings
- Limited/no dental care
- Frequent sugar intake
- No access to fluoridated water or tablets.

Lower-risk Group

None of the above.

Diagnosis of Caries

As caries can be arrested or even reversed, early diagnosis is important (Table 2.7).

- Good eyesight (and a clean, dry, well-illuminated tooth).
- A blunt probe should only be used to horizontally remove plaque away from the fissures as a sharp probe may actually damage the lesion. Use of explorer is not advised because the sharp tips of an explorer may damage small lesions with intact surfaces. Probing can cause fracture and cavitation of incipient lesion. It may spread the organism in the mouth. Explorer is considered useful to remove plaque and debris and check the surface characteristics of suspected carious lesions. Gentle pressure just required to blanch a fingernail without causing any pain or

Table 2.7 Diagnosis of decay (helpful hints)

	Healthy	*Decalcified*	*Decay*
Visual examination	Normal tooth color	White spot	Black/brown
Clinical examination	Hard	Hard	Soft
Radiographic examination	Normal	Normal	Radiolucent

damage is considered ideal. All surfaces of a tooth are cleaned of debris and plaque.

- Bitewing radiographs are useful in the detection of occlusal and proximal caries.

PREVENTIVE DENTISTRY

This branch of dentistry includes methods like:

- Plaque control methods
- Fluoride regime
- Dental sealants and varnishes
- Diet modification and good nutrition
- Patient education.

CARIES PREVENTION

A lot of research has been directed towards methods to prevent caries. These can be categorized into the following headings:

- Reduction of decay-causing bacteria
- Health promoting dietary practices
- Exposure to fluoride sealing susceptible tooth defects
- Proper frequency of dental visits
  Or
- Mechanical plaque control
- Chemical methods
- Diet restriction and modification
- Replacement therapy.

Mechanical and Chemical Plaque Control Methods

Plaque can be kept under control via various mechanisms. The goal is to remove plaque effectively at least once daily. The technique selected should be based on the individuals' needs and abilities.

Brushing: Two basic types of brushes are available-manual and automatic. Vigorous scrubbing of the teeth should not be attempted and the patient should be made cautious of the damage caused by it. Over a period of time, this may lead to gingival recession and cervical abrasions. A medium or a small head with medium bristle strength should be used. They should be replaced on time. There are different methods of tooth brushing which are advised by the dental professional according to the patients' needs.

- Charters method
- Bass method
- Modified stillman method.

Interdental Brushes: These are in the shape of cones used by patients with wide and broad interdental spaces. Single tufted brushes can be used in areas of malaligned teeth. Wooden sticks are triangular in shape and are used by patients with gingival recession.

Dental Floss: This is a nylon or Teflon tape which aids in removal of plaque/food particles from the interdental areas. It can either be circular (floss) or flat (tape). They can be waxes or unwaxed and come in different colors. Other interdental aids available nowadays are tuft end brushes, bridge cleaners, automatic flosses and perio aid.

Antiplaque Agents: These are delivered to the oral cavity through vehicles. They may be in the form of mouth rinses, dentifrices, sprays, chewing gums etc. These are antimicrobial agents who inhibit bacteria associated with disease, reduce existing plaque and prevent its further formation and inhibit acid production.

Chlorhexidine Mouth Wash

This is the most effective antiplaque agent. It is a bactericidal and fungicidal antiseptic. It has both hydrophilic and hydrophobic properties. It is a bisbiguanide which is more effective against Gram positive bacteria. It is available as 0.2% chlorhexidine gluconate mouthwash 10 mL daily for one week per month or for 2–3 weeks straight and repeated every 2–3 months, for nearly a year and a 1% gel (Corsodyl). Unwanted effects include staining of teeth with prolonged use, disturbance in taste and reversible parotid swelling. Its main use is in the treatment of gingivitis, but it has also been demonstrated to be effective in reducing dental caries. The target groups are mainly pregnant women and mothers of infants.

Xylitol

Xylitol is a normal part of everyday metabolism. Pure xylitol is a white crystalline substance that looks and tastes like sugar. It is slowly absorbed. Xylitol is a 5 carbon sugar that cannot be used by bacteria, as it leads to cell death. It also causes reduction in lactic acid production which leads to reduction in remineralization. The effect is long lasting. It is part of normal everyday metabolism and is distributed throughout nature. Sources are fruits, berries, corncobs, etc. The side effects are diarrhea, if taken in large amounts (Table 2.8).

Toothpastes

These contain ingredients which help in removing food residues from the tooth surfaces (Table 2.9). Present day toothpastes contain fluorides.

Table 2.8 Mechanism of action of xylitol

Mechanism of action
• Prevents *Streptococcus mutans* from binding to sucrose • Increases the concentration of amino acids and ammonia, thus neutralizing the plaque acids • Increases salivary flow • Enhances remineralization

Table 2.9 Constituents of toothpastes

Ingredient	*Function*
Sodium monofluorophosphate/sodium fluoride	Main ingredient of toothpastes, helps in providing fluoride and caries reduction
Anticalculus agent (sodium pyrophosphate)	Decreases calculus formation
Desensitizing agents (strontium or potassium chloride/formaldehyde)	–
Antibacterial agent (triclosan)	–
Humectants	Prevents drying
Abrasives (calcium carbonate)	–
Preservatives	–
Flavoring and binding agents	–

They also help in reducing calculus formation. Brushing should be done twice daily and should start as soon as the first teeth erupt in the oral cavity.

FLUORIDE THERAPY

Fluoride is a mineral that is present in all natural waters to some extent. It is the ionic form of the element fluorine. It has a high affinity for calcium, therefore, is very compatible with teeth and bone. Fluoride is released from dental plaque during the acidic conditions of eating.

Mechanism of Action

Topical

- It slows demineralization
- Enhances remineralization.

The pH in the oral cavity falls within seconds of ingestion of dietary sugars and can stay like that for up to nearly two hours. This lowering down of the pH leads to demineralization of the tooth surface. When pH returns to normal/neutral, remineralization can occur (Table 2.10).

Systemic

- Increases enamel resistance by the development of fluorapatite thus improving the crystal size
- Decreases enamel solubility

Pre-eruptive = Systemic fluoride benefits
Posteruptive = Topical fluoride benefits

Fluoride also continues to alter the structure of the enamel crystals, thus making them less acid soluble. It is more effective in decreasing smooth surface caries than pit and fissure caries.

Antibacterial

- Disrupts enzyme systems—fluoride inhibits bacterial metabolization of carbohydrates to produce acid and affects the bacterial production of adhesive acids (Hamilton, 1990).
- Concentrates in plaque.

To summarize the anticaries functions of fluoride:
- Prevents demineralization
- Enhances remineralization
- Alters the action of the plaque bacteria
- Helps in posteruptive maturation of enamel
- Decreases enamel solubility

Absorption of Fluoride

Fluoride is absorbed from the stomach and attains its peak level after one hour. The required amount is absorbed through the intestines and travels

Table 2.10 Mechanism of action of fluorides

Demineralization	*Remineralization*
Frequent exposure to acids	Exposure to fluoride
Frequent carbohydrate intake	Removal of plaque
Presence of plaque	Balanced and nourishing diet
Decreased salivary flow	Limited exposure to carbohydrates

via the blood stream. Excretion is via the kidneys, skin and faces. Traces of fluoride can also be found in breast milk and saliva. Only a small amount of fluoride crosses the placenta.

METHODS OF FLUORIDE DELIVERY

Topical (are applied directly to the teeth) methods:
- Fluoride varnishes
- Topical application of foams and gels
- Fluoridated toothpastes
- Fluoridated mouth rinses.

Systemic Fluoride Methods

- Water and community fluoridation
- Milk
- Salt
- Dietary fluoride supplements.

Other professionally applied fluoride solutions can be:
- Prophylactic pastes which contain stannous fluoride with zirconium sulphate as an abrasive. These are used during professional teeth cleaning.
- Fluoride solutions like NaF 2% and stannous fluoride 8%
- Fluoride gels like APF.

Professionally Applied Acidulated Phosphate Fluoride Gels

These gels are recommended for children aged 6 years and above or adults with smooth surface caries. A 4 minute application of the acidulated phosphate fluoride (APF) and tray method is most effective. Such treatment is recommended 2–6 times a year for caries active patients.

Method of Application

Dry the teeth. Leave the tray with the fluoride gel on the teeth for 4 minutes. Instruct the patient not to rinse, eat or drink for the next 30 minutes.

Fluoride Varnishes

As an alternative to the APF gels, fluoride varnishes may be used. More fluoride is incorporated into the outer enamel with a fluoride varnish treatment. These are professionally applied. They are available as 5% Na or 226000 ppm fluoride resin. Fluoride varnish like Duraphat is applied directly to the lesions to aid arrest. They should be applied site specifically. When applied on the teeth, the fluoride is held in contact with the enamel, until the varnish wears off.

Advantages

- Safe and easy to apply
- Requires little patient co-operation
- No gaging as a tray is not used
- Fluoride levels remain low because the varnish wears off over a matter of days
- Ideal for young children who tend to swallow other topically applied fluorides.

Application of Fluoride Varnish

Using gentle finger pressure open the mouth, remove excess saliva and plaque and isolate the desired teeth after drying them. Apply a thin layer of varnish to all surfaces of the teeth. Instructions to be given include a soft diet for the rest of the day, not to floss or brush until the next morning.

Home Delivered Fluoride Solutions

- *Fluoride containing rinsing solutions:* These are contraindicated in children less than 7 years of age as they may swallow it. They are prescribed as 0.2% weekly/fortnightly or 0.05% daily. The most commonly used is Sodium fluoride (NaF). They are recommended for children and adults with smooth surface caries.
- *Irrigation devices:* These deliver a pulsating stream of water or chemical agent to the teeth and gingiva. These can be used at home or professionally applied in the dental clinic. They help in keeping the sub gingival bacterial levels to a minimum.
- *Fluoridated toothpastes:* A pea sized dab or a small smear of toothpaste is recommended for young children. Children should be supervised while brushing until they are 7 years of age. Three main types of fluoride have been approved by the FDA as safe and effective use in dentifrices:
    1. Sodium fluoride (for use in paste)
    2. Sodium monofluorophosphate (holds fluoride in a complex form)
    3. Stannous fluoride (reduces gingivitis but causes staining).

Dental Pit and Fissure Sealants

They are used as a means to protect the occlusal surfaces of the teeth from dental decay which remains a significant problem even with optimum water fluoridation. Placement of sealants should be accomplished as soon as possible following the eruption of the permanent molars. The most common type of fissure sealant is composite resins used with an acid etch technique. These materials do not require any drilling or preparation of the tooth prior to its placement. Slight chemical and physical modification of the enamel surface makes it more receptive to bonding. They should be carefully applied to the susceptible teeth for the maximum benefit.

Indications

- Children with physical handicap
- Those with extensive caries in the primary teeth.

Types

Sealants can be classified according to their:
- Polymerization method (light cure or self-cure)
- Color (clear or tinted)
- Filled or unfilled
- Resin system (Bis-GMA or urethane diacrylate).

Method of Application

Isolate the tooth after drying and prophylaxis. Etch with 30–50% phosphoric acid for 20–30 sec. Wash thoroughly, and dry well. Apply the pit and fissure sealant. After the application of the sealant and its polymerization, evaluate the sealant for retention and occlusion. If there is any deficiency of the material or bubbles are present, apply more material and cure it.

Water Fluoridation

The safe and recommended concentration of fluoride in water is 1 ppm (parts per million). This can be either school water fluoridation or community level (Table 2.11). Fluoridated water is the most effective method as it provides both topical and systemic benefits of fluoride (Table 2.12). It benefits everyone in the community regardless of their socioeconomic status or compliance as a dental patient. Caries reduction following water fluoridation is usually 40–50% for primary teeth and 50–60% for permanent teeth. This still remains the most cost-effective and beneficial method.

Table 2.11 Various fluorides

Method	*Frequency/Duration*	*Dosage*
Community of water fluoridation	Lifetime consumption	0.7–1.2 ppm
Fluoride tabs/drops	Preschool–8th grade	Varies by age
Mouth rinses	School year	0.05% NaF (daily) 0.2% NaF (weekly)
Toothpaste	Lifetime	0.24% NaF 0.76% MFP 0.4% SNF2
APF/tray gel	1–2 times a year	1.2% APF
Fluoride varnish	2–4 times a year	0.2% NaF

Table 2.12 Recommended daily fluoride supplementation (For children who live in areas with water supplies containing less than 0.3 ppm fluoride)

Age	<0.3 ppm	0.3–0.6 ppm	>0.6 ppm
6 months–3 years	0.25 mg/day	–	–
3–6 years	0.50 mg/day	0.25 mg/day	–
6–16 years	1.00 mg/day	0.50 mg/day	–

Source: Adapted from American Pediatric Dentistry Handbook, 1999

Advantages

- No additional effort is required by the individual
- Low cost
- Very effective in reducing interproximal caries.

Fluoridation with milk and salt have also been tried successfully. Salt fluoridation is a cheap and effective way in rural communities where water fluoridation is not present. 2.5–7 ppm in milk have been tried.

SAFETY AND TOXICITY OF FLUORIDE

Fluoride has been proven to be safe and effective when used in appropriate recommended dosages. But like any other substance, if used in large quantities can have adverse effects.

Chronic exposure to fluoride even at very low concentrations can lead to fluorosis in developing teeth. Acute exposure can lead to poisoning and even death.

Fluorosis (Mottling)

This occurs due to long term or excess use of fluoride. Clinically, it manifests as a permanent intrinsic white to brown discoloration of the enamel. It can vary from faint white opacities to severe pitting. Fluorosis occurs due to the increase in the porosity of the outer third layer of enamel. There has been an increase in its prevalence due to ambient fluoride available. Fluorosis is measured by Dean's Index (Mild to severe).

Fluoride Toxicity

Safely tolerated dose of fluoride is 1 mg/kg body weight.
Certainly lethal dose of fluoride is 16–32 mg F/kg (Hodge and Smith)
15 mg F/kg (Whitford)
32–64 mg F/kg (Laura and David Mitchell)

The probable toxic dose is 5 mg F/kg body weight. Patient should be hospitalized at this time as death can occur within 4 hours. Symptoms of overdose are nausea and vomiting.

Treatment of Fluoride Overdose

Determine the patient's weight and estimate the amount of fluoride ingested. If less than 8 mg F/kg, then give large volumes of milk and observe. If the ingested amount is more than 8 mg F/kg body weight refer to a hospital immediately. Gastric lavage and IV calcium gluconate can also be given, if there is cause for any delay.

Note on Caries Vaccine

Vaccine is defined as the suspension of attenuated or killed microorganisms administered for the prevention or treatment of an infectious disease. The primary IgG that affects dental caries is IgA. Routes of administration can be oral, systemic, gingivo-salivary, and active or passive immunization.

Note on Ozone in the Prevention of Dental Caries

Ozone treatment has been shown to help in the elimination of bacteria associated with dental caries. It can also lead to the reversal of the lesion. It is delivered to the tooth surfaces for about 30–40 sec followed by remineralization solutions and fluoride rinses. It is effective in pit and fissure caries, smooth surface caries, root and cervical caries.

Note on Nova-Min Technology

Nova-Min is a man-made mineral which leads to the formation of hydroxyapatite crystals. It is odorless, colorless and biocompatible. It promotes remineralization and strengthening of the teeth by reversing the time and age effects on the teeth as well reducing decay. When Nova-Min is exposed to saliva, it releases calcium and phosphate ions which become available to the body's own remineralization process and combine with the naturally occurring ions in the saliva to produce hydroxyapatite.

Note on Lasers in Preventing Dental Caries

CO_2 laser causes increased acid resistance of the enamel. Lasers cause an irregular and rough surface of the enamel thereby, increasing the bond strength between the resin and the enamel.

PREVENTION

Oral Health and Health Care Healthy People 2010

"Oral diseases and conditions may have a significant impact on general health.....Oral health care is an important, but often neglected, component of total health care. Regular dental visits provide an opportunity for the early diagnosis, prevention, and treatment of oral and craniofacial diseases and conditions for persons of all ages, as well as for the assessment of self-care practices".

In the past decade, there has been a shift toward improved diagnosis and treatment of noncavitated incipient lesions as well as prevention and arrest of these lesions. Changes have been observed not only in the prevalence of dental caries but also in the distribution and pattern of the disease in the population.

Some of the changes that have taken place in the past decade influencing caries/oral disease prevention are:

- Changes in the disease levels of the populations
- Changes in patient understanding and requests
- Advances in dental materials and equipment
- Understanding of the caries pathogenic process.

The most important part in the treatment of oral disease is its prevention. The preventive approach model recognizes that caries is a chronic process that has episodes of activity and inactivity and that with early recognition of the disease process, before cavitation, intervention will stop and even reverse the disease process.

The need for prevention arises from a mix of various factors like:

- Treatment is intensive
- Cost of treatment is high
- Disease causes pain and suffering
- Disease process can compromise nutrition and speech.

Goals of Prevention

- Early detection of the incipient lesion
- Identification of high-risk patient/patient assessment
- Reduce the number of cariogenic bacteria in the mouth
- Limitation of the carious activity.

Preventive dental care should begin in infancy, within the first year of life before teeth first appear, and continue throughout life. Even before teeth erupt, parents can clean infants' gums after feeding.

Levels of Prevention

Primary Prevention

This can be defined as action taken prior to the onset of a disease which removes the possibility that a disease will occur. In other words, it aims at reducing the occurrence of a disease in a population. This is accomplished by health promotion and specific preventive measures like water fluoridation and diet control. This is aimed at healthy individuals. This also includes:

- Patient education
- Diet control and motivation

- Identification of caries susceptibility
- Fluorides
- Plaque control measures
- Periodic follow ups.

True primary prevention prevents the occurrence of the disease by avoiding disease determinants. In tooth decay, this can be related to reducing the reservoir of bacteria, reducing transmission and reducing colonization of cariogenic bacteria.

Reservoir → Vector → Receptor

Reducing the reservoir can be achieved by use of stannous fluoride and chlorhexidine.

Reducing transmission can be achieved by avoiding shared utensils, cleaning pacifier in mouth, etc. Reducing colonization can be done by following optimum oral hygiene methods like brushing with fluoridated tooth paste, diet control (reducing the frequency of carbohydrates) and topical fluoride application (e.g. fluoride varnish). Primary disease prevention may be achieved with early intervention and anticipatory guidance which includes informing parents of the conditions that create caries and cavities; its natural progression; and its prevention.

Secondary Prevention

This can be defined as the action which halts the progress of a disease at its incipient stage and prevents any further complications. In other words, it aims at reducing the number of existing cases of an illness or dysfunction. The measures under this category are:

- Early detection and preventive resin restoration
- Prevention of the loss of tooth structure
- Prevention of loss of pulp vitality.

Secondary prevention prevents the occurrence of the disease by maintaining a state of balance between disease and oral health. A state of optimal oral health is not absence of activity, but rather a balance of activity. The teeth are in a constant state of demineralization (loss of mineral) and remineralization which is an ongoing process. When demineralization exceeds remineralization, the earliest signs of tooth decay ("white spot") begin; however, at this point, it is reversible. Remineralization can occur, when there is a balance between diet, oral hygiene and fluoride exposure and such measures should be instituted at this point.

When individuals and children have not benefited from primary prevention measures and anticipatory guidance, and caries activity has progressed to the point that there is tooth destruction, the following concepts are employed:

- *Disease suppression:* This is suppression of the dental caries activity before restoring the teeth. It involves diet control to reduce frequency of the number of acid attacks on teeth, fluoride applications to increase remineralization and resistance to attack and gross caries excavation to decrease bacterial load.

- *Disease arrest:* Once caries activity has been suppressed, affected teeth will have lost original contour of the tooth structure ("cavity") but will be dark or glossy in appearance and will not need to be restored, unless it is an issue of function or esthetics. (Arrested Caries).

Tertiary Prevention

This includes the measures taken to limit or prevent the loss of a unit, to minimize suffering caused by existing departure from good health and to promote patients adjustment to irremediable conditions. In other words, it helps in disability limitation and rehabilitation and helps the individuals to deal with the effects of the disease and to prevent further recurrence.

Failure of Early Intervention

Tooth decay in the primary teeth, has significant functional and disease progression consequences:

- *Disease:* Disease in the primary teeth will spread to the incoming permanent teeth. It impacts all the new teeth as they become available. Children that have untreated, active oral disease are at an increased risk for more generalized, severe tooth decay.
- *Child:* Early childhood tooth decay in the primary teeth, if not treated, results in chronic pain and infection. It may also lead to inability to eat.
- *Dentition:* Loss of primary teeth impairs mastication, affects the development of the craniofacial system, and results in loss of arch space for the succeeding permanent teeth to erupt into the proper position in the oral cavity.

DENTAL HEALTH EDUCATION

This should be given by all the health professionals (Table 2.13). The Health Education Authority in the UK has published a policy document laying four points:

1. Restrict sugar containing foods to mealtimes.
2. Clean teeth and gums thoroughly twice daily with a fluoridated tooth paste.
3. Attend the dentist regularly.
4. Water fluoridation is beneficial.

Dental health education can be given in many ways via the mass media, community health programs which can be planned and targeted towards a particular group, or one to one in a clinical environment which is most beneficial, as individuals relate better to their doctor.

Table 2.13 Guides for patient education

- Listen carefully to the patient as they might have different needs
- Explain the complex relationship between plaque, caries and sugar
- Assess the motivation and try to relate it to their needs
- Keep the instructions simple
- Positive re-enforcement

Diet Analysis

Dietary factors play a very important role in the prevention of dental caries. There is little evidence in differentiating between the cariogenic potential of white sugar, brown sugar, fructose, dextrose. But sucrose remains the main source of decay due to its availability and frequency of consumption and ability to facilitate production of extracellular polysaccharide in plaque. A dietary analysis is undertaken to assess the patient's current intake of caries causing food to assess the need for dietary counseling. A food diary should be maintained by the individual for a week, including a weekend, detailing everything they eat. It should include all meals, any snacks or supplements and any fluoridated measures. This is then studied and used to show any dietary habits of the individual that can or is having an adverse effect on his oral health.

Diet Counseling

Efforts should be directed towards a decrease in the amount and frequency of foods which are acidogenic (Table 2.14). These should be tailored according to the individual's needs. They are most useful in patients with high caries activity, and suspected dietary erosions. Flour and starch do not necessarily have decay causing properties, but when combined with sugar like in cookies, the potential for caries activity and risk increases (Tables 2.15 and 2.16).

Table 2.14 Diet counseling

Discourage these snacks	*Encourage these snacks*
Soda	Milk and vegetables
Any sweetened drinks	Sugar free drinks
Candy and gum containing sugar	Yogurt and vegetable dips
Cakes and sweet rolls	Unsweetened juices and nuts
Cookies and chips	Fruits, cheese and eggs
Crackers	Popcorn and sandwiches
Jellies/jam	Sugar free gum

Table 2.15 Dietary recommendations

- Drink and eat sweets less often
- When/if you drink or eat decay causing foods, have them at mealtime (because you get an acid-attack at each meal anyway)
- Eat snacks all at once
- Encourage consumption of foods which are rich in protein, and enhance mastication, salivary flow and oral clearance
- Encourage consumption of milk and water instead of sugary acidic drinks

Table 2.16 DMFT

DMFT index
D = decayed
M = missing
F = filled
T = teeth
DMFT applies to permanent teeth
DMFS applies to permanent tooth surfaces
DMFT/DMFS applies to primary dentition
Components of DMF can be used to determine:
$\frac{D}{DMF}$ = Index of treatment need
$\frac{F}{DMF}$ = Index of restorative provision (also known as Care Index)
$\frac{M}{DMF}$ = Index of treatment failure

Goals of Diet Counseling (Ref: DCNA, October 2006)

- Discourage foods like soda, sweetened drinks, sugar containing gums, candy, cakes, chips, jellies.
- Encourage foods like milk, vegetables, fruits, cheese, yoghurt, eggs, sandwiches, sugar free gum. Remember to choose foods according to age especially for children.
- Tell the patients to eat sweets less or to have them at mealtimes as you get an acid attack at each meal anyway.
- Eat all the snacks at one time to decrease the number of acid attacks on the teeth.

- Rapidly clear cariogenic foods from the oral cavity by brushing or by protective means (xylitol)
- Increase use of less fermentable and artificial sweeteners as an alternate to sucrose:
  - Saccharine (Sweet and Low)
  - Xylitol
  - Sorbitol
  - Aspartame (NutraSweet and Equal)
  - Mannitol.

ORAL HYGIENE INSTRUCTIONS

This should be done for all the patients. The dentist should provide helpful suggestions for plaque removal according to the individual's needs and dexterity. Parents should be involved in the oral hygiene instructions (OHI) for children, until the child is 7 years of age. Flossing or other interproximal cleaning aids instructions should begin between the ages of 8–10 years. Flossing instructions should be included depending on the child's manual dexterity. The clinician may use pamphlets and other educational materials for demonstration. OHI is the best tool in the primary prevention of periodontal disease.

INDICES

Community Periodontal Index

The community periodontal index (CPI) is a quick, easy method for assessing and describing the overall periodontal status of a community (Table 2.17). The CPI, which is promoted by the World Health Organization and used throughout the world, evaluates three indicators of periodontal status - gingival bleeding, calculus, and periodontal pockets. It does not evaluate clinical loss of attachment. Until recently, the CPI was known as the community periodontal index of treatment needs (CPITN). Changing patterns of periodontal treatment, however, have invalidated the treatment needs portion of the original index. For this reason, the index is now used to evaluate periodontal status rather than periodontal treatment needs.

All patients 18 years and older should be routinely screened for periodontal disease during the exam appointment. This screening does not replace thorough periodontal charting when complex periodontal treatment is being considered.

A specially designed periodontal probe is used for screening. The probe features a 0.5 mm balled end and a colored band extending 3.5–5.5 mm from the tip. Gentle pressure should be used to avoid pain and discomfort.

Table 2.17 Community periodontal index

Score	Indicators
0	No disease
1	Bleeding
2	Calculus
3	4–5 mm pockets
4	6 mm or deeper pocket

CONCLUSION

The popular proverb "prevention is better than cure" fits right into this branch of dentistry. It is imperative that, we as dentists should focus and treat not only those who require treatment, but also treat those who are likely to fall under this category.

BIBLIOGRAPHY

1. Anderson M. Chlorhexidine and xylitol gum in caries prevention. Special Care in Dentistry. 2003;23:173-6.
2. Beltran ED, Burt BA. The pre-and posteruptive effects of fluoride in the caries decline. J Public Health Dent. 1988;48:233-40.
3. Billers IR, et al. Enamel loss during a prophylaxis polish in vitro. J Int Assoc Dent. 1980;11:7-12.
4. Birkhed D. Behavioral aspects of dietary habits and dental caries. Caries Res. 1990;24:27-35.
5. Burt BA a CDC. Fluoridation of drinking water to prevent dental caries. MMWR Morb Mortal Wkly Rep. 1999;48:933-40.
6. Consensus: Oral health effects of products that increase salivary flow rate. J Am Dent Assoc; 1988.pp.116-757.
7. Donly, KJ. Fluoride varnishes. J Calif Dent Assoc. 2003;31:217-19.
8. EAM Kidd. Essentials of dental caries: The disease and its management, Wright. 1987.
9. Edmondson IMS. Food composition and food cariogenicity factors affecting the cariogenic potential of soods. Caries Res. 1990;24:60-71.
10. Eklund SA. Dentistry, Dental Practice, and the Community. 4th edn. WB Saunders Co. 1992.
11. Featherstone JD. Caries balance: the basis for caries management by risk assessment. Oral Health Prev Dent. 2004;2:259-64.
12. Hamilton IR. Biochemical effects of fluoride on oral bacteria. J Dent Res. 1990; 69:660-67.
13. Holve S. Fluoride varnish applied at well child care visits can reduce early childhood caries. IHS Primary Care Provider. October 2006.
14. Kanellis M, et al. *Streptococcus mutans* suppression in preschool children using 1% chlorhexidine gel. Abstract at http://confex.com/iadr/2004Hawaii/techprogram/abstract_39586.htm.

15. Mitchell L, Mitchell DA. *Oxford* Handbook of Clinical Dentistry- 3rd edn. 1999.
16. Ramos-Gomex FJ, et al. Implementing an infant oral care program. J Calif. Dent. Assoc. 2002;30:752-6.
17. Ripa LW. Sealants revisited: an update of effectiveness of pit and fissure sealants. Caries Res. 1993;27:77-82.
18. Scheer M, Phipps K. Compliance with chlorhexidine and xylitol among high-risk mothers. Abstract, J Public Health Dent. 2003;63(Suppl 1):38.
19. Stamm JW, Bohannan HM, Graves RC, Disney JA. The efficiency of caries prevention with weekly fluoride mouthrinses. J Dent Educ. 1984;48(11):617-26.
20. The Oral Health Survey of American Indian and Alaska Native Dental Patients: Findings, Regional Differences and National Comparisons. DHHS, IHS Division of Oral Health; 1999.
21. Wagoner WF, Siegel M. Pit and fissure sealant application: updating the technique. JADA. 1996;127:351-61.
22. Weintraub JA. Fluoride varnish for caries prevention: comparisons with other preventive agents and recommendations for a community-based protocol. Special Care in Dentistry. 2003;23(5):180-6.
23. World Health Organization. Fluorides and oral health. Geneva: The World Health Organization; 1994.

ADDITIONAL RESOURCES

1. National Head Start Oral Health Resource Center
   www.mchoralhealth.org/HeadStart/materials/

CHAPTER **3**

ISOLATION AND SOFT TISSUE PROTECTION IN DENTISTRY

Priyanka Jain

INTRODUCTION

Dentistry is the art and science to restore and maintain health and functional comfort of the natural dentition along with satisfactory esthetic appearance. All restorations should fulfill the established requirements of physiology and health with regards to both surface and functional characteristics. The components of the oral environment like the tongue, lips, cheek, the facial/lingual sulci and the floor of the mouth present some obstacle to the mechanical treatment of the tooth. Consistent and adequate management and control of the soft tissue is critical. In adhesive dentistry, this control will make the difference between an excellent restoration and a clinical failure.

Effective soft-tissue management is a required skill for any dentist. Successful control of the soft tissue has always challenged dentists in creating indirect restorations. For the purposes of restorative procedures, soft tissue control refers to the clinical management of the marginal gingival tissues, crevicular fluids, and localized bleeding to create a clean and visible operating field. This enables clinically acceptable dental impressions and the successful use of adhesive dental materials. Many ceramic and indirect composite materials require the use of adhesive materials for cementation. No fluids or blood should be present on the tooth preparation because any sort of contamination will negatively affect the bond strength of the material and cause the restoration to fail. Therefore, proper soft-tissue management is critical and essential during cementation.

Good soft-tissue management is also important when placing direct resin restorations, including Class II, Class III, Class IV, and Class V type dental fillings. Because composite resins are held in place by the use of adhesive bonding, no blood or fluids should contaminate the operating field during the placement of the resin material. This chapter will talk about various techniques and materials used in soft-tissue management, which will lead to a better final restoration.

Sources of Moisture in the Clinical Environment

Moisture: These can be from various sources, like:

- Saliva
- Blood—from inflamed gingival tissues and iatrogenic damage
- Gingival crevicular fluid—from inflamed gingival tissues
- Water—from the rotary instruments and water from triplex syringe
- Dental materials—from the materials that we use during treatment like etchant, irrigant solutions, etc.

Control of the Field of Operation

The Tongue

Movements of the tongue should be minimized during treatment so as to avoid injury during the procedure. But the tongue cannot be totally immobilized, hence retraction is done away from the field of operation (Table 3.1). At the same time the retraction of the tongue should not initiate a gaging reflex. Therefore, this may be accomplished with a vacuum tip extension or a mouth mirror. Wooden tongue blade, a cotton roll or an automaton, (a mechanical device designed to clamp under the chin with an extension into the mouth to depress the tongue or to hold the cotton rolls in an attempt to keep the saliva away from the surface of the teeth), may also be used. The selection of the type of retraction required is determined by the length of the procedure, the agility and thickness of the tongue and the strength of the cheek muscles. The selection should be done keeping the patients comfort in mind. Utmost care is required in the placement of the selected device as the soft tissues of the oral cavity can bruise quite easily. The chair side assistant can hold the vacuum tip, and the mouth mirror or the tongue blade firmly in place by exerting adequate pressure without causing any discomfort or harm to the patient.

Table 3.1 Importance of adequate isolation, retraction and moisture control

Patient related factors	*Dentist related factors*
• Comfortable for the patient during the procedure • It also protects the patient from swallowing or aspirating any foreign body/material • It also helps in avoiding damage to the soft tissues during the length of the procedure	• Allows greater visibility and accessibility of the operating field • Allows greater convenience and efficiency to the operator and infection control by reducing the aerosol production. It also prevents the contamination of the cavity preparation/root canal

Lip and Cheek Retraction

Retraction of the lips and cheek is very essential for the proper exposure of the operating field. Partial retraction can be accomplished by opening the mouth and stabilizing the mandible but for complete retraction, mechanical aids are required. This provides good visibility and prevents the tissues from being traumatized during the various operative procedures.

Facial/Lingual Sulci and the Floor of the Mouth

Although these areas are relatively stable but sometimes, they do encroach on the operating field. This is most common while working on the cervical areas of the mandibular molars.

METHODS OF ISOLATION

The techniques of isolation in the oral environment can be classified as direct and indirect methods and/or surgical and nonsurgical methods (Table 3.2).

Table 3.2 Classification of the methods of gingival tissue displacement

Nonsurgical/atraumatic	*Surgical*
Mechanical • Retraction crown – Modified temporary crown • Modified impression techniques – Copper band impression technique • Mechanical retractor – Gingival protectors – Matrices and wedges – Rubber dam • Retraction cord (twisted/knitted/braided) without astringent/vasoconstrictor • Retraction strips • Retraction paste without a hemostatic agent *Mechanico-chemical* • Retraction cord with hemostatic agent (vasoconstrictor or astringent) • Retraction paste with hemostatic agent (with vasoconstrictor or astringent)	• Rotary gingival curettage • Surgical methods – Gingivoplasty – Gingivectomy – Periodontal flap procedures • Electrosurgery • Laser – CO_2 – Diode – Nd:YAG – Argon laser

Direct Methods

- Rubber dam
- Cotton rolls
- Suction devices—high volume evacuators, saliva ejectors (low volume evacuators)
- Gingival retraction cords
- Lasers
- Rotary curettage
- Electro surgery.

Indirect Methods

- *Comfortable positioning of the patient in a relaxed environment:* The patient should be comfortably seated and the surroundings should be pleasing and relaxed. All these help in reducing the anxiety levels of the patient and thus reduces salivation.
- *Local anesthesia:* This helps in reducing the discomfort for the patient during treatment and controlling moisture by decreasing salivation. The vasoconstrictor also helps in reducing bleeding during the procedure.
- *Anti-anxiety drugs:* These are used in patients to help reduce the amount of salivation in whom no any mechanical form of device is useful.

Aids for Retraction and Protection

Tongue Guards

On application they create a wall between the tongue and the operating field with an adjustable space. They are usually metallic (autoclavable) or plastic (disposable).

Tongue Depressors

These suppress the elevation of the tongue during the actual procedure. They are wooden and disposable. They can be used in combination with a mouth mirror in cases of a large tongue.

Cheek and Lip Retractors

These are designed to fit half of the upper and the lower lip including the corners of the mouth. Their use is two fold. They can be used to retract the lips and the cheek outwards and backwards thus exposing the facial surfaces of the teeth. These are may be used for photographic purposes. For retraction of the facial surfaces of one quadrant only, smaller retractors are also available which fit only one lip and the adjacent corner of the mouth.

Mouth Props

These are rigid devices made of rubber and are a useful aid during preparations on the posterior teeth. They help the patient in keeping the mouth open comfortably. They have blunt corners and serrations on their surfaces which helps them to stabilize on the occlusal surfaces of the teeth. A mouth prop is inserted in between the teeth of opposite jaws on the non-working side between the maxillary and the mandibular teeth leading to increased mouth opening (as they are placed more posteriorly). They are then stabilized by asking the patient to bite on it. The device should not be pushed too posteriorly as it may put strain the patients masticatory muscles. They should be disengaged periodically to allow the patient to relax his muscles. They can be either as block types or ratchet types.

Ideal characteristics of a mouth prop
- Should be stable
- Should be easily removable
- Should be sterilizable or disposable
- Comfortable for the patient
- Easily adaptable and adjustable

Saliva Ejectors/Low Volume Ejectors

These remove the saliva and water that collects in the floor of the mouth during the procedure but have little capacity in picking up any solids. These may be used in conjunction with cotton rolls and rubber dam. The tip should be smooth and nonirritating. Saliva ejectors are usually single use and are made of disposable plastic which can be shaped by bending with the fingers to improve fluid control. They are placed in a position/area least likely to interfere with the operators work.

Types of Saliva Ejectors

- *Svedopter:* This is a saliva ejector with a tongue retractor and protects the tongue and the floor of the mouth. It does not give lingual access to mandibular teeth and cannot be used if tori are present. If made of metal, it can cause soft tissue bruising and can sometimes initiate gag reflex.
- *Hygrofomic saliva ejectors:* These are used in the same manner as Svedopter but are more comfortable in use and give access to the lingual aspect of the mandibular molars. They are used in conjunction with absorbent cotton.
- *High volume ejectors:* These are used for suctioning water and debris from the mouth when high speed hand pieces are used. They are made of plastic and are disposable. Metal ones are also available which

may be re-used. They are straight or slightly angled depending on the requirement. The tip of the evacuator is placed distal to the tooth being operated upon so as not to block the operators view. They should be placed before the positioning of the hand piece and the mouth mirror.

Advantages of Saliva Ejectors

- Quadrant dentistry is facilitated
- There is no dehydration of the tissues
- Improved accessibility and visibility for the operator.

Cotton Rolls

These may be used in conjunction with other methods like the saliva ejector. They prove useful and effective to control small amounts of moisture and retract soft tissues at the same time. But cotton rolls only provides moisture control for a short period of time and are not effective if large volumes of fluid are present. They also become ineffective during active tongue movements and in the presence of shallow sulci which makes their placement and retention difficult.

Absorbents

Like cotton rolls, absorbents are helpful for short durations. They have to be used in conjunction with saliva ejectors. They do not prevent contamination of the area and do not prevent debris from accumulating. They need to be replaced when wet and cannot be used with high speed hand pieces. They can be manually rolled or prefabricated.

Throat Shields

These are indicated when rubber dam is not being used to prevent the patient from swallowing/aspirating any foreign object. This is very important while working on a tooth in the maxillary arch. Gauze (5 into 5 cm) is spread and unfolded over the tongue and the posterior part of the mouth which helps in recovering small objects.

Cellulose Wafers/Parotid Shield

These are used in conjunction with cotton rolls in cases of the facial aspect of the posterior teeth to absorb the saliva excreted by the parotid gland.

Rubber Dam: Rubber dam was first introduced in 1864 by SC Barnum, a New York dentist. Rubber dam ensures appropriate dryness of the teeth and improves the quality of clinical restorative dentistry.

Advantages

The rubber dam is the most successful mode of isolation of the operating field. Its salient advantages are:

- It provides a totally dry and clean field.
- It also provides maximum access and visibility by the control of moisture and retracting the soft tissue.
- It prevents the moisture contamination of the restorative materials used during treatment thus improving the functional properties of these materials.
- It prevents the patient from swallowing/aspirating small instruments, burs, debris during the procedure.
- Rubber dam increases the operator's efficiency and productivity.

Disadvantages

- Time consuming and patients may object at times
- Cannot be used in case of extremely malpositioned teeth
- Cannot be used in children suffering from asthma, some upper respiratory infections or mouth breathing problems.

Rubber Dam Set

Rubber dam may be presented as a *raincoat* that keeps the tooth dry and held on by a *button* (clamp) and kept straight by a *coat hanger* (frame). It is advisable to administer local analgesia where a clamp may impinge on the gingiva.

Rubber Dam Sheets: These come in different colors according to the thickness of the sheet like green, blue and black to provide good contrast with the surrounding and may be flavored for the children. They are made from natural latex . A rubber dam sheet has a shiny and a dull side, the shiny side is less reflective and faces the occlusal surface. The sheet thickness varies from thin, medium, heavy, extra heavy, special heavy. They are available as rolls or sheets in thickness of 0.006"to 0.01" (thin, medium, heavy, extra heavy) (Table 3.3).

Table 3.3 Rubber dam sheets

Gauge	*Thickness*
Thin	0.0006 inch
Medium	0.0008 inch
Heavy	0.010 inch
Extra heavy	0.012 inch
Special heavy	0.014 inch

Rubber Dam Template (Stamp): These have positions of the teeth marked on them and are used to transfer them to the rubber dam sheet for holes to be punched.

Rubber Dam Punch: This is used for making holes in the dam. It has a rotating metal disc bearing 5 to 6 holes of different sizes according to size of teeth and a sharp pointed plunger .5–2.5 mm in diameter.

Rubber Dam Clamps: These are used for anchoring and securing the sheet to the teeth to be isolated. They come in different shapes and sizes according to the teeth and also come differently for deciduous and permanent teeth. They can either be with wings or without wings (used mainly for the deciduous dentition). The clamp has four prongs that rest on the mesial and distal line angle of the tooth and two jaws connected by a bow.

Types of Retainers/Clamps

- *Winged retainers:* These are clamps with wing like projections on the outer aspect of their jaws to provide extra retraction of the rubber dam from the field of operation (Table 3.4). The wings are passed through the punched holes in the dam and the dam and the retainer are placed together on the concerned tooth. After placement, the dam is slipped carefully over the wings onto the tooth.
- *Wingless retainers:* These are clamps having no wings. The retainer is first placed on the tooth and the dam then stretched over the clamp onto the tooth.

Rubber Dam Clamp Forceps: This is used for the placement and removal of the retainers from the tooth. There are two types of retainer forceps available namely Stokes brewer and Ash type.

Rubber Dam Frame/Holder: This supports the edges of the rubber dam sheet. A rubber dam frame can either be plastic or metal. They are used to maintain the borders of the rubber dam in position.

Types of Rubber Dam Holder

- *Young's holder:* This is a U-shaped metal frame with small metal projections for securing borders of the rubber dam.
- *Ash pattern:* Most suitable for children.
- *Swenska N-Ø frames:* Are suitable for taking radiographs with the dam.

Table 3.4 Clamps

Recent advances in rubber dam clamps
• Handi dam • Cushioning metal clamp jaws • Insta dam • Fiber optic clamps • Liquid dam

Rubber Dam Napkin: This is placed between the sheet and the patient's skin to prevent direct contact with the rubber dam sheet thus reducing the risk of allergies. This also acts as a cushion, and absorbs saliva at the corner of the mouth.

Waxed Dental Floss: This is tied around the clamp before it is carried to the oral cavity to prevent accidental aspiration of the clamp.

Wedget: This is an elastic used to secure the dam around the teeth farthest away from the clamp to improve the interdental contacts and to prevent aspiration of the clamp.

Certain Factors to Keep in Mind During the Application of Rubber Dam

- The proximal contacts should be tested with the help of dental floss before the application of the ruler dam sheet.
- The retainer selected should be stable as the movement of the retainer can injure the gingiva and the tooth resulting in postoperative pain and sensitivity.
- To prevent gingival trauma, the jaws of the retainer should not extend beyond the mesial and the distal line angles of the tooth.
- The retainer should be tied with the dental floss to prevent its aspiration.
- While punching holes in the rubber dam sheet, they should be placed at an adequate distance from each other. Insufficient spacing between the holes can force the narrower dimension of the sheet to slip to the mesial or distal of the papilla rather than encompassing it which can interfere in the field of operation.
- A lubricant (petroleum jelly) should be used to protect the lips and the corners of the mouth from the abrading action of the rubber dam sheet.

CONTROL OF THE OPERATING FIELD IN DIFFERENT QUADRANTS

Mandibular Right Quadrant

The assistant can control the tongue movements with the help of a suction tip used for evacuating saliva. The tip is usually beveled and the bevel faces the tooth under treatment. The tip should be placed at the lingual/palatal surface of the teeth slightly posterior to the tooth under treatment. The extension of the same suction tip will additionally aid in depressing the tongue. In cases where the tongue is very agile or large, the dental assistant can use a mouth mirror in his left hand and lay it firmly on the tongue or place it under the right side of the tongue to retract it to the opposite side of the mouth. The operator can approach the oral cavity from the 8 o'clock to

9 o'clock position thus utilizing the area at the right anterior of the mouth and at the same time using a mouth mirror in his left hand with positive pressure away from the teeth, to control the lips and the cheek movements.

Mandibular Left Quadrant

The suction tip may be placed at the extreme left corner of the mouth, with the beveled surface facing the buccal surface of the teeth thus aiding in the retraction of the lips and the cheek away from the operating field. A cheek retractor may be used in cases of cheeks with excess buccal pad of fat or strong musculature. The operator can approach the operating field (using the reverse mirror position) from the 11 o'clock position. For easier access the patients head can be turned slightly towards the right.

Maxillary Right Quadrant

A vacuum tip may be positioned on the palatal surfaces of the right maxillary teeth. The mouth mirror can be rested against the tongue and the mandibular incisors to aid the patient in keeping the mouth open. The tongue should be pressed downwards with slight pressure to prevent its elevation during the procedure. The dentist can hold the mouth mirror in his left hand for vision while the instruments to be used during the procedure are held with the thumb and the two fingers. The tips of the third and the fourth are used for support and to retract the cheek if and when required.

Maxillary Left Quadrant

The suction tip may be placed on the occlusal surface anterior to the tooth being worked on. The assistant can rest the mouth mirror on the mandibular anterior to aid in keeping the mouth open. The mouth mirror is held in the left hand while the right hand holds the instruments with the thumb and the first two fingers as the case with the mandibular right quadrant. But in cases where access is very difficult like with the facial surfaces, the mirror may be used to retract the cheek to facilitate direct vision.

Maxillary Anterior Teeth

The suction tip may be placed at the palatal surface of the teeth anterior to the one being operated upon with the beveled side against the palatal surfaces near the incisal edges of the teeth being prepared. The approach is from the 11 o' clock position using indirect vision with the mouth mirror placed in a reverse manner for a palatal view of the surface. If the facial surfaces are to be treated, then 9 o' clock approach is recommended with the suction tip on the facial surface of the anterior teeth or on the palatal, depending on the flow of the water supply.

Mandibular Anterior Teeth

The suction tip may be placed in the trough formed by the lower lip and the facial surfaces of the lower anterior teeth. The lower lip is gently stretched out and away from the teeth to form the desired trough. In cases where the facial surfaces are desired for the procedure, the suction tip is placed on the lingual side of the teeth, thus retracting the tongue at the same time.

During the dental treatment procedure, the main concern is to keep the tongue and the cheek away from the field of operation and to prevent the water from accumulating and hindering the vision and causing discomfort to the patient. The assistant should avoid placing the suction tip near the soft palate as this may stimulate a gag reflex. A firm placement of the tip on the gingiva, or tongue is probably the best rule to follow.

GINGIVAL RETRACTION

Atraumatic/Nonsurgical Methods

Harmony and compatibility between a restoration and the periodontium that surrounds the teeth is essential and crucial to the success of any restorative procedure. Displacement of the gingival tissue is essential for obtaining accurate impressions for the fabrication of fixed restorations, particularly when the finish line is at, or just within, the gingival sulcus. This is also true when dealing with the restoration of the cervical lesions due to their proximity to the periodontal tissue. For all the above mentioned operative procedures, the most important in soft tissue management is the gingival displacement (Table 3.5).

Gingival displacement may be defined as the deflection of marginal gingiva away from the tooth. This is performed to create sufficient lateral and vertical space between the prepared finish line and the gingival tissue to allow the injection of adequate bulk of the impression material into the expanded crevice. The displacement of the gingiva is also required during the preparation of the tooth cervically and even while placing and finishing the restoration located cervically. This is done to avoid trauma to the periodontal tissue. This can be accomplished by means of:

- Chemical–hemostatic medicament
- Mechanical methods
- Surgical methods-electro surgery and gingival curettage
- Lasers.

Mechanical Retractors

Gingival Protector

This can be used to displace soft tissue to protect gingiva from rotary instruments during tooth preparation and finishing. A crescent-shaped

Table 3.5 Recommendations for nonsurgical gingival displacement in different clinical situations

Procedure	*Factor*	*Situation*	*Technique*
Tooth preparation	Location of the margin	• Removal of caries extending subgingivally	• Using gingival protector or cervical rubber dam clamp. In case of deep inaccessible subgingival lesions surgical gingival retraction can be done
		• Subgingival margin encroaching the biological width	• Re-establish the biological width surgically/ orthodontically
Impression taking	Gingival condition	• Gingival bleeding	• Use astringent applicator to control the bleeding
		• Gingival sulcus depth	• Single-cord technique is preferred if the gingival sulcus is shallow. Double-cord retraction technique is preferred in cases with deep gingival sulcus
		• Gingival thickness	• Excess gingival bulge or hypertrophied gingival tissue may be removed with electrocautery/laser
	Number of prepared teeth	• Single	• Single-cord impression technique can be used
		• Multiple	• Double-cord impression technique/retraction paste technique can be used
	Impression material	• PVS/polyether	• Thoroughly wash the gingival sulcus after the use of aluminum sulfate compounds, aluminum chloride, ferric sulfate, as they are may alter the setting of the impression material

tip on an adjustable ball-joint is attached to a metal handle which can be rotated to an angle according to the required tooth's surface, thereby achieving gingival fit. Such protectors can be used for veneer preparations, finishing veneer margins (porcelain/resin), cervical (facial) subgingival caries, and/or for the removal and checking the marginal fit of crowns. These tips are autoclavable thus preventing cross-contamination.

Wooden Wedges

Wooden wedges can be placed interproximally to mechanically depress the gingiva, thus providing retraction. Matrices with gingival extension can also displace the gingival tissue when placing interproximal restorations.

Rubber Dam

Heavy, extra heavy and special heavy gauges of rubber dam with proper interseptal dimensions may be used when a limited number of teeth in one quadrant are being restored or in cases where the preparations do not extend very far subgingivally. During impression taking, the sulfide compounds utilized in the manufacturing of latex can inhibit the polymerization of polyvinyl siloxane (PVS) impression material. Hence, rubber dam should be avoided when this material is used.

Retraction Strip

The material used in a retraction strip is chemically extracted from a biocompatible polymer (hydroxylate polyvinyl acetate) that creates net-like strips without debris or fragments. These can be easily shaped and adapted into the sulcus without local anesthesia, and are highly effective for absorption of intraoral fluids such as blood, saliva, and crevicular fluid. These sponge-like strips expand with absorption of fluids and exert pressure on gingival tissues to cause displacement.

Retraction Cords

Cords can be fabricated from cotton yarn or purchased commercially in a variety of forms. Unfortunately, their effectiveness is limited because the use of pressure alone will not control sulcular hemorrhage. Therefore, they usually have some hemostatic agent (vasoconstrictor or astringent) premixed in them to prevent bleeding (Table 3.6). The chemicals used along with retraction cords (gingival displacement medicaments) can be broadly classified into vasoconstrictors and astringents. If properly used, these can be used for isolation especially in cases of treatment of mandibular cervical lesions (Table 3.7). They improve the accessibility and visibility and also restrict the use of excess restorative material. Most importantly, they produce the lateral displacement of gingiva without blanching it. They are manufactured in three forms:

1. Braided
2. Twisted
3. Knitted.

Choice of the type of retraction cord to use depends on the operator's preference. The cord may be packed with a special instrument called FISCHER packing instrument. Sufficient diameter of the cord should be used for adequate displacement.

Table 3.6 Retraction cords

Desirable qualities of a cord include
• Dark color (to maximize contrast with the tissues, tooth, and cord) • Be absorbent (to allow the uptake of the liquid medicaments) and • Be available in different diameters (to accommodate the varying morphologies of the gingival sulcus)

Table 3.7 Various retraction cords

Braided cords	*Knitted cords*
• Easier to place	• Easy to place too
• Impregnated with astringent and is stable	• Expands when wet
• Minimal soft tissue damage and no tear during placement	• Minimal tearing at the cutting ends
• Serrated in nature	

Advantages of Retraction Cords

- Effective in controlling gingival hemorrhage and retracting gingival tissues at the same time
- Can be used as an adjunct to other methods
- Can be used in cases where rubber dam application is not possible like in cervical preparations.

Disadvantages of Retraction Cords

- Only effective in controlling small amounts of fluids
- May need local anesthetic prior to placement
- Can be difficult to insert
- Can cause gingival damage if not inserted properly.

Vasoconstrictors

These include epinephrine and sympathomimetic amines . Epinephrine-impregnated retraction cords contain 0.2–1 mg of racemic epinephrine per inch of cord depending on the diameter and the brand. The epinephrine is used in the concentration of 0.1% and 8%. The amount absorbed depends on its concentration in the cord, length of cord used, amount of vascular bed exposed, and duration of the cord application. For patients falling under the category of contraindications for epinephrine, a cord impregnated with some other agent must be substituted.

Sympathomimetic amines capable of producing local vasoconstriction with minimal systemic side effects include tetrahydrozoline HCl, (0.05%); oxymetazoline, (0.05%); and phenylephrine HCl, (0.25%). Retraction cord can be dipped in these to assist in hemostasis. Newer hemostatic agents such as the tetrahydrozoline and oxymetazoline have a more acceptable pH and are recommended.

Astringents

These act primarily by precipitation of protein and inhibiting transcapillary movement of plasma proteins. They have relatively low cell permeability and act generally as irritants in moderate concentrations and as caustics in higher concentrations. These are:

Aluminum Sulfate Compounds (Aluminum Potassium Sulfate [Alum] and Aluminum Sulfate): Alum is safer and has fewer systemic effects than epinephrine. Cords saturated with 100% alum can be safely left in the sulcus for as long as 20 minutes without any adverse effect. The concern in using aluminum sulfate (it differs from alum) is that they can inhibit/retard the setting reaction of additional reaction impression materials.

Aluminum Chloride: This is one of the most commonly used astringents in the concentration of 5–25%. Aluminum chloride is the least irritating of the medicaments used for impregnating retraction cords, but they are capable of disturbing the setting of PVS impression materials . The inhibitory effect can be greatly reduced by thoroughly rinsing the preparation with water after the treated cord is removed.

Ferric Sulfate: This provides good hemostasis on exposed connective tissue. This astringent is provided in solution form only, generally in the concentration of 13–20%. During tissue hemorrhage, the solution should be rubbed into the bleeding areas with an applicator (dento-infusor) or a soaked cotton pellet. Ferric sulfate can also modify the accuracy during impressions because it disturbs the setting reaction of polyvinyl siloxanes. The drawback of using this agent is that due to its iron content, ferric sulfate stains gingival tissues a yellow-brown to black color for several days after being used as a retraction agent.

Techniques for Retraction Cord Placement

Two procedures widely used for placing the retraction cord are the single-cord and the double-cord techniques. The technique to be used is based on the clinical situation.

Single-Cord Technique

This technique is indicated when making impressions of one to three prepared teeth with healthy gingival tissues, especially when the prepared margins are at or above the tissue. In this technique, a single cord is placed in the sulcus and removed before the impression is taken. This provides displacement about the width of the cord. The main disadvantage of this is that in a deep sulcus, however, the tissue can collapse over the top of the cord. This often causes the impression material to tear on removal. Though commonly practiced, this technique is often unsatisfactory.

Double-Cord Technique

This technique can be used with single or multiple preparations. It is especially useful for making impressions when tissue health is compromised. The double-cord technique employs two cords, one placed above the other. A thin cord such as silk suture is first packed under the preparation margin to control gingival seepage and hemorrhage. This cord is typically left in place for the impression. The second, larger cord is impregnated with hemostatic agent and placed above the first cord for a minimum of 4 minutes and removed before the impression is taken.

The main advantage of this technique is that the first cord remains in place within the sulcus, thus reducing the tendency of the gingival cuff to recoil and displace partially set impression material. This not only helps to control gingival hemorrhage and exudates but also overcomes the problem of the sulcus impression tearing because of inadequate bulk. Another advantage of the double-cord technique is that the first cord acts as a sulcus liner, preventing tearing of the epithelium and subsequent bleeding. However, the main disadvantage of this technique is that failure to remove the first cord can cause gingival inflammation. Furthermore, if the deeper cord is left in place the impression material may stick to it and cause the impression to tear upon removal.

Retraction Paste

These are the cordless retraction materials. They are available in a paste-like form and supplied with a specialized dispenser. These cordless retraction materials displace the gingiva when injected into the sulcus. Because of the passive technique used to place these pastes, they are significantly less traumatic to the tissue than the conventional retraction cord. The main drawback of these is that the amount of retraction offered by these pastes is limited, especially with extremely subgingival margins and its high cost. These pastes are also available with hemostatic agents such as aluminum chloride and a mild, natural astringent to control the seepage of fluid.

SURGICAL METHODS OF GINGIVAL RETRACTION

Rotary Curettage

This is a troughing technique, wherein a portion of the epithelium within the sulcus is removed to expose the finish line. It should be done only on the healthy gingival tissue. No bleeding on probing, and a minimum of 3 mm deep sulcus are the main criteria for this technique. The main drawback of this technique is that due to poor tactile sensation while doing this, this can prove to be potentially damaging to the periodontium.

Electrosurgery

This is the surgical retraction of the sulcular epithelium using an electrode to produce gingival retraction. This technique may be used in areas of inflammation in gingival tissue where the retraction cord cannot be used and in cases where there is gingival proliferation around the prepared finish line. It cannot be used in patients with cardiac pacemakers.

Lasers

A laser is a device that converts electrical power from the wall into coherent, monochromatic and collimated light capable of changing a target substance, such as human tissues. The tissues are modified due to thermal effects produced by the light. *LASER* is an acronym for **L**ight **A**mplification by **S**timulated **E**mission of **R**adiation. The first laser in dentistry was introduced in 1982 by the Directed Energy, Inc. and Pfizer who introduced the carbon dioxide (CO_2) gas laser for dentistry. Lasers are identified by the active medium that they use to create their energy, such as gases, types of rods, dye types, or the wavelength of the diode they use. They are of three types:
1. *Solid State (rod style):* Er:YAG, YSGG
2. *Gas:* Carbon dioxide, Argon
3. *Semiconductor:* Diodes.

Laser procedures are divided into two categories: soft tissue procedures and hard tissue procedures (Table 3.8). Soft tissue procedures consist of certain treatment procedures for the gingiva, such as muscle attachment, reshaping of gingival tissues, and crown lengthening. Hard tissue laser procedures incorporate tooth decay procedures and dental fillings, etc.
The main types of lasers used in dentistry are:
- Diode laser (810 nm–980 nm)
- CO_2 (carbon dioxide, 10600 nm)
- YAG family (2100 nm–2940 nm) i.e. Er:YAG (erbium yttrium aluminum garnet), ErCr:YSGG (erbium chromium yttrium selenium gallium garnet), and Hol:YAG (holmium yttrium aluminum garnet). These feature predominantly as hard tissue lasers. Nd:YAG (neodynium, yttrium aluminum garnet) is an effective dental laser wavelength in soft tissue procedures.

These lasing media produce wavelength specific light, which is selectively absorbed in certain tissues. YAG lasers have an absorption peak in water; therefore the water component of tissues is volatilized before breakdown of structure. Diode and Nd:YAG lasers have an absorption peak

Table 3.8 Use of lasers in dentistry

Soft tissue procedures for which lasers can be used
• Gingivectomy, Gingivoplasty, Operculectomy
• Recovering dental implants
• Treating inflammation around implants
• Troughing for impressions
• Treating aphthous ulcers
• Incising and draining abscesses
• Fibroma removal and biopsies
• Sealing lymphatics in the surgical area
• Frenectomy
• Reducing sulcular oral bacteria and other flora
• Recontouring interproximal tissue
• Accelerating healing for split lips
• Soft tissue debridement
• Reducing hyperplasia

in pigmented tissue and, therefore, are good for periodontal tissue lasing and coagulation.

The YAG range is recommended for cavity preparation and hard tissue removal, whereas the diode CO_2 and Nd:YAG lasers are useful for soft tissue procedures.

A hard tissue laser is wavelength specific to water and, therefore, can be used clinically on both hard and soft tissues. However, care must be taken to avoid unwanted interactions on root surfaces. For many cosmetic and periodontal indications, a soft tissue laser is more efficient. Treatment with soft tissue laser is different from conventional methods because the patient's acceptance is greater. The laser is more efficient and sometimes faster. There is less postoperative discomfort for the patient, and the bacteria levels in affected areas are reduced. Additionally, there is virtually no collateral damage to healthy tissue, and anesthesia is not necessarily required. Overall, laser dental procedures are safer, and there is a decreased healing time.

Advantages of Lasers

Laser has many advantages over traditional surgical instruments. Dental laser surgery has also proven to be highly effective and pain-free. The use of laser technology prevents infections and protects the surrounding healthy tissues. In addition to this, the duration of this procedure is very short as compared to traditional surgery and there are absolutely no risks associated with this type of dental treatment. The operator can control the energy applied to the optical resonator, and can vary the beam diameter on the target tissue. The operator can also control pulsing or continuous lasing, pulse duration and pulse relaxation times. These will all control the target tissue effects. Laser dentistry facilitates minimal healing time after complicated operations. Some other minor problems such as benign tumors can also be treated with the help of laser. The treatment is highly precise and totally effective.

Laser dentistry is now applied to many dental procedures including implants and tooth extraction. Different parameters are used for different types of procedures to prevent complications. Laser dental surgery is a highly accurate treatment which causes little or no pain. Implants are especially well-placed using this technique with greatly reduced chances of developing infections or other complications.

SOME CLINICAL APPLICATIONS

Soft Tissue Management for Direct Resin Restorations and Bonded Indirect Restorations

All the materials and techniques described above can be used when placing a direct composite restoration and during cementation of a bonded indirect restoration. The clinician must identify the area and the places where tissue/fluids may present an issue during a bonding procedure. Retraction cord may be used for Class III and Class V composite resin restorations as the nature of the decay associated with these restorations brings them in close proximity of the gingival tissues. During cementation of the porcelain veneers and/or anterior all ceramic crowns, gingival tissues must be retracted again to properly isolate this area so that the restoration is bonded correctly.

Soft Tissue Management for Final Impression Taking

Double-Cord Technique

This is used for deflection of the soft tissue to get the accurate details of the margins of the tooth preparation (refer to retraction cord placement).

Single Retraction Cord Technique

This technique can work well with tooth preparations that terminate supragingivally or at the tissue height. Often, this technique will work well, provided the soft tissue and the related fluids in the area are controlled and the prepared teeth have healthy gingival tissues.

Soft Tissue Control via Soft Tissue Alterations

In clinical where the soft tissue is too bulky and, or too inflamed to enable visualization of the preparation margin, the use of electrosurgery or laser surgery enables the clinician to see where to place the margin of the final restoration. Gingivectomy with either an electrosurgery or laser can be the solution while dealing with excessive and/or irritated soft tissue.

Chemical Management of Soft Tissue and Crevicular Fluids

Bleeding is managed chemically in most of the cases. Ferric sulfate, aluminum chloride, and epinephrine are the most commonly used. Since ferric sulfate may leave a black organic residue on the tooth preparation, it may prove to be a problem while placing an all-ceramic restoration or composite resin restorations. Therefore, aluminum chloride, while not quite as effective as ferric sulfate can be used for controlling localized bleeding. Aluminum chloride leaves no dark residue on the restoration. This makes it the chemical of choice when the final restoration is made of an all-ceramic or indirect composite. Epinephrine stops localized bleeding through vasoconstriction. When used with a local anesthetic in a 1:50,000 concentrations, it can be highly effective at controlling localized bleeding for a short period by directly infiltrating into the desired area.

Soft Tissue Management for Various Procedures

Intraoral Examination Procedure

Low volume suction may be used to remove the saliva build up, gauze can be used to dry the teeth and soft tissue to visualize them better. Triplex syringe can be used to dry small amounts of moisture from the tooth surfaces.

Prophylaxis

Low volume suction may be used to remove the saliva build-up during the procedure.

Topical Fluoride Application

During fluoride application, low volume suction may be used to remove the saliva build up during and after the procedure.

Fissure Sealant Application

During this procedure, rubber dam is the first choice for optimal moisture control and to isolate the working field. Cotton rolls are the second option to isolate the working field. Triplex syringe may be used to dry small amounts of moisture from the tooth surfaces and high volume suction may be used to remove the water which is used to wash away the etchant during the procedure.

Simple Restorative Procedures

As during the fissure sealant application procedure, rubber dam is the first choice for optimal moisture control and to isolate the working field. Cotton rolls are the second option to isolate the working field. Triplex syringe can be used to dry small amounts of moisture from the tooth surfaces and high volume suction is used to remove the water used during the procedure.

Endodontic Procedures

Rubber dam is the only choice for complete and optimal moisture control and to isolate the working field. High volume suction is used to remove the solutions used to rinse the root canal(s) during the procedure.

Alginate Impression Taking

Low volume suction and the triplex syringe are used.

CONCLUSION

A healthy relationship between restorations and their surrounding periodontal structures should be the goal of a dentist. Several techniques have proven to be relatively predictable, safe, and efficacious in the management of the gingival tissue in restorative dentistry. No scientific evidence has established the superiority of one technique over the other. The selection of any one of the various methods of soft-tissue management to control the operative site may solely depend on the clinical situation and the preference of the operator.

BIBLIOGRAPHY

1. Baharav H, Laufer BZ, Langer Y, et al. The effect of displacement time on gingival crevice width. Int J Prosthodont. 1997;10(3):248-53.
2. Bennani V, Schwass D, Chandler N. Gingival retraction techniques for implants versus teeth: current status. J Am Dent Assoc. 2008;139(10):1354-63.
3. Benson BW, Bomberg TJ, Hatch RA, Hoffman W Jr. Tissue displacement methods in fixed prosthodontics. J Prosthet Dent. 1986;55(2):175-81.
4. Bowles WH, Tardy SJ, Vahadi A. Evaluation of new gingival retraction agents. J Dent Res. 1991;70(11):1447-9.
5. Conrad HJ, Holtan JR. Internalized discoloration of dentin under porcelain crowns: a clinical report. J Prosthet Dent. 2009;101(3):153-7.
6. Ferrari M, Cagidiaco MC, Ercoli C. Tissue management with a new gingival retraction material: a preliminary clinical report. J Prosthet Dent. 1996;75(3): 242-7.
7. Hansen PA, Tira DE, Barlow J. Current methods of finish-line exposure by practicing prosthodontists. J Prosthodont. 1999; 8(3):163-70.
8. Nemetz H, Donovan T, Landesman H. Exposing the gingival margin: a systematic approach for the control of hemorrhage. J Prosthet Dent. 1984;51(5):647-51.
9. O'Mahony A, Spencer P, Williams K, Corcoran J. Effect of 3 medicaments on the dimensional accuracy and surface detail reproduction of polyvinyl siloxane impressions. Quintessence Int. 2000;31(3):201-6.
10. Phatale S, Marawar PP, Byakod G, et al. Effect of retraction materials on gingival health: A histopathological study. J Indian Soc Periodontol. 2010;14(1):35-9.
11. Shen C. Impression materials. In: Anusavice KJ, Ed. Phillips' Science of Dental Materials. 11th edn. St Louis, MO: Saunders; 2003.pp.205-54.
12. Tyas M. Cotton pellets and gingival retraction cords. Clinical notes No. 2. Aust Dent J. 1984;29(4):279.
13. Wassell RW, Barker D, Walls AW. Crowns and other extra-coronal restorations: impression materials and technique. Br Dent J. 2002;192(12):679-90.
14. Woody RD, Miller A, Staffanou RS. Review of the pH of hemostatic agents used in tissue displacement. J Prosthet Dent. 1993;70(2):191-2.

CHAPTER 4

DENTAL RADIOGRAPHY

Priyanka Jain

INTRODUCTION

The use of X-rays is an integral part of clinical dentistry, with some form of radiographic examination necessary on the majority of patients. As a result, radiographs are often referred to as the clinician's *main diagnostic aid.*

A radiographic image is formed by a controlled burst of X-ray radiation which penetrates oral structures at different levels, depending on varying anatomical densities, before striking the film or sensor. Teeth appear lighter because less radiation penetrates them to reach the film. Dental caries, infections and other changes in the bone density, and the periodontal ligament, appear darker because X-rays readily penetrate these less dense structures.

It is possible for both tooth decay and periodontal disease to be missed during a clinical exam, therefore, radiographic evaluation of the dental and periodontal tissues is a critical segment of the comprehensive oral examination.

Radiation Dose Measurement

Most important measurement in this category is the assessment of the detrimental effects of the radiological procedures (Table 4.1). The absorbed dose may be measured for different types of radiation. The absorbed dose is adjusted by a quality factor (Q) specific to the type of radiation, to assess the detrimental effect on the tissues.

The equivalent dose reaching a particular organ is measured and multiplied by the weighting factor for that organ. Adding up the values for all the organs/tissues involved in the exposure, gives us the value that represents the risk of harm from that exposure. When referring to the dose for a particular procedure, the effective dose is the one which is usually quoted.

Table 4.1 Dose measurements

Dose	*Comments*	*Unit*
Radiation absorbed dose	This is a measure of the amount of energy absorbed from the radiation exposure per unit mass of tissue	Gray (Gy) = 1 joules absorbed/kg
Equivalent dose (Equivalent dose = radiation absorbed dose multiplied by Q)	A measure which allows comparison between different types of radiation in regard to their absorbed doses in the body	Sievert (Sv)
Quality factor (Q)	Represents the biological effects of each type of radiation like X-rays, gamma rays and beta particles	Q for X-ray = 1, alpha particles = 20 Therefore, equivalent dose = radiation absorbed dose
Effective dose (Equivalent dose multiplied by the tissue weighting factor)	Each body tissue is affected differently by radiation. Therefore, effective dose allows doses from different investigations of different parts of the body to be compared, by converting all doses to an equivalent whole body	Sievert (Sv)
Weighting factor (W)	Measures the risk of the tissue being damaged by radiation e.g. the higher the damage, the higher is W	

Sources of Radiation Exposure

The public is exposed to radiation from both natural and man-made sources. Radiation exposures can either be a full body radiation or a specific area.

Natural sources include cosmic rays from energetic subatomic particles, photons from sun, airline travel, terrestrial or gamma rays from external sources such as rocks, soil and internal sources radionuclides which are inhaled or ingested. Together background, radiation from cosmic and terrestrial sources amounts to about annual effective dose of 2.4 mSv worldwide. Gamma rays alone contribute to nearly 87% of radiation.

Man-made radiation or artificial background radiation include medical and dental diagnostic radiation which amounts to roughly over one billion medical X-ray examinations worldwide in a year (this contributes to nearly 12% of the total exposure), consumer and industrial products from domestic water supply, tobacco, combustible fuel and nuclear explosions fallout and radioactive wastes.

BIOLOGICAL EFFECTS OF RADIATION

X-rays interact with living tissues and can cause biological changes which are mediated directly by excitation of atoms or indirectly as a result of chemical changes occurring near the cells. As a result, affected cells may be damaged or killed. These can be classified as genetic or somatic effects (Flow chart 4.1). Genetic effects involve chromosomal damage or mutation in the reproductive cells and will affect future generations. Somatic effects involve damage to other tissues and result in changes in the present lifetime of the individual (e.g. radiation burns, leukemia). These are hazardous, as the effects are painless, latent and cumulative.

Factors Affecting Radio Sensitivity

- Dose or the amount of radiation. The higher the dose, the greater is the effect
- The rate of exposure
- The higher the oxygen level in irradiated cells, greater is the damage.

Flow chart 4.1 Effects of radiation on the body

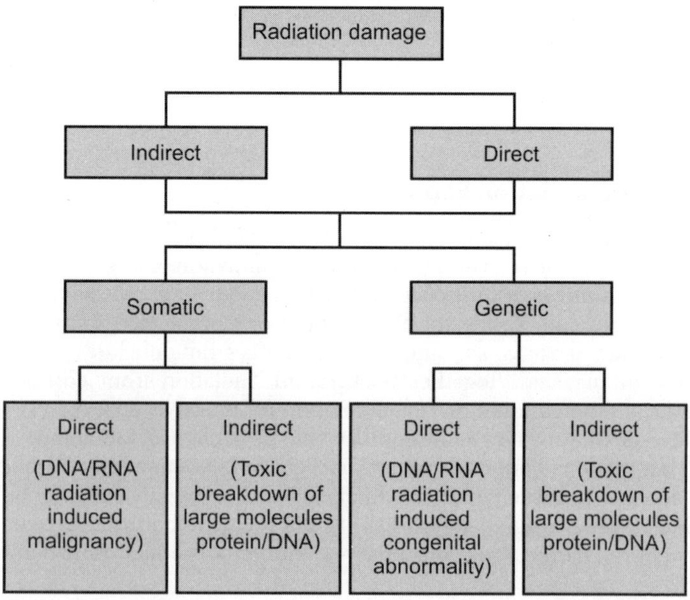

Radiation can have two types of effects on the body:

1. *Deterministic:* These effects are certain to happen if a high dose is given. The severity of response is dose dependent to the dose which means that when the dose is large enough, effects can occur in all people. But at the same time, response cannot be determined below a certain dose threshold, e.g. oral effects after radiation therapy, whole body radiation leading to radiation sickness, reddening of the skin, and development of cataracts.
2. *Stochastic:* The probability of occurrence is proportional to the dose which means that these effects may happen and there is no dose threshold. For example, radiation induced cancer and congenital abnormalities.

Radiation effects are dependent or influenced by various factors like:

- Total dose given
- Total area covered by the procedure
- Type of tissue irradiated
- Dose rate
- Age of the patient

The frequency of taking radiographs in dentistry is also based on various factors like:

- Patient's oral hygiene
- Caries activity
- Dental history
- Reliability of patient
- ADA guidelines which states that full-mouth series should be taken at 1–5 years and bitewings at 6 months to 3 years and panoramic at 1–5 years.

RADIATION PROTECTION AND SAFETY

Dose Limitation

Ionizing radiation is the subject of considerable safety legislation designed to minimize the risks to radiation workers and to patients. The *International Commission on Radiological Protection (ICRP)* regularly publishes data and general recommendations based on the following general principles:

- No practice shall be adopted, unless its introduction produces a positive net benefit *(Justification)*. Therefore, the benefit from the exposure should exceed the risk of harm to the patient.
- All exposures shall be kept *as low as reasonably practicable* (ALARP), taking economic and social factors into account *(Optimization)*. The dentist should reduce unnecessary radiation exposure to the patient and the staff.

- The dose equivalent to individuals shall not exceed the limits recommended by the ICRP *(Limitation)*. The patient should not be exposed to high doses (Table 4.2).

For the purpose of radiation protection and dose limitation, the ICRP has divided the population into three groups:

1. Patients.
2. Radiation workers (classified and non-classified).
3. General public.

Radiation Workers

Radiation workers are those people who are exposed to radiation during their work. This exposure carries no benefit and only risk. The ICRP further divides these workers into two subgroups depending on the level of occupational exposure:

1. *Classified workers:* They receive high levels of exposure to radiation at work and thus require compulsory personal monitoring and health checks.
2. *Nonclassified workers:* This compromises most dental staff. They receive low levels of exposure to radiation at work (as in the dental surgery).

General Public

This group includes everyone who is not receiving a radiation dose either as a patient or as a radiation worker, but who may be exposed inadvertently, for example, someone in a dental surgery waiting room.

Dose Limits

The present occupational exposure limits are based on the fact that no individuals will have deterministic effects and that the probability for stochastic effects is as low as reasonably and economically practical (Table 4.3).

Methods of Monitoring Radiation Dose

There are three main devices for monitoring radiation dose:

Film Badges

These are generally worn on the outside of the clothes, at the level of the reproductive organs, for 1–3 months before being processed. They are the most common form of personal monitoring device. They are simple and relatively inexpensive. They provide a permanent record of dose received by measuring the type and energy of radiation encountered but do not give any indication of exposure.

Table 4.2 Suggested guidelines for radiation protection

	Precautions	Reasons
Patient	X-ray should operate at 70 kV	• This produces the best combination of optimum energy, tissue penetration and image contrast
	Aluminum filtration	• Results in decreased patient exposure with no loss of information. This also absorbs most of the low energy X-rays that would otherwise be absorbed by the skin
	Rectangular collimation	• This reduces the width of the beam to a minimum to cover the film, thus decreasing exposure
	Films/screens	• Films of speed lower than film E should not be used to reduce the exposure time • Extraoral radiographs should be taken using cassettes with rare earth intensifying screens, as these amplify the X-ray signal within the cassette and reduce the dose required
	Source to skin distance	• Should be 40 cm rather than shorter distances of 20 cm
	Film holders	• Recommended for periapical and bitewing radiographs with collimated beam (ADA 2006)
Clinical judgment	X-rays should only be taken, if they are justified following a thorough clinical examination. Radiographs should only be prescribed after an evaluation of the patient's needs that includes a health history review, a clinical dental history assessment, a clinical examination, and an evaluation of susceptibility to dental diseases (ADA 2006)	• Unnecessary radiographs increases the amount of dose
Radiographic technique	Radiographs should be taken as accurately as possible by using film holders and beam aiming devices	

Contd...

Contd...

	Precautions	Reasons
Quality assurance (Quality assurance may be defined as any planned activity to ensure that a dental surgery will consistently produce high quality images with minimum exposure to patients and personnel, *ADA 2006*)	The main areas that form the basis of a QA program are: • Personnel and training • Image quality (Department of Health, UK, 2001), the recommended method of assessing image quality is to compare the radiograph with a good quality reference film and to subjectively rate the quality • Working procedure • X-ray equipment • Audit • Dark room	• Reduce the number of repeat X-rays • Reduce the cost of the procedure • Increase efficiency • Minimum radiation exposure • Determine the sources of error and their correction • Produce images of high quality
Continuing education	Practitioners should remain informed about safety updates and the availability of new equipment, supplies and techniques that could further improve the diagnostic quality of radiographs and decrease radiation exposure	
Protecting the personnel	• Try not to hold the film during exposure. Always use a film holder • Do not stand in the line of the primary beam • Stand behind a lead barrier (2 mm thickness)	
Public	• Warning/informative signs to indicate hazardous radiation • Patients should not be allowed to wait in corridors next to the X-ray room	

Table 4.3 Recommended annual dose limits

Recommendation	*According to ICRP*
Occupational dose limits	• 50 mSv annual effective dose limit and 100 mSv in a 5 year cumulative effective dose limit (regarding stochastic effects) • 150 mSv equivalent dose limits to lens of the eye and 500 mSv annual equivalent dose limits to skin and extremities (regarding deterministic effects)
Public dose limits (nonoccupational)	• 1 mSv annual effective dose limit, not to exceed annual average of 1 mSv over 5 years (regarding stochastic effects) • 15 mSv equivalent dose limits to lens of the eye and 50 mSv annual equivalent dose limits to skin and extremities (regarding deterministic effects)
Pregnant women (embryo-fetus)	• 2 mSv equivalent dose limit after the pregnancy has been declared

Source: From International Commission on Radiological Protection (ICRP): Radiation protection, ICRP Publication 60, 1990

Thermoluminescent Dosimeters (TLD) (Badges and Extremity Monitor)

These are used for personal monitoring of the whole body and/or the extremities, as well as measuring the skin dose from particular investigations. Personal monitors consist of a yellow or orange plastic holder, worn like the film badge. The lithium fluoride which is present in these badges is reusable and read-out measurements are easily automated and rapidly produced. The disadvantage is that, they do not give any permanent record and are relatively expensive to use.

Ionization Chambers

Image Quality: The unacceptable films should be collected over a period of time, (week) and analyzed. This is called film reject analysis (Tables 4.4 and 4.5).

RADIOLOGICAL INTERPRETATION AND DIAGNOSIS

The role of radiographs in dentistry is multifactorial. They help in the clinical examination phase, in confirming a diagnosis or rejecting it, during treatment planning, actual treatment and follow-up treatment. But at the same time, radiographic examination and diagnosis has its own limitations.

Table 4.4 Radiograph rating

Rating	*Quality*	*Basis*
1	Excellent	No errors of patient preparation, exposure, positioning, processing or film handling
2	Diagnostically acceptable	Some errors of patient preparation, exposure, positioning, processing or film handling, but which do not detract from the diagnostic utility of the radiograph
3	Unacceptable	Errors of patient preparation, exposure, positioning, processing or film handling, which render the radiograph diagnostically unacceptable

Source: From National Radiological Protection Board 1994 Guidelines on Radiological Standards for Primary Dental Care. Doc. NRPB, 5, No. 3

Table 4.5 Minimum targets for radiographic quality

Rating	*Percentage of radiographs taken*
1	Not less than 70%
2	Not greater than 20%
3	Not greater than 10%

Source: From National Radiological Protection Board 1994 Guidelines on Radiological Standards for Primary Dental Care. Doc. NRPB, 5, No. 3

It is a blind tool and we need to justify its use. It cannot replace clinical examination and needs further investigation to properly achieve a diagnosis.

Ideal radiograph should have the following properties:

- Image is the same size and shape as the object
- Image has good detail, good density and contrast
- Anatomical accuracy of radiographic images
- Proper coverage of the area of interest

Mandibular molar periapical X-ray film (either parelling or bisecting angle technique) comes closest to satisfying these requirements.

The Importance of Radiographic Interpretation

Radiographic interpretation is an essential part of the diagnostic process. The ability to evaluate and recognize what is revealed by a radiograph helps us to detect diseases, lesions and conditions which cannot be identified clinically and arrive at a definitive diagnosis.

INTERPRETATION AND DIAGNOSIS

Interpretation refers to an explanation of what is viewed on a radiograph, while diagnosis refers to the identification of disease by clinical examination or analysis. In other words, radiographic interpretation is one of the steps in reaching a diagnosis.

Principles of Radiographic Interpretation

The area of interest should be completely visible at proper angulations. All the boundaries of the area of interest must be seen with the normal structures around it. Knowledge and familiarity of all the normal anatomical landmarks as well as all various pathological conditions that may affect the area of interest is very important. The radiograph should be viewed by an appropriate person and under good viewing conditions.

Ideal Viewing Condition

Viewing should be attempted in a darkened room or the ambient light in the room should be reduced. All intraoral radiographs should be mounted in a holder. Light from the view-box should be of equal intensity across the viewing surface and the film should fit properly on the view box. A magnifying lens should be used for a more detailed examination of small and delicate areas of the film.

Thumb Rule in Radiographic Interpretation

The dentist should always keep in mind that the radiograph is a two dimensional image of a three dimensional structure/object. Therefore, we must apply the Clark's rule, while interpreting teeth on the buccal or lingual sides. The rule states that the most distant object from the cone of the tube head (lingual) moves towards the direction of the cone.

SLOB—same lingual opposite buccal

Oblique projections may be required for anatomically complicated areas. The key steps in radiographic interpretation are:

- Visualization or image analysis
- Perception and observation
- Integration of information and its interpretation.

IMAGE ANALYSIS

The importance of image analysis is to use a systemic approach to identify all the normal anatomy present in an image.

L—Localize

O—Observe

G—General considerations
I—Interpret
C—Correlate.

Localize and Observe

Localize or generalize the lesion/condition on the radiograph. Ensure that the radiograph is of the person being examined; check the date and the name of the patient. The right and left markers should be identified and marked accordingly. Each and every shadow/artifact visible should be accounted for and evaluated to ascertain, whether it is a feature of the normal anatomy on the radiograph, is a pathologic lesion or a superimposition of structures. The embossed dot on the periapical film is used to identify the right and the left sides and the normal anatomical landmarks are used to identify the jaw and the area.

In cases of intraoral images, under good viewing conditions, all the normal anatomical landmarks (including the bone) are identified. In cases of any doubt of any changes in the appearance of these landmarks, they should be compared against another image of acceptable quality having the same corresponding area of interest. The next step is to examine the alveolar process and its height in relation to the teeth (loss of height may indicate periodontal disease). After that the dentition and its associated structures should be examined. The number, sequence, appearance, root structure, enamel length, presence of crowns, interproximal caries, restorations on the teeth, pulp chambers, root resorption, etc. should all be examined in thorough detail.

In cases of extraoral radiographs, a more systemic approach should be adopted. A step by step analysis of all the radiographic characteristics of the pathology helps the dentist in improving upon the accuracy of his interpretation.

Localize

- Identify the location and limit of the pathology and describe it. This helps the dentist in assigning the pathology to various categories as some may be localized and some may be generalized. If the pathology appears to be generalized, then systemic abnormalities like metabolic or endocrinal conditions can be considered. In case of the lesion being localized, next important thing to examine is whether it is present unilaterally or bilaterally.
- Ascertain the position of the lesion. Is the lesion involving the soft tissue or has it penetrated the bone? If it is in the bone, is it enlarging and affecting the adjacent anatomical structures?
- Next, establish whether it is present singularly or is multifocal? This also helps the dentist in assigning the lesion to the appropriate category.

The size of the lesion does not aid in arriving to a diagnosis but at the same time, it helps in the differential diagnosis.

Observe

- Any unaccountable shadows/artefacts should be thoroughly examined, for example shadows in crowns, cervical area, roots, periapical area, and integrity of the bone.
- The outline of the lesion should be established—whether it is an ill-defined border or a well-defined border? If the borders are well-defined, then the next step is to determine whether they are punched out, sclerotic, corticated or has a soft tissue capsule around it which can be seen as a radiolucent line at the periphery of the lesion. An ill-defined border should be described along with the surrounding structure which is invaded upon or is blending with it (this tells us the rapidity of growth of the lesion). The shape of the lesion (circular, unilocular, multilocular) should also be assessed.

General Considerations

As mentioned before in the text, a radiograph is a two dimensional projection of a three dimensional object/structure (width and height but not the depth). Cervical burnout is misinterpreted as proximal caries which occurs due to less density and more penetration of rays.

Pulp exposure should never be diagnosed or determined from radiograph only. The proximity to the pulp can ascertain from the radiograph but again these findings should be correlated clinically in the patient's mouth.

Interpretation

Study the features of teeth and bone. Displacement of teeth is more common with slow growing lesions. The direction of displacement is also important. Widening of the periodontal ligament membrane occurs in a lot of conditions. Determine, if the widening is uniform or irregular. Determine the presence/absence of the lamina dura also. The surrounding bone and its density along with the pattern of its trabecular also helps in arriving at a diagnosis. Changes in the bone to look for are in the density, changes at the margin, changes inside the lesion and its effect on the surrounding tissues and finally changes within the structure.

Correlation

The final step is to correlate all of the radiographic features to reach a radiographic differential diagnosis. To achieve a proper diagnosis, we have to correlate the radiographic findings with clinical examination, patient's history and other diagnostic aids. There are four possible outcomes that the dentist can reach:

1. *True positive:* The disease is present and is identified.
2. *False positive:* The disease is absent on the radiograph but is identified by the dentist.
3. *True negative:* The disease is absent and is thus not identified.
4. *False negative:* The disease is present but not identified or detected.

FILMS USED IN TAKING RADIOGRAPHS

There are two types of film used in dentistry:

1. *Direct exposure film:* This is used intraorally. It is exposed when X-rays come in contact with it. The film is sealed in a light-tight packet. There are two types of direct exposure film: D-speed, also called ultra speed, and F-speed, which is called insight.
2. *Screen film:* This is used for extraoral radiographs. Screen film is especially sensitive to the effects of light from an intensifying screen. Using the screen-film combination allows a very large reduction in the amount of radiation needed to expose the film (30–60 times less radiation than that required by direct exposure film).

Other types of films used are:

- *Intraoral films:* These are used for:
  - Bitewing films which depict the crowns of both maxillary and mandibular teeth on one film
  - Periapical films, which show the entire length of the teeth in either the maxillary or mandibular arch
  - Occlusal films, which are usually exposed at approximately right angles (perpendicular) to the occlusal plane and show broad areas of the teeth and bone.
- Extraoral films
- Films with slow speed like A, B, C speed
- Films with fast speed like D ultra-speed, K ekta speed, F ultra ekta speed
- Hyper speed films like G which is 800 speed film
- Single use film packet
- Double use film packet
- Screen films
  - Sensitive to blue light like calcium tungstate
  - Sensitive to green light like rare earth screens
- Nonscreen films.

Film Speed and Size

The speed of a film represents the amount of radiation required to produce a radiograph of acceptable density (Table 4.6), (density is the degree of

Table 4.6 Film sizes

Type of film	*Size*	*Use*
Intraoral	# 0	Used in children for both periapical (PA) and bitewing (BW) films and also used for patients with small mouths
	# 1	Used for adult anterior periapical with the paralleling technique
	# 2	Used for adult posterior periapical and bitewings and for children with larger mouths, also used in anterior region of adults for periapical films taken with bisecting-angle technique and are also used for occlusal films in children
	# 3	Used for extra-long bitewing films; one film covers all teeth on one side of the mouth
	# 4	Used for occlusal films (primarily adults)
Extraoral	5″ x 12″ and 6″ x 12″	Both of these films are used in panoramic radiography. Some machines use 5″x 12″ and others use 6″ x 12″
	8″ x 10″	This size is used for cephalometric films, skull films and tomograms (TMJ)
	5″ x 7″	This size is not often used. It may be used for lateral oblique jaw films

darkening of the film). As the speed of the film increases, the amount of radiation needed to properly expose it decreases.

Intraoral Films

- D-speed (ultra speed) was once the most common intraoral film speed used, but it is now gradually being replaced by F-speed film. Technically, this slower film produces sharper images, improving the diagnostic ability of the film.
- *F-speed (Insight):* This film has large silver halide crystals requiring less radiation for exposure resulting in a 60% reduction in the patient exposure when compared to D-speed film.

Extraoral Films

The speed of extraoral film is increased with an increase in the size of the silver halide crystals. In general, the faster the film, the less sharp the radiographic image will be. Extraoral films are always used with intensifying screens. Like films, screens have different speeds. The overall speed of an extraoral film system (film plus screen) is determined by the combined speeds of the film and the screen.

VARIOUS RADIOGRAPHIC TECHNIQUES

Intraoral Views

Periapical View

This view is intended to show the area around the root of the tooth. Normally, the entire tooth is seen, showing the internal resorption, allowing the identification of root problems, interproximal caries, and the condition of the bone surrounding the teeth. This film is also used in endodontic treatment of a carious tooth.

This can be achieved by two methods:

1. *Paralleling technique:* The film is placed parallel to the tooth and a film holder is used. This produces the most accurate and reproducible image with no image distortion. There is no coning off the image. Rectangular collimation used reduces the radiation dose to the patient. The crowns of the teeth and the periodontal bone levels are well depicted with no superimposition of the zygomatic buttress on the maxillary molars. The image shows little or no magnification. A long cone periapical is taken to assess periodontal pocketing around the lower incisors.
2. *Bisecting angle:* This technique is an alternative to the paralleling technique. The paralleling technique is routine periapical radiography, but there are some instances when it is very difficult to use due to patient anatomy or lack of cooperation. In these situations, the bisecting angle technique may be used. The film can be held in the mouth with the thumb or index finger or a film holder may be used. The film is placed against the back of the tooth and the tube head is aligned at 90 degrees to the line bisecting the tooth and the film.

   This technique is most useful in areas with limited space like patients with shallow palate. The most common disadvantage of this view is that it can lead to elongation or foreshortening of the image due to the in accurate judgment of the vertical angulation of the tube. The advantages of the bisecting angle technique are that it is comfortable to use, as the film is placed in the mouth at an angle to the long axis of the teeth, therefore, the film doesn't impinge on the tissues as much. There are no anatomical restrictions, as the film can be angled to accommodate different anatomical situations.

Anatomical variations situations which might require using the bisecting angle technique are patients with shallow palate, a large palatal torus, a shallow or tender floor of the mouth and a short lingual frenum (tongue-tie). This type of dental imaging can lead to more distortion because as the film and teeth are at an angle to each other (not parallel), it is harder to position X-ray beam. A film holder is often not used, as it is difficult to visualize where the X-ray beam should be directed and therefore, the film is less stable.

Bitewing View

This used where there is a need to project the crowns of the teeth in both the arches in the same image. This also allows the dentist to assess the associated alveolar bone levels of the teeth. The patient is asked to bite on a paper tab stuck on the film packet. The tube head is positioned at 90 degrees to the arch in a horizontal plane for the beam to pass between the contact points of the teeth. Vertically, the beam is angled slightly downwards to avoid the overlapping of the contact areas and to account for the curve of monsoon on the occlusal plane. This is mainly used to detect interproximal caries.

Occlusal View

This view displays the occlusal surfaces of the teeth with their relationship to the alveolar bone. It is also used to identify the extent of larger pathological conditions, to locate an object in the buccolingual direction, to show the developing dentition in impacted maxillary canine in children and to image patients with trismus (inability to open the mouth).

- *Maxillary/upper standard occlusal view:* This is the most common occlusal radiograph taken in the maxillary arch. This is used to detect pathology and unerupted or supernumerary teeth in the palate. The film is placed in the patient's mouth by asking the patient to bite gently against it, so that the film lies against the occlusal surfaces of the upper anterior teeth. The tube head is angled 60–70-degrees downwards and beam is aimed horizontally through the bridge of the nose.
- *Mandibular/lower standard occlusal view:* This view depicts clearly the lower incisors and their surrounding bone levels. Therefore, this is used for assessing pathology that extends beyond the scope of a periapical radiograph.
- *Upper vertex (true) occlusal view:* This view is no longer used due to the high dose of radiation required for this. This was used previously to detect the position of any unerupted or supernumerary teeth relative to the dental arch.
- *Lower true occlusal view:* This view is used to detect and assess mandibular fractures and cysts and tumors in the anterior mandible. This view can also be used to detect salivary calculi in the submandibular duct and to assess the buccolingual displacement of symphyseal and parasymphyseal fractures of the mandible.
- *Upper oblique occlusal view:* The posterior teeth and their surrounding bone and the antral floor can be depicted clearly in this image. This is used for imaging pathology in these areas, detecting and assessing dentoalveolar fractures and roots displaced into the antrum.
- *Lower oblique occlusal view:* This view is used in conjunction with lower true occlusal for detecting the salivary calculi in the submandibular

duct. It can also be used to detect any pathology in the posterior part of the body of the mandible.

The principle of parallax can be used to gather information about the position of an unerupted tooth relative to the dental arch. *Parallax* technique works on the basis that when two projections are taken, those objects further away from the tube move in the same direction, as the tube and those closer to the tube move in the opposite direction. The acronym SLOB—same lingual opposite buccal is generally used to remember this. In the horizontal plane, this can be performed by using two periapical views and two occlusal views. In the vertical plane, an occlusal plus a peri apical or a panoramic and a periapical with an occlusal is used.

Extraoral Views

Panoramic View

This is also referred to as dental panoramic tomogram (DPT) or orthopantomogram (OPG/OPT). It displays all the oral structures and is made with a specific device called orthopantomogram. This technique allows the simultaneous and comparative study of the joints, and the dentoalveolar arches. An image of the dental arches is produced by the technique of tomography for producing images of a section of an object. The X-ray tube and the film are rotated producing blurring of the structures on either side of the center of rotation. A horseshoe shaped focal plane called the focal trough (the section of the object in focus on the tomogram) is produced during exposure. The indications for this view are assessment of third molars, assessment of fractures of the mandible, assessment of antral pathology, planning implants, in orthodontic treatments, assessment of bone heights, bony disorders of the temporomandibular joints (TMJ) and assessment of bony lesions of the arches. The panoramic film is the most common extraoral film used in dentistry. It does not provide the detail that intraoral films do, but it gives an overall view of the entire dentition, both maxillary and mandibular. It is very helpful for third molar extractions.

Extraoral Views of the Mandible Other than Orthopantomogram

Posteroanterior (PA) View of the Mandible/Jaw: This view is used to assess fractures and pathology in the posterior part of the mandible and the condyles. They are also used to evaluate trauma and developmental problems.

Oblique Lateral View: This can be used to image the ramus and the body of the mandible. The lateral oblique jaw film can be used to image the third molar region in adults and to show the developing posterior dentition in children. This view is also used to image posterior maxilla.

Reverse Towne's View/Projection: This is used to assess the condyles.

Transcranial View: This provides information on the components of this joint, including the head of the condyle, the glenoid fossa and the articular eminence.

Oblique Lateral for the Posterior Maxila

Occipitomental View: This is used to assess the sinuses and fractures of the zygomatic complex, orbits and coronoid process. This can also be used to assess middle third facial injuries and nasoethmoidal fractures.

Submentovertex View (SMV): This is used for the assessment of the zygomatic arches and to assess pathology in the palate and the skull. This view is contraindicated, if there is any possibility of a fractured cervical spine.

Lateral Cephalometric View: It clearly shows both the soft profile (face) and bony structures on the same film. This film is used routinely by orthodontists in developing treatment plans for their patients. It is also used by oral surgeons for evaluating trauma and conditions requiring surgical correction.

RECENT ADVANCES IN RADIOGRAPHIC TECHNIQUES

Digital Imaging

This technique uses a conventional X-ray machine but the film is replaced by a sensor with a charge coupled device (CCD). The receptors convert the image into digital data. Digital imaging incorporates computer technology in the capture, display, enhancement, and storage of direct radiographic images. The first direct digital imaging system, Radiovisiography (RVG), was invented by Dr Frances Mouyensand in 1984.

Digital radiography is the latest advancement in dental imaging (Table 4.7). There are two main types of digital radiography:

1. *Direct digital imaging (produces the image immediately on the monitor post-exposure):* There are different types of digital imaging according to the films—extraoral (cephalometric, panoramic and tomographic which can be used to view available bone in a facial-lingual view for implant planning) and Intraoral (periapical and bitewings).
2. *Indirect digital imaging:* The main *advantages* of this technique include superior enhancement of images, low radiation dose, three dimensional reconstructions of the images, alleviates the need for conventional processing, efficient storage, can be used for teleradiology purposes, is highly helpful in patient education and acceptance of treatment plans and options.

Table 4.7 Recent advances in radiographic techniques

Various radiographic techniques	
Intraoral views	• Periapical (paralleling and bisecting angle) • Bitewing • Occlusal (upper and lower standard occlusal, upper true and lower true occlusal, upper and lower oblique occlusal)
Extraoral views	• Panoramic • Oblique lateral (maxillary and mandibular) • Posteroanterior view of the mandible • Reverse towne's projection • Occipitomental • Submentovertex • Lateral cephalometric
Digital imaging	
Conventional tomography	
Computed tomography (CT)	
Magnetic resonance imaging (MRI)	
Ultrasonography	
Cone beam computed tomography	
Sialography	
Temporomandibular imaging	

The *disadvantages* include cost factor, medico legal issues (the ability to manipulate the images for fraudulent purposes), cross-infection control (the intraoral sensor can not be sterilized), the bulk of the sensor, some loss of image resolution compared to the film and a large amount of disc space is required for storage. This technique is used in almost all dental specialties for the detection of tumors, detection of metastatic hard tissue lesions, as a follow-up upon trauma or surgery, to check the healing of the periapical lesions after endodontic treatment, during instrumentation, for implant assessment and analysis, detection of caries and periodontal diseases, and detection of any perforation to the surrounding soft tissue like maxillary sinus and many other uses.

Conventional Tomographic View

This view is used to reproduce cross-sectional views of the maxilla and the mandible. The indications for this technique are for implant assessment and planning and assessing the buccolingual expansion of pathology. This also helps to determine the position of impacted/supernumerary teeth.

Computed Tomography

This view depicts both the soft tissues and the bone. It is indicated in assessing mid facial trauma; blow out fracture of the orbital floor and bony lesions.

Magnetic Resonance Imaging

This view gives excellent soft tissue detail and is commonly used for tumor staging and assessment of intracranial diseases. This is also particularly useful in detecting the internal derangement of the temporomandibular joint. The main advantage is that there is no ionizing radiation used in this technique. This is contraindicated in patients with pacemakers, cochlear implants and in the first trimester of pregnancy.

Ultrasonography

This is useful for superficial soft tissues like lymph nodes and salivary glands. It can be used to distinguish between solid and cystic masses and can be used to guide fine needle aspiration. It does not use any ionizing radiation. It can also be used to break up calculi.

Cone Beam Computed Tomography

This is the most recent and expensive advancement in digital radiography. A scan in the area of interest is taken, and the resulting image is displayed as image slices and/or 3-dimensional (3-D) images of the area.

OTHER RADIOGRAPHIC TECHNIQUES IN THE HEAD AND NECK

Sialography

This technique involves the introduction of a radiographic contrast medium into the ductal system of the salivary glands (parotid or submandibular). The image is then captured. This is indicated for the assessment of the structure of the gland and to detect the presence of any calculi in them. It is contraindicated in patients with known allergy to iodine containing compounds or those who have any infections in the gland.

Temporomandibular Imaging

These include the TMJ arthrography (contrast medium is injected into the joint space) to determine the disc position and to detect any disc perforations and adhesions, transpharyngeal view, transcranial view and transorbital view.

RADIOGRAPHIC ERRORS AND ARTEFACTS

An artefact is any optical density that is not an anatomical landmark or an unwanted density on the radiograph that interferes with diagnosis (Table 4.8). Films with errors should be avoided, as retake will lead to unnecessary radiation exposure to the patient, waste film and time (money) and interfere with accurate interpretation and diagnosis.

Radiopaque Artefacts

These can be dental appliances, body piercings, jewelry or eye glasses left in the mouth during exposure. They will appear as radiopaque artefacts superimposed over the dental image. To correct this error, all these items should be removed before placing of the film.

There are three time periods during which artefacts/errors can occur:

1. Technique and projection errors.
2. Exposure errors.
3. Processing errors.

Technique and Projection Errors

- *Patient preparation errors:* These could be blurred image, pressure mark or a radiopaque artefact.
- *Film placement errors:* These include double image, dot artefact, distortion, crown not shown, area of interest not shown clearly, reversed film, apices cut off, black line, etc.
- *Projection errors:* Incorrect vertical and horizontal angulation.

Exposure Errors

- Blank image
- Low density image
- High density image
- Image with high and low contrast.

Processing Errors

- *Chemical errors:* These include light image, dark image, blank image, reticulation, black spot or patch, black line, white spot or patch, yellowish brown discoloration.
- *Film handling errors:* These include writing lines, developer cut off, fixer cut off, overlapped film, finger nail artefact, smudged or scratched film, static electricity.

Table 4.8 Radiographic errors

Error	*Reason*
Blurred image	Caused mainly by the movement of the film, patient or X-ray tube head during exposure. This can be corrected by explaining to the patient and reminding him to remain motionless during exposure
Pressure mark	Marks from the incisal edge and cusps of the teeth (mostly in the pediatric occlusal radiograph) may appear as black or white on the radiographic film. To correct this error, ask the patient to bite gently on the film
Double image	When an exposed film is re-exposed, the resulting film will have 2 superimposed images
Reversed film	This error is seen as a low density with herringbone, tire-track or dotted pattern. This is a result of directing the X-ray through the lead foil side of the film back
Dot artefact	The identification (embossed) dot produces a circular radiolucent artefact on the final radiograph which may interfere with interpretation of the apical areas of the teeth
Apices cut off	Occurs when the film is not positioned apically enough to record the entire tooth
Crown not shown	This is when the film is not extended enough occlusally
Area of interest not shown	This happens when the film is not placed correctly enough to cover all the structures in the area of interest or if film is not centralized enough
Incorrect vertical and horizontal elongation	X-ray tube head is positioned at too shallow an angle with respect to the teeth or the film could have been bent in the mouth by excessive pressure from the patient's finger supporting the film packet
Coning-off/ alignment artefact	X-ray tube head is placed too high and is not aiming directly at the film packet, thus resulting in a partial image on the resultant radiograph
Blank image	The film that did not receive any radiation and appears clear
Underexposure	Exposure time is too less probably due to incorrect exposure setting on the timer or faulty timer. The film appears pale in nature
Under development	Developer solution is too cold, too dilute or too old. The film could have been left in the developer solution for too short a time
Over exposure	Usually the exposure time is too great due to either a faulty timer or incorrect exposure setting
Over development	The developer solution may be too hot, or too concentrated. The film could have been left in the developer for too long
Fogged film	Occurs due to any light leakage in the darkroom, faulty safe lighting or poor film storage. It can also occur by the use of old films, as a result of poor stock control

Contd...

Contd...

Error	*Reason*
Reticulation	This error occurs when the film is subjected to a sudden temperature change between the developer and water and appears as cracked film
Black spot or patch/black line	Developer contamination
White spot/patch	Contamination of the fixer solution before processing
Yellowish brown discoloration	Insufficient washing or exhausted solutions. There is hyporetention of the remaining thiosulphate from the fixer solution
Writing lines and finger nail artefacts	These may appear as black or white. Finger nail artefact is due to the rough handling of the film and appears as a black or white crescent shaped mark. These are also known as kink marks
Blank white border	Occurs when the film is not completely immersed in the fixer solution
Blank black border	When the film is not completely immersed in the developer solution
Smudged or scratched films	When the film is touched by fingers contaminated by any of the processing solutions, smudges can be seen on the film. If the film is scratched due to careless handling, white lines appear on the film

Unique Radiographic Appearances

Appearance on the radiograph	*Associated conditions*
Ground glass appearance	• Fibrous dysplasia • Hyperparathyroidism
Cotton wool appearance	• Paget disease (osteitis deformans) • Periapical cemento-osseous dysplasia • Gardner syndrome (osteoma) • Gigantiform cementoma
Sunburst radioopacities	• Osteosarcoma • Intraosseous hemangioma
Onion-skin appearance	• Proliferative periostitis • Ewing sarcoma • Langerhans cell disease

CONCLUSION

The use of X-rays is an integral part of clinical dentistry, with some form of radiographic examination necessary on the majority of patients.

BIBLIOGRAPHY

1. FGDP (UK)- RCS 1998 Selection criteria for dental radiography.
2. Napier ID. Reference doses for dental radiography. British Dental Journal. 1999; 186(8):392-6.
3. National Council on Radiation protection and measurements: Limitation of exposure to ionizing radiation, 1993.
4. National Radiological Protection Board 1994 Guidelines on Radiology Standards for primary dental care. Doc. NRPB, 5, No. 3.
5. Sources and effects of ionizing radiation, volume 1: sources, New York, 2000. UNSCEAR, UN Publication.
6. White SC, Pharoah MJ. Oral radiology: principles and interpretation, 6th edn. Mosby Elsevier, 2009.

CHAPTER 5

RADIOGRAPHIC DIAGNOSIS OF CARIES

Balaram Naik, Priyanka Jain

INTRODUCTION

Almost since the discovery of X-rays by William Conrad Roentgen in 1895, radiography has been used to detect the effects of dental caries on dental hard tissues. Radiography has been primarily used for the detection of lesions on the proximal surfaces of teeth, which are not clinically visible for inspection. Radiographs are useful in the detection of caries because of the nature of the disease process. Demineralization and destruction of hard tooth structures result in a loss of tooth density in the area of the lesion. The decreased density allows a greater penetration of X-rays in the carious area, and as a result, the carious lesion appears as a radiolucency on a dental radiograph (Fig. 5.1). Radiolucent structures permit the passage of the X-ray beam and appear dark or black on a dental radiograph. A dental examination for caries cannot be considered complete without radiographs. It enables the dental professional not only to evaluate the extent and severity of a carious lesion seen clinically, but also to identify carious lesions that are not visible clinically. Caries can reach a large size before it presents clinical problems and a good diagnostician must find and treat the caries before that stage is reached.

Carious lesions are detectable radiographically when there has been enough demineralization to allow it to differentiate from normal. On average they have around 50–70% sensitivity in detecting carious lesions. 40% demineralization is required for definitive decision on caries.

The degree of radiolucency seen on a dental radiograph is determined by the extent and severity of the destruction seen as a result of the caries process. Caries is always farther advanced clinically than what is seen on a dental radiograph. Radiography is an important supplement to clinical examination for detecting dental caries. In cases when the surface is fully intact (when there is no breakdown) clinical examination may not be able to diagnose the demineralization process beneath the surfaces including the occlusal surfaces.

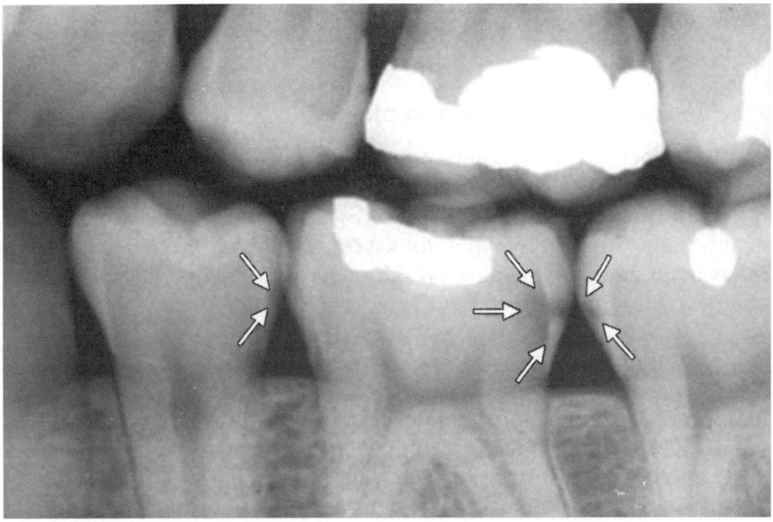

Fig. 5.1 Radiograph showing radiolucency

RADIOGRAPHIC DIAGNOSIS AND TECHNIQUES

- *Posterior bitewing views:* This is used mainly for the premolar and molar view. This is the most important view for caries. Anterior bitewings can be used for periodontal assessments.
- *Periapical views:* Paralleling technique must be used to see caries best.
- *Panoramic view:* This is often not suitable to see incipient caries as it lacks sufficient details but can be used to view occlusal caries.
- *Lateral oblique:* Not used in the diagnosis of caries.
- Any radiograph that shows the teeth.

The bitewing film is primarily used for caries diagnosis, but the periapical film is also helpful. The difference in angulation between the two films gives two different perspectives and can prove helpful in diagnosing recurrent caries around existing restorations. Approximately 40–50% demineralization is required for radiographic detection of a lesion. The actual depth of penetration of a carious lesion is actually deeper than it appears on the radiograph. Radiographic diagnosis of dental caries is fundamentally based on the fact that as the caries process proceeds, the mineral content of enamel and dentin decreases with a resultant decrease in the attenuation of the X-ray beam as it passes through the teeth. This is recorded on the image receptor as an increase in radiographic density. This increase in radiographic density must be detected by the clinician as a sign of a carious lesion. Many different factors can affect the ability to accurately detect these lesions such as exposure parameters, type of image receptor, image processing, display system, viewing conditions and ultimately the training and experience of the human observer (Table 5.1).

Frequency of Taking Radiographs

The frequency of radiographic procedures can be determined clinically only and by taking a complete dental history. Factors such as oral hygiene, fluoride exposure, diet, history of caries and age are very important in determining this. Radiographs for caries should be taken at 1–3 years intervals in adults depending on the mentioned factors. In caries prone children, this frequency can be as early as 6–12 months.

Using Intraoral Films

Radiographic examinations in dentistry include bitewing projection, IOPA radiographs using paralleling technique and dental panoramic tomogram. Size 2 adult films are used for the bitewing projection from 7 years upwards. The use of a single film of size 3 results in overlapping contact points and cone-cut images. In smaller children, size 0 maybe used instead of size 2. Digital imaging can be used for this purpose. The disadvantages associated with digital imaging are that the surface area of the sensor used is smaller than a conventional size 2 intraoral film used, which results in fewer teeth being displayed on the resultant image. Also, the stiffness and increased thickness of the sensors may result in projection errors and re-takes. The *bitewing* radiograph, a radiograph that shows the crowns of both the upper and lower teeth on the same film, is the radiograph of choice for the evaluation of dental caries. In order for a bitewing radiograph to be considered diagnostic for the evaluation of dental caries, the following criteria should be met.

Table 5.1 Factors affecting appearance of caries on radiographs

Buccolingual thickness of tooth	The thicker the tooth, the more difficult it is to see the extent of the caries
Limitations of two-dimensional film	The extent of carious involvement cannot be seen in a buccolingual (cheek to tongue) direction
X-ray beam angle (horizontal or vertical)	This is important when trying to identify and diagnose recurrent caries, since changes in angulation can cause the superimposition of the existing restoration with the carious lesion. Overlap due to improper horizontal angulation makes it very difficult to diagnose early interproximal caries
Exposure factors	Caries detection is improved with a lower kVp setting, which provides a higher contrast. If the overall density of the film is too light or too dark, the diagnostic potential of the film becomes limited. Excessive filtration will have the same effect as kVp. Density of the radiograph is affected by the exposure times

Diagnostic Bitewing Criteria

- *Exposure and processing:* Proper film exposure and processing techniques must be used.
- *Open contacts:* Interproximal areas must demonstrate open contacts; a thin radiolucent line should be seen between the contacts of adjacent teeth.
- *Occlusal plane:* The occlusal plane should be positioned horizontally along the midline of the long axis of the film.
- *Premolar placement:* The premolar bitewing should demonstrate the distal contact areas of both the maxillary and mandibular canines.
- *Molar placement:* The molar bitewing should be centered over the second molar.
- *Errors:* The bitewing should be free of technique errors (e.g. cone cuts, film bending and backwards placement of a film).

CARIES CLASSIFICATION

The radiographic appearance of dental caries can be classified according to the location of the caries on the tooth. Caries involving the interproximal, occlusal, buccal, lingual and root surfaces may all be seen on a dental radiograph. In addition, recurrent and rampant caries may also be viewed on dental radiographs. Caries viewed on a dental radiograph can be classified according to the depth of penetration the lesion exhibits through the enamel and dentin as *incipient, moderate, advanced* and *severe.* I = Incipient (Stage I), M = Moderate (Stage II), A = Advanced (Stage III), S = Severe (Stage IV).

Haugejorden and Slack 1975 Classification

C-1: Enamel caries less than halfway through the enamel (incipient caries).

C-2: Enamel caries penetrating at least halfway through the enamel.

C-3: Caries at the dentinoenamel junction (moderate lesion).

C-4: Dentin caries halfway to the pulp (severe lesion).

INTERPROXIMAL CARIES

The term *interproximal* means between two adjacent surfaces. Caries found on the smooth surfaces between two teeth is termed *interproximal caries.* On a dental radiograph, interproximal caries is typically seen at or just below (apical to) the contact point. This area is difficult, to examine clinically and visually. As caries progresses inward through the enamel of the tooth, it assumes a triangular configuration; the apex (or point) of the triangle is seen at the dentinoenamel junction (DEJ). As caries reaches the DEJ, it spreads laterally and continues into dentin. Another triangular configuration is seen in dentin, this time the base of the triangle is found along the DEJ and the apex is pointed toward the pulp chamber.

Incipient Interproximal Caries

An incipient interproximal lesion (Fig. 5.2) extends less than halfway through the thickness of enamel. The term incipient means beginning to exist or appear. An incipient lesion is seen as a notch on the outer surface of the enamel only in the caries susceptible zone. This is usually not restored unless the patient has high caries activity. This can be treatment with Fluoride. The outline of the caries is poorly demarcated and diagnosis can easily be missed.

Moderate Interproximal Caries

A moderate interproximal lesion (Fig. 5.3) extends greater than halfway through the thickness of enamel, but does not involve the DEJ. A moderate lesion is seen in enamel only. It can appear as a triangle with a broad base towards the outer surface, as a diffuse radiolucent image or as a combination of both.

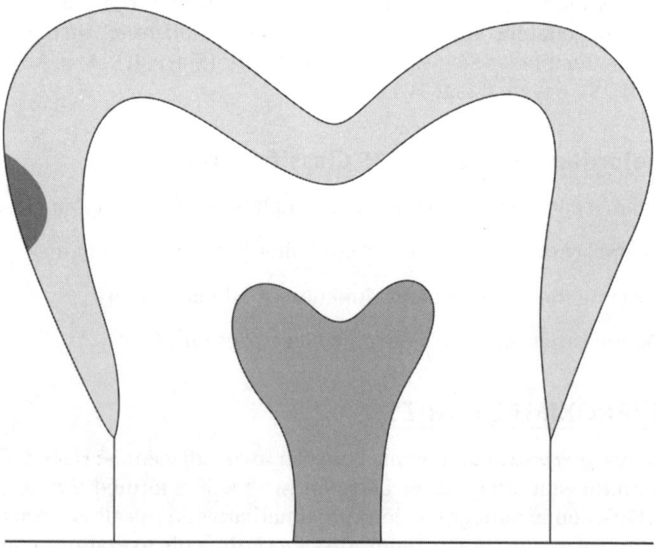

Fig. 5.2 Less than half the thickness of enamel

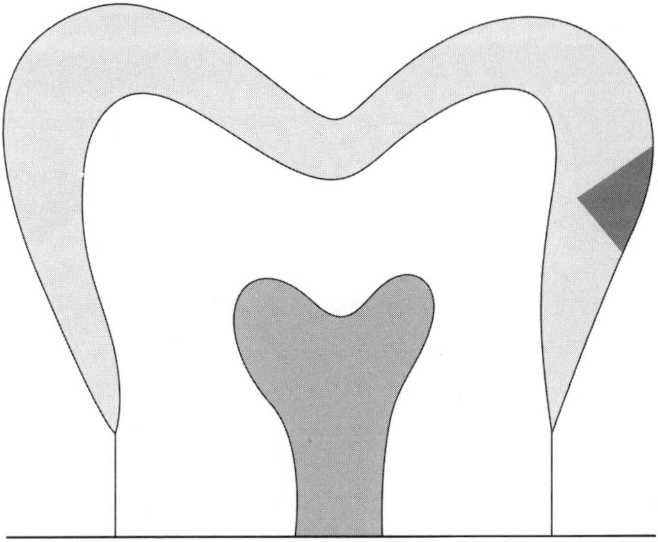

Fig. 5.3 Greater than half the thickness of enamel and does not involve dentinoenamel junction

Advanced Caries

An advanced interproximal lesion (Fig. 5.4) appears as a radiolucent triangular zone extending to the DEJ or through the DEJ and into the dentin, but does not extend through the dentin greater than half the distance toward the pulp. An advanced lesion affects both enamel and dentin.

Severe Caries

A severe interproximal lesion (Fig. 5.5) extends through enamel, through the dentin and greater than half the distance towards the pulp. A severe lesion involves both the enamel and dentin and may clinically appear as a cavitation (or hole) in the tooth. There are undermined enamel fractures under masticatory load leaving a large cavity.

False Interpretations

The presence or absence of a carious lesion on the same set of radiographs can prove to be very confusing even to the most experienced dentists. Various morphological structures like pits and fissures, cervical burnout, dental anomalies like hypoplastic pits can mimic the appearance of a carious

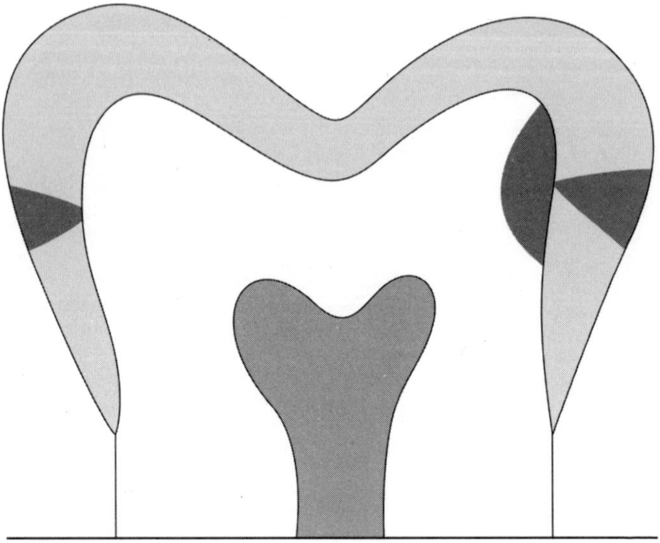

Fig. 5.4 Involves enamel and the dentinoenamel junction and less than half the distance to the pulp cavity

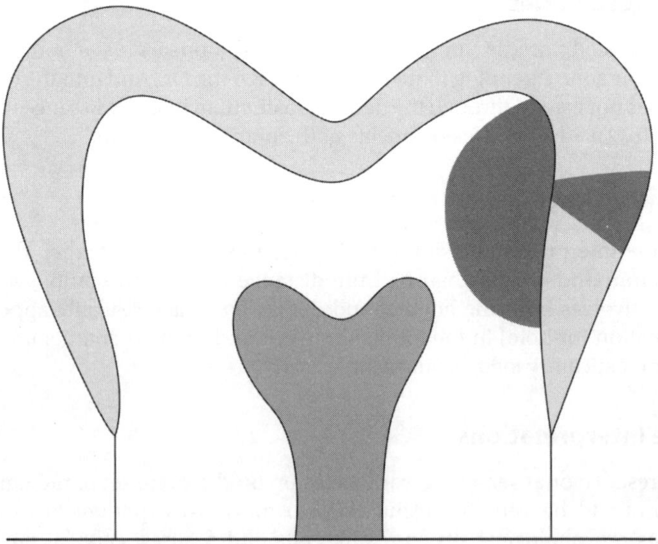

Fig. 5.5 Dentine penetrated more than half the distance to the pulp cavity

lesion. Proximal lesions extending only in enamel cannot be detected by radiography. A lesion extending into the dentin in the radiograph is easier to detect. Such false-positive diagnoses calls for a more conservative approach to caries diagnosis and treatment.

OCCLUSAL CARIES

The term *occlusal* refers to the chewing surfaces of the teeth. Caries that involves the pit and fissure surfaces of the posterior teeth is termed *occlusal caries*. This may also occur at the base of a pit or fissure with no clinical signs. A thorough clinical examination is the method of choice for the detection of occlusal caries. Because of the superimposition of the dense buccal and lingual enamel cusps, early occlusal caries is difficult to see on a dental radiograph; consequently, occlusal caries is not seen on a radiograph until there is involvement of the DEJ. Occlusal carious lesions can be classified as incipient, moderate and severe.

Incipient Occlusal Caries

Incipient occlusal caries cannot be seen on a dental radiograph and must be detected clinically with an explorer instead. The caries start on the walls of the pits and fissures and tend to spread perpendicular to the DEJ. The only detectable change is a fine gray shadow at the DEJ.

Moderate Occlusal Caries

Moderate occlusal caries extends into dentin and is seen as a very thin radiolucent line. This stage induces specific changes helping in a definitive diagnosis. A broad base thin radiolucent zone is located in the dentin with minimal or no changes in the enamel of the occlusal surface of the tooth.

Severe Occlusal Caries

Severe occlusal caries extends into dentin and is seen as a large radiolucency. This is readily observed both clinically and radiographically. The radiolucency extends under the enamel of the occlusal surface of the tooth. Severe occlusal caries appears as a cavitation (or hole) in a tooth. However, pulp exposure cannot be determined. The deeper the occlusal caries, the easier it is to determine on the radiograph.

False Interpretations

False positive diagnoses for occlusal caries include superimposition of the image of the buccal pit with or without an associated composite restoration. A false positive diagnosis may result in a sound surface being damaged.

Therefore, when there are no clinical signs and symptoms and only a false positive radiological diagnosis, it is always advisable to observe and monitor these cases and withhold any treatment procedures.

BUCCAL AND LINGUAL CARIES (CERVICAL CARIES)

These carious lesions often occur on the enamel pits and fissures of the teeth. They are round when small and as they enlarge, they become elliptical. They have sharp, well-defined borders. It is often difficult to differentiate between buccal and lingual caries on a radiograph. When superimposed on DEJ, these lesions mimic occlusal caries. The trick to diagnose them from occlusal caries is to look for well-defined noncarious enamel around the radiolucency which surrounds the buccal or the palatal lesion.

As the names suggest, buccal caries involves the buccal tooth surface, while lingual caries involves the lingual tooth surface. Because of the superimposition of the densities of normal tooth structure, buccal and lingual caries is difficult to detect on a dental radiograph and instead, is best detected clinically. The radiolucent outline will be more clearly defined on the lingual side due to the smaller film-object distance.

When viewed on a dental radiograph, caries that involves the buccal or lingual smooth surfaces appears as a small, circular radiolucency. Projection effect may make the caries appear enlarged. This can easily be mistaken for interproximal caries. In order to determine the location of the lesion, a clinical examination with an explorer is necessary.

ROOT SURFACE CARIES (CEMENTAL CARIES)

Root surface caries only involves the roots of teeth. The cementum and dentin located just below the cervical region of the tooth is involved. No involvement of enamel is seen. This is also known as cemental caries. This occurs with advanced gingival recession on exposed dentin. Bone loss precedes the caries process and result in exposed root surfaces. This can also occur with food packing, open contacts and over eruption of teeth. These lesions are often detected clinically and radiographs are not necessary.

Clinically, root surface caries is easily detected on exposed root surfaces with the most common locations being the exposed roots of the mandibular premolar and molar areas.

On a dental radiograph, root surface caries appears as a cupped-out or crater-shaped radiolucency just below the cementoenamel junction (CEJ) but coronal to the bone height. Early lesions may be difficult to detect on a dental radiograph. Root caries are usually found in older individuals with chronic recession or periodontitis.

False Interpretations

A surface may appear to be carious as a result of the cervical burn out and may mimic root caries. The true carious lesion can be differentiated by the absence of an image of the root edge and by the appearance of a diffuse rounded inner border where the tooth substance has been lost.

RECURRENT CARIES/SECONDARY CARIES

The radiolucency depends on the amount of demineralization and the extent of the restoration.

Secondary or *recurrent caries* occurs adjacent to/under a pre-existing restoration. Caries occurs in this region because of inadequate cavity preparation, defective margins or incomplete removal of caries prior to the placement of the restoration. High caries incidence and poor oral hygiene also play a part.

On a dental radiograph, recurrent caries appears as a radiolucent area just beneath a restoration, and is most often seen beneath the interproximal margins of a restoration. Radio-opacity of the restoration may often hide much of the carious lesion on the radiograph, and thus may sometimes be confused with lining.

RAMPANT CARIES

The term rampant means growing or spreading unchecked. Rampant caries is advanced and severe caries which affects numerous teeth in the dentition and is typically seen in children with poor dietary habits, high carbohydrate diet or in adults with a decreased salivary flow. This mainly affects the mandibular anterior teeth. Nursing bottle syndrome is a type of rampant caries but is increasingly becoming rare.

RADIATION CARIES/DRUG RELATED CARIES

This results from xerostomia caused by head and neck radiation therapy and is usually seen as a radiolucent shadow at the necks (cervical caries) of teeth. It tends to spread mesially and distally in patients with poor oral hygiene. This can be controlled by fluoride therapy.

ARRESTED CARIES

This is seen on the proximal surfaces of teeth as a vague radiolucent notch where the adjacent tooth is lost. It is rarely seen in pits and fissures and can easily be mistaken as a cervical burnout.

CONDITIONS RESEMBLING CARIES ON RADIOGRAPHS

A number of radiolucencies that involve the crown and roots of teeth may be confused with dental caries. *Restorative materials, abrasion, attrition* and *cervical burnout* may all resemble dental caries on a radiograph (Table 5.2). The dentist must remember that the final diagnosis of caries is made only after the clinical and radiographic findings are corroborated. Both the clinical examination and interpretation of radiographs are mutually contributory aids in making the diagnosis of dental caries.

Restorative Materials

Materials such as composites, silicates and acrylics, may appear radiolucent and resemble dental caries on a radiograph. The appearance of an anterior cavity preparation restored with these materials differs from the appearance of interproximal caries and can be identified by the well-defined, smooth outline (Fig. 5.6).

In addition, a careful clinical examination helps the dental professional determine the difference between a restorative material and dental caries.

Abrasion

This refers to the wearing of tooth structure from the friction of a foreign object. Tooth brush abrasion affects the root surface of a tooth and may be confused with root surface caries.

On a dental radiograph, tooth brush abrasion appears as a well-defined horizontal radiolucency along the cervical region of a tooth (Fig. 5.7). Clinically, the areas affected by abrasion appear as hard, highly polished defects in dentin and should not be confused with root caries that appears brown and leathery.

Table 5.2 Conditions resembling caries on radiographs

Condition	*Appearance on radiograph*	*Resembles*
Restorative materials	Well-defined, smooth outline	Interproximal caries
Abrasion	Well-defined horizontal radiolucency along the cervical region of a tooth	Root surface caries
Attrition	Shallow concavities	Incisal/occlusal caries
Cervical burnout	Collar or wedge-shaped radiolucency on the mesial and distal root surfaces	Root caries, arrested caries

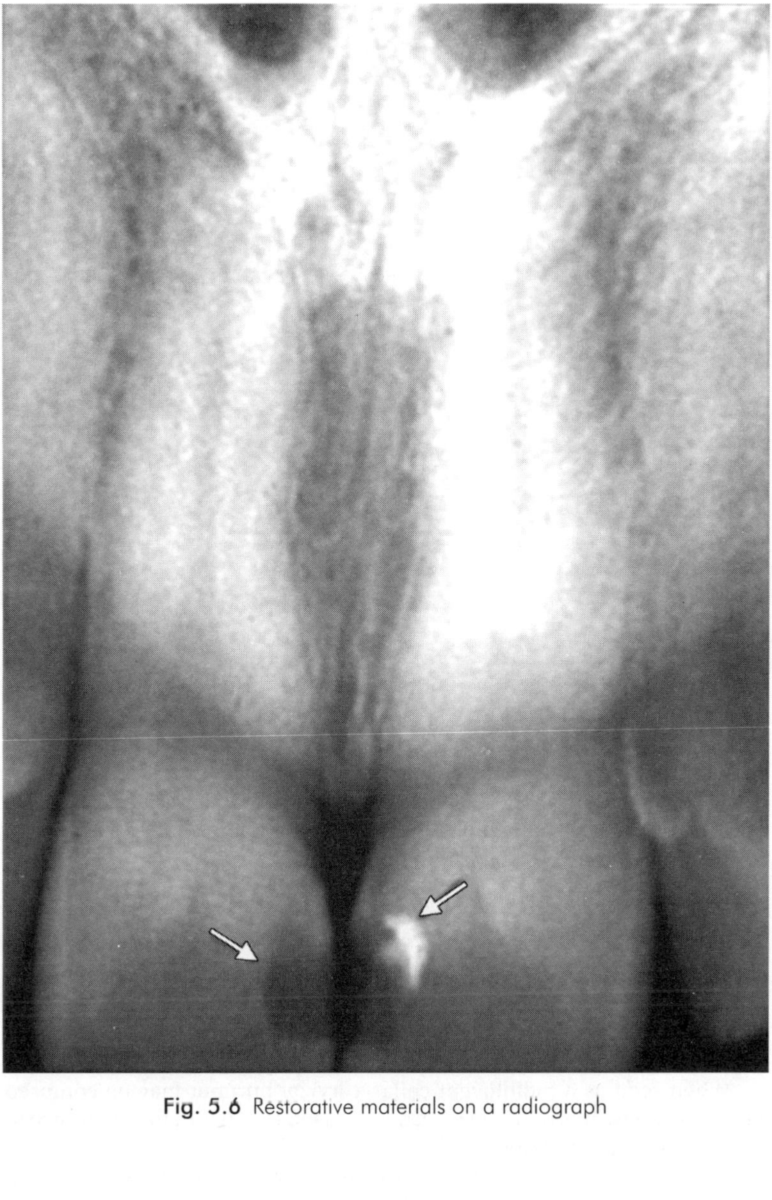

Fig. 5.6 Restorative materials on a radiograph

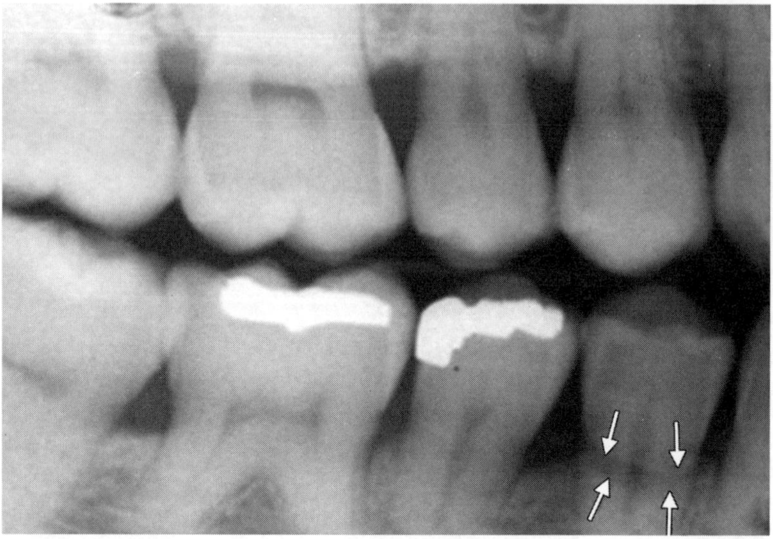

Fig. 5.7 Abrasive tooth surface

Attrition

The mechanical wearing down of teeth may be mistaken for dental caries on a radiograph. Attrition may be seen on the incisal or occlusal surfaces of deciduous or permanent teeth (Fig. 5.8). When the incisal or occlusal enamel is worn away, the underlying dentin wears away rapidly, and shallow concavities may form. These concavities may resemble occlusal or incisal caries on a dental radiograph. Clinical examination enables the dental professional to distinguish attrition from caries.

Cervical Burnout

A radiolucent artifact seen on dental radiograph may also be confused with dental caries. Cervical burnout appears as a collar or wedge-shaped radiolucency on the mesial and distal root surfaces near the CEJ of a tooth (Fig. 5.9).

When seen as a radiolucent collar, cervical burnout may be confused with root caries. This radiolucent artifact is seen because of the difference in densities of adjacent tissues.

Posteriorly, this radiolucency usually disappears when another film of the region is examined. Caries does not occur on the root of the tooth unless there is loss of alveolar bone and gingival tissue due to recession or

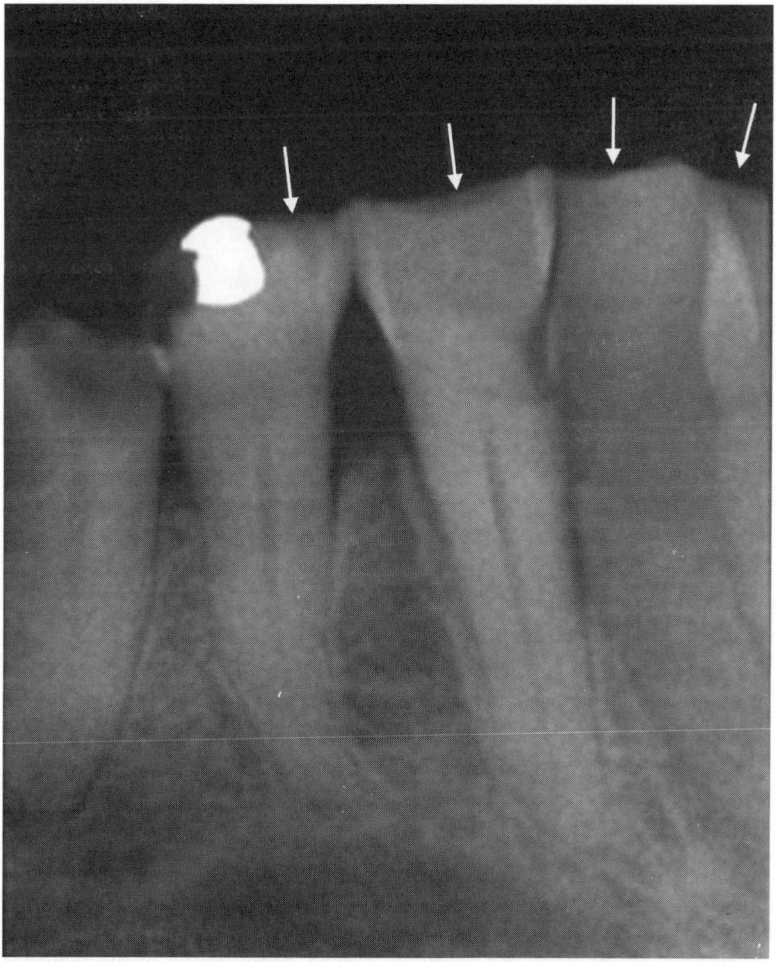

Fig. 5.8 Attrited tooth surfaces

periodontitis. Posteriorly, the invagination of the proximal root surfaces allow more X-rays to pass through this area, resulting in a more radiolucent appearance on the radiograph. X-rays directed at a different angle usually pass through more tooth structure and the radiolucency disappears. Anteriorly, the space between the enamel and the bone overlying the tooth will appear more radiolucent than either the enamel or the bone-tooth combination.

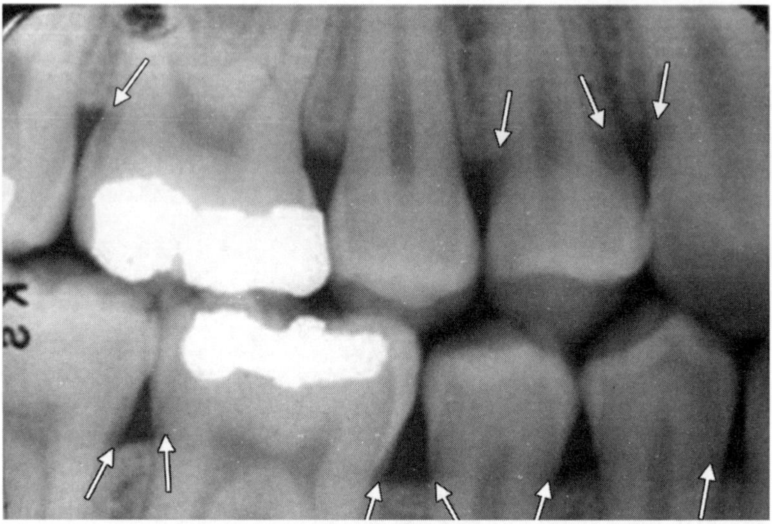

Fig. 5.9 Cervical burnout

MACH BAND EFFECT

This is an optical illusion giving appearance of increased radiolucency at the junction of differing tissue densities, such as enamel and dentin. If you block off the enamel with a fingernail, the radiolucency will disappear due to the Mach band effect. If the radiolucency persists, it may be caries.

CONCLUSION

It is imperative to keep in mind that the lesion detected in the radiograph is merely a result of the bacterial activity on the tooth surface and radiographs alone cannot reveal whether the lesion is active or arrested. Radiography is a valuable supplement to a thorough clinical examination of the teeth for detecting caries.

BIBLIOGRAPHY

1. Fejerskov O, Kidd EAM. Dental Caries: The Disease and Its Clinical Management, 1st edn, Blackwell, 2003.
2. Selwitz RH, Ismail AI, Pitts NB. Dental caries, Lancet. 2007;369:51-9.
3. White S, Pharaoh M. Oral Radiology: Principles and Interpretation, 6th edn, 2009.

CHAPTER 6

RADIOGRAPHIC DIAGNOSIS OF PERIODONTITIS

Priyanka Jain

INTRODUCTION

Radiography plays an important role in determining the extent of periodontal disease and therapy. They provide information about the integrity and status of the periodontium and a permanent record of the condition of the bone throughout the course of the disease.

The clinical and the radiographic examinations are complimentary to each other. The clinical examination should include periodontal probing, gingival index, mobility charting, and an evaluation of the attached gingiva. Radiographs are an adjunct to the diagnostic process.

LIMITATIONS OF RADIOGRAPHS

Radiographs show two dimensional representations of three-dimensional structures. At times, radiographs may not adequately show the severity of disease. Early destructive bone lesions sometimes are not radiographically detectable. Buccal and lingual alveolar bone is particularly difficult to evaluate because of superimposition (Table 6.1). In addition to the radiographic findings, the clinician should also rely on clinical examination, including sulcular depths, tooth mobility, and appearance of the attached gingiva in order to decide on the diagnosis and treatment plan. Radiographs do not show the soft-tissue to hard-tissue relationship and thus do not provide any information about the depth of soft tissue pockets. Furthermore, in cases of over-erupted teeth or severe attrition cases, bone level cannot be measured from the cemento-enamel junction (CEJ) is taken as the reference point for bone level measurements). Due to superimposition, the details of the bony architecture may be lost on the radiographs. Additionally, they also do not demonstrate incipient disease, (a minimum of 55–60% demineralization must occur before radiographic changes are apparent).

Table 6.1 Radiographic assessment of periodontal conditions and features of interest on radiographs

- Amount of bone present (bone levels)
- Condition of the alveolar crests
- Bone loss in the furcation areas (even/angular)
- Furcation involvement
- Calculus
- Root morphologies
- Width of the periodontal ligament space
- Local irritating factors, like calculus and poorly contoured restorations
- Open interproximal contacts
- Pathologic considerations, like periapical lesions and root resorption

Table 6.2 Clinical features not evident on radiographs

- Gingival inflammation
- Gingival bleeding
- Gingival redness
- Gingival recession
- Gingival enlargement
- Bleeding on probing
- Tooth mobility

Only a careful clinical examination, combined with a proper radiographic diagnostic technique will help in determining the presence and extent of periodontal disease. Since gingivitis is a lesion of soft tissue only, no radiographic changes will be seen on the radiograph (Table 6.2).

In addition to all these, radiographs also do not show any evidence of past disease. Inaccuracies in beam angulation and exposure may result in overlap and cervical burnout, thus compromising the detection of the disease process.

RADIOGRAPHIC TECHNIQUES FOR PERIODONTAL DISEASE

The radiographic projections normally used in the detection of periodontal diseases are bitewing radiographs and periapicals.

Conventional Bitewing Radiographs

Bitewing radiographs show the interproximal surfaces of the teeth and the crest of the alveolar bone of both the maxilla and the mandible on the same film. They show least distortion. While the horizontal bitewings are used primarily to detect interproximal decay, vertical bitewings (whereby the film is placed with its long axis at 90 degrees to the placement for horizontal bitewing), provide some information on the patient's periodontal status. They provide a good view of the interproximal bone and may prove useful in cases with minor bone loss (Table 6.2). The height of the interproximal alveolar bone margin relative to the cemento-enamel junction can also be observed. Also, subgingival calculus deposits may be detected. However, the value of bitewing radiographs in the diagnosis of periodontal diseases is limited by the fact that only the coronal sections of the roots of the teeth are observed, and they are limited to the molar-premolar regions. For intact arches, two vertical bitewings per posterior sextant are required.

In younger individuals, careful observation of the alveolar bone height around first permanent molars may help detect those individuals at risk of early-onset forms of periodontitis (juvenile periodontitis and rapidly progressive periodontitis). However, radiographs should be used only as a supplement to a careful clinical examination using a periodontal probe around such sites (up to 30 percent of bone may be lost before it is evident radiographically).

Conventional Periapical Radiographs

In the diagnosis of periodontal diseases, periapical radiographs can provide useful information that cannot be obtained through examination of the soft tissues alone (Table 6.3). Long cone paralleling projections preferably with rectangular collimators should be used. Full mouth surveys of paralleling periapical radiographs have been considered to be a "gold standard" for periodontal diagnosis and treatment planning. They allow the assessment of the full length of the roots and the periapical area. In the anterior region, a periapical projection with paralleling technique is recommended. Periapical projections in the posterior teeth are often not recommended due to the presence of hard palate which can present a distorted view between the teeth and the height of the alveolar bone.

Table 6.3 Differences between horizontal and vertical bitewings

	Advantages	*Disadvantages*
Horizontal bitewings	Good for early detection, as it produces good reproducible image	Apices are not seen, so the bone levels cannot be estimated accurately
	Several teeth can be viewed on one film	Cannot help in the detection of endoperio lesions
Vertical bitewings	Several teeth can be seen on one film	Cannot be used to detect deeper bony defects
	Deeper bony defects can be detected	Tooth apex is not visible on the radiograph

Structures on the Radiographs and their Significance

Teeth

- *Clinical crown-root ratio:* This refers to the ratio between the length of the root that is surrounded by bone and the remainder of the tooth.
- *Presence of calculus:* Both subgingival and supragingival calculus deposits can be observed on periapical radiographs.
- *Presence of root resorption:* Internal or external root resorption can be detected.
- *The contours and margins of restorations:* The relationship between interproximal overhangs and/or poorly contoured restorations, and loss of periodontal bone can be screened by radiographic examination.
- *Fractures of the root:* A tooth with a horizontal or vertical root fracture can present with periodontal symptoms.

Bone

The pattern of bone loss around individual teeth can be determined only through examination of radiographs. Periapical radiographs, using the long cone paralleling technique, provide the most accurate representation of the height of the bone in relation to the CEJ, and to the actual length of the tooth. Various features of bone loss that can be determined by radiographs like:

- *Pattern of bone loss:* Is the bone loss horizontal or vertical?
- *Extent of bone loss:* Is the bone loss generalized/localized to certain teeth?
- Severity of bone loss
- *Furcation involvement:* Is there any evidence of radiolucency in the furcation areas?
- *Lamina dura:* Whereas its presence indicates good supporting bone, its presence does not always signify pathology.
- *Periodontal ligament space:* A widening of the periodontal ligament space may indicate that the tooth is subject to occlusal forces or is mobile. It may also be an early sign of pulpal inflammation. In such cases, a careful clinical examination is necessary to make a diagnosis.

Advantages of periapical projection in determining periodontal status:

- Teeth apices can be visualized
- Long cone paralleling technique gives a good reproducible image of high quality.

Disadvantages of periapical projection:

- Full mouth periapicals are required to assess the periodontal status of an individual. This requires multiple films, hence, more exposure to the individual.

Conventional Panoramic Radiographs

Panoramic radiographs provide a general view of the oral structures, and are useful for screening bone loss patterns in general. They are not suitable for accurate assessment of the degree of bone loss associated with individual teeth, as there is severe distortion. Superimposition of structures does not allow proper assessment of certain areas of the mouth like the mandibular incisor area. In contrast to intraoral radiographs, such as periapical films and vertical or horizontal bitewings, panoramic radiographs provide a considerable amount of information about the periodontium that cannot be obtained by any other noninvasive means. Panoramic radiographs may also reveal some form of dental abnormality unrelated to periodontal disease, but may not reveal alveolar bony defects as accurately as periapical radiographs.

Advantages of Panoramic Radiographs

- Single exposure is convenient
- Entire dentition is seen in one film
- Apices can be seen.

Disadvantages of Panoramic Radiographs

- Image quality is poor than the periapical radiograph
- Less accurate.

Digital Panoramic Radiography versus Conventional Intraoral Radiography

The ability to manipulate the panoramic images, such as zooming in and changing contrast, is a useful feature in assessment of bony defects and root morphologies, and open (access) flap debridement surgeries. This helps in anticipating the shape, depth and extent of bony defects as compared to viewing conventional intraoral radiographs. The ability to zoom in and magnify defects and to adjust the contrast and brightness allows for greater and improved "visualization" of bone levels and intrabony defects (Table 6.4).

Table 6.4 Prichard's criteria for radiographs

Prichard's four criteria for radiograph with good angulation suggests that:
1. The radiograph should show the tips of the molar cusps with little or none of the occlusal surface showing.
2. Enamel caps and pulp chambers should be distinct.
3. Interproximal spaces should be open.
4. Proximal contacts should not overlap, unless teeth are out of line anatomically.

Digital Intraoral Radiography

Digital intraoral radiograph for periodontal assessment is less encouraging but nonetheless generally positive. There are two approaches to digital imaging, *direct digital imaging and indirect digital imaging*. "Direct" is achieved by using a solid state sensor to detect X-rays. For intraoral use, these sensors are bulky and inflexible, and require a cable connection. These sensors must convert X-ray detection to electronic signals for subsequent electronic processing to produce usable images. These direct digital images can be of high quality.

Indirect digital imaging involves a latent image being acquired using a photostimulable phosphor plate, and then after the latent image is captured on this plate, the image is scanned by laser to produce a usable image. There are various advantages of indirect digital imaging over direct digital imaging. The plates can be the same sizes as intraoral conventional X-ray films and so all conventional intraoral clinical approaches can be used. Also there is no need for a cable, patient tolerance is greater, and the expense is less. However, depending on the approach, the image quality may not be as good as with the direct imaging. Direct imaging produces immediate images which is not necessarily so with indirect digital imaging. Further, the flexibility of the plate means that image distortion due to plate bending can occur, as with film bending in conventional radiography.

Digital Subtraction Radiography

Digital subtraction radiography (DSR) in periodontology basically allows the detection of small changes in alveolar bone, which might otherwise go undetected. For this purpose, serial radiographs need to be taken with the best possible reproducible projection geometry. Bite blocks must be made and attached to the film holders and the film holder must be reproducibly aligned to the X-ray beam collimating device. Once, standardized serial periapical radiographs have been produced, then there are various methods to determine the changes (+ indicating more bone/more bone density, - indicating less bone/less bone density) between two radiographic images.

The main issue in DSR is that periodontally involved teeth are often mobile and can be displaced by the bite block. Also, the custom bite block does not fit post-therapy and thus, the serial images cannot be aligned and the altered tooth positions in the serial images cannot be corrected for. The problem of storage of these bite blocks also may prove difficult.

Cone-Beam Computed Tomography

Conventional computed tomography (CT) does not offer any favorable cost-benefit, dose exposure or therapeutic advantage in periodontal practice. Cone-beam geometry allows for reduced dose of radiation. This, in combination with "fast" receptors and the reduced cost of manufacturing the machines, has allowed for the introduction of cone-beam CT into dental/oral imaging. One difference between cone-beam CT and conventional CT is that the cone-beam produces increased scatter on images making cone-beam CT unsuitable for soft tissue, a major benefit of conventional CT, which in fact is of great use in dental/oral radiography. Because the cone-beam geometry allows for a large volume of tissues to be scanned with a single sweep resulting in a digital image, cone-beam CT is also known as *digital volume tomography* (DVT).

Exposure factors also play a role in increasing the diagnostic yield from the radiographs. Beam energy of 80 kVp is used and a film that is slightly light is used for examining the cortical margins of the bone.

NORMAL RADIOGRAPHIC ANATOMY

Normal, healthy alveolar bone has characteristic appearance on radiographs. The bone height is within 2 millimeters of the (CEJ). The crestal bone is a continuation of the lamina dura of the teeth, and is continuous from tooth to tooth. Between the anterior teeth, the alveolar crest is pointed and between the posterior teeth, the lamina dura and the crestal bone form a box, with sharp angles. The alveolar crest is parallel to a line connecting the adjacent CEJ between the posterior teeth.

The periodontal ligament space varies along the length of the roots. The alveolar crest is continuous with the lamina dura of the adjacent teeth. The periodontal ligament space is always slightly wider around the cervical portion of the tooth root. When viewing the lamina dura and the periodontal ligament, only the interproximal portions are visible. The buccal and lingual areas are not seen in the radiograph. Widening of the periodontal ligament space and loss of lamina dura may be interpreted as resorption of the alveolar bone. The overall height of the alveolar crestal bone in relationship to the cemento-enamel junction gives evidence of whether loss of bone has occurred. Bony changes cannot be radiographically detected, until they are advanced.

Pattern of the Bone Loss

When the crest of the bone is still parallel with a line between the cemento-enamel junctions of two adjacent teeth, it is called *horizontal bone loss*. It is usually caused by inflammation. It may be mild, moderate or severe depending on the extent. Mild loss is 1–2 mm loss of the supporting bone, moderate is greater than 2 mm loss and anything beyond that is termed as severe loss. When the amount of remaining bone is fairly and evenly distributed throughout the dentition, it is described as generalized horizontal bone loss. If confined to a specific area, localized horizontal bone loss is used. Horizontal bone loss radiographically appears as decreased alveolar marginal bone around adjacent teeth. With horizontal bone loss, both the buccal and lingual plates of bone, as well as interdental bone are resorbed. Clinically, horizontal bone loss is characterized by suprabony pockets, which occurs, when the epithelial attachment is coronal to the bony defect.

Irregular reduction in the height of crestal bone is termed *angular or vertical bone loss*. With vertical bone loss, there will be greater bone loss on the mesial surface of one tooth than on the adjacent tooth. These defects develop when the bone loss progresses down the root of the tooth resulting in the deepening of the clinical periodontal pocket. Usually, inflammation and trauma from occlusion are combined in causing the destruction and irregular shape of the bone. Vertical bone loss is usually localized to one or two teeth. Radiographically, it presents as a vertical deformity that extends apically along the roots of the affected tooth. They can be of two types:

1. *Interproximal crater:* This is a two walled small sausage shaped bony defect at crest of interdental bone. They are more common in the posterior teeth due to the broad buccal-lingual dimensions in these areas.
2. *Infrabony defect:* This is the vertical defect along root of tooth. The initial appearance is widened periodontal ligament space. Vertical bone loss, resulting from infrabony defects, occurs when the walls of the pocket are within a bony housing. Periodontal disease can cause a vertical defect to extend apically from the alveolar margin. This vertical defect may be one, two, or three walled, based on loss of the cortices. It is described as three walled when both lingual and buccal cortical plates remain, two walled when one of these plates have been resorbed and one walled when both plates have been resorbed or lost.

Furcation Exposure

The furcation is where multiple tooth roots divide at the trunk of the tooth. The furcation is a normal structure usually filled with bone. Furcation exposure results from intraradicular (between the roots) bone loss due to advanced periodontal disease. Bone loss from periodontal disease may extend into the furcation of multirooted teeth (molars and pre-molars). It is initially seen as widening of the periodontal ligament space at the crest of the furcation. As the lesion advances, the bone loss progresses apically. It is sometimes difficult to determine whether the intraradicular space is involved, unless there is a radiographic radiolucent area in the region of the furcation. Lack of radiographically detectable furcation involvement is not confirmation of the absence of periodontal destruction. Advanced furcation exposures, where both cortical plates are resorbed, are easily recognized on radiographs.

Types of Furcation Exposure

- *Class I (incipient)*: Furcation involvement exists, when the tip of a probe can just enter the furcation area. Bone partially fills the area where the roots meet. Radiographically, there is a decreased density of the bone at the furcation.
- *Class II (definite):* Furcation exposure exists, when the probe tip extends horizontally into the area where the roots diverge, but it does not exit on the other side. Radiographically, there will be bone loss at the furcation.
- *Class III (through-and-through):* Exposure lesions exist secondary to advanced periodontal disease with extensive osseous destruction. In these cases, alveolar bone has resorbed to a point that an explorer probe passes through the defect unobstructed. Radiographically, there will be an area of complete bone loss.

RADIOGRAPHIC CHANGES SEEN IN PERIODONTAL DISEASE

Radiographs do not reveal minor destructive changes in the bone. Therefore, slight radiographic changes can mean that the disease has progressed beyond the early stages. Radiographs are an indirect method for determining bone loss, as they show the amount of bone remaining rather than the amount lost. Also, the amount of bone lost is the difference between the physiological bone level and the height of the remaining bone. Periodontal disease causes inflammatory lesions in the marginal bone with both osteoblastic and osteoclastic activity. Osteoclastic activity will cause changes in the morphology of the crestal bone with the initial response being the destruction of bone. Chronic lesions will show some osteosclerosis.

Periodontitis clinically, is presented by pocket formation or gingival recession and radiographically, there is rounding of the alveolar margin (Table 6.5). There is also a loss in the continuity of the lamina dura at the level of the alveolar margin. The earliest radiographic sign of periodontitis is a loss of definition of the crestal bone. The alveolar crest loses its distinct sharp appearance and becomes blunted. The bony margin becomes diffuse and irregular, and may show areas of localized erosion. In the incisor regions, there will be a blunting of the alveolar crests. In the premolar and molar regions, there may also be loss of the normally sharp angle between the lamina dura and the alveolar crest.

The direction of bone loss can be horizontal or vertical (angular).

- *Horizontal bone loss:* Clinically, horizontal bone loss is typified by suprabony pockets, which occurs when the epithelial attachment is coronal to the bony defect.
- Radiographically, the *vertical bone defect* is generally V shaped and sharply outlined. It is immediately adjacent to the root surface of

Table 6.5 Classification of periodontal diseases

Types of periodontal diseases (according to Highfield)
• Gingival diseases • Chronic periodontitis • Aggressive periodontitis • Periodontitis as a manifestation of systemic disease • Necrotizing periodontal disease • Abscesses of periodontium • Periodontal-endodontic lesions

the affected tooth, and the adjacent bone has a normal radiographic appearance.

- Alveolar dehiscence exists, when the alveolar cortical bone is resorbed along the entire length of the root. Radiographically, there will be a radiolucency surrounding the effected root.

GINGIVAL DISEASES

Both plaque induced and nonplaque induced gingival diseases can be diagnosed on the basis of clinical findings and the results of further investigations without the need for radiographs. If the clinical records (chartings and study casts) are comprehensive and accurate, the stability of the periodontium can be assessed without the need for radiographs, although radiographs should of course reveal further alveolar bone loss, but such radiographic evidence would in normal clinical circumstances only be a confirmatory finding of new or recurrent periodontitis.

Chronic Periodontitis

Both localized and generalized chronic periodontitis are characterized by pocket formation and/or gingival recession, both of which are clinically detectable without radiographs. Chronic periodontitis can be said to be localized, if less than 30 percent of available sites display clinical attachment loss, and generalized, if more than 30 percent of sites display clinical attachment loss. This differentiation is made more on the basis of clinical findings and although radiographs may be used but they may mislead. Chronic periodontitis can be further characterized by various degrees of severity on the basis of measures of clinical attachment loss. Therefore, for the assessment of the severity of chronic periodontitis, radiographs are not required, although radiographs may be used, but are not essential.

The manner in which radiographs may mislead in the assessment of extent of the disease is that the chronic periodontitis may have been treated and while the radiographs may show the extent of the number of interproximal sites, or teeth, with bone loss, however, it is the presence or absence of the clinical signs apparent only on clinical examination which indicate extent of current chronic periodontitis. Similarly, in the determination of the severity of chronic periodontitis from the estimation of alveolar bone heights shown on conventional radiographs, the chronic periodontitis might have been previously successfully treated and so the assessment of severity is an assessment of the severity of the previous chronic periodontitis and not of the current status.

The diagnosis of chronic periodontitis is made on the basis of periodontal pockets and/or recession. In some clinical situations, restorations may impede the accessibility of the periodontal probe into a pocket and/or may obscure the CEJ and so compromise the clinical assessment of the presence and severity of chronic periodontitis. In such a situation, radiographic evidence of alveolar bone loss may be helpful. Similarly, subgingival calculus or root surface malformations may impede the passage of the periodontal probe. In these situations, radiographic evidence of alveolar bone loss may be helpful, as it may direct the attention of the examining dentist to probe carefully sites or teeth with evident radiographic bone loss.

Aggressive Periodontitis

Both localized and generalized aggressive periodontitis share the common features of chronic periodontitis, pockets and/or recession. However, there is or has been rapid attachment loss and bone destruction and, in some cases, a familial aggregation can be elicited, and apart from the periodontitis, the patients are otherwise clinically healthy. The differentiation between *localized* (first molar/incisor presentation with interproximal clinical attachment loss on at least two permanent teeth, one of which is a molar and involving no more than two teeth other than first molars and incisors) and *generalized* (interproximal clinical attachment loss affecting at least three permanent teeth other than first molars and incisors), needs to be made clinically and radiographs may not be required. The diagnosis should not be made on the basis of radiographs alone, and given that the key feature is clinical attachment loss, radiographic examination may not be required for the diagnosis of aggressive periodontitis, although the localized form may present with a very characteristic "mirror image" pattern of bone destruction.

Periodontitis as a Manifestation of Systemic Disease

Periodontitis as a manifestation of systemic disease proposes only those diseases in which the periodontitis is a manifestation of the disease process and does not include disease states or medications which modify existing periodontitis. Periodontitis as a manifestation of a disease process can be diagnosed and characterized on the basis of the findings from a clinical examination.

Necrotizing Periodontal Diseases

Necrotizing periodontal diseases are divided into *necrotizing ulcerative gingivitis,* (an infection characterized by gingival necrosis presenting as "punched-out" papillae, with gingival bleeding and pain, a characteristic foetid breath and pseudomembranes covering the ulcerations, which bleed readily on being disturbed) and *necrotizing ulcerative periodontitis* (there is not only necrosis of gingival tissues, but also necrosis of periodontal ligament, and alveolar bone). Both of these diagnoses are established on the basis of the symptoms and the clinical signs, and radiographs may not be required.

Abscesses of Periodontium

Abscesses affecting periodontal tissues can be divided into *gingival abscess,* (a localized prevalent infection that involves the marginal gingiva or interdental papilla), *periodontal abscess,* (a localized purulent infection within the tissues adjacent to a periodontal pocket), and *pericoronal abscess,* (a localized purulent infection within the tissue surrounding the crown of a partially erupted tooth). A periodontal abscess may lead to the destruction of periodontal ligament and alveolar bone, whereas a gingival abscess and a pericoronal abscess probably will not give rise to radiographically detectable bone loss. Conventional radiographs may, therefore, allow for the differentiation between a gingival abscess and a periodontal abscess, but clinical findings alone should be sufficient to allow for this differentiation. Periodontal abscesses may result from conditions such as root fractures or cemental tears which may not be apparent radiographically. Radiographs can aid in sometimes determining the underlying cause for the diagnosis.

Periodontitis Associated with Endodontic Lesions

A primary periodontal lesion which mimics an endodontic lesion is still just solely a periodontal lesion and so is not a "perio-endo" lesion. Similarly, an endodontic lesion with a sinus draining through the periodontal ligament, which after successful endodontic therapy completely resolves without the need for any periodontal therapeutic intervention, is only an endodontic lesion and is not a "perio-endo" lesion. When the practitioner needs to combine the periodontal and endodontic pathologies, it is termed as a combined periodontal-endodontic lesion. For this diagnosis, the standard conventional intraoral radiographic exposures for diagnosing periapical periodontitis, usually periapical radiographs, are required. The use of

Table 6.6 Radiographs in periodontal diagnosis

Diagnosis	*Radiographs required for establishing diagnosis*
Gingival diseases	Not required
Chronic periodontitis	Not required, may supplement the clinical examination
Aggressive periodontitis	Not required but in some cases radiographs may display rapid bone loss
Periodontitis as a manifestation of periodontal diseases	Not required
Necrotizing periodontal diseases	Not required
Abscesses of the periodontium	Not required
Periodontitis associated with endodontic lesions	Required for endodontic diagnosis
Developmental or acquired deformities and conditions	Required for tooth related problem

guttapercha cones inserted into any sinus opening to trace the origin of a draining lesion is a very useful approach at the time of exposing a paralleling periapical radiograph in the diagnosis of combined lesions.

CONCLUSION

Radiographs do not play a major role in periodontal diagnosis but are hugely useful in guiding periodontal treatment planning decisions. Radiographs should be prescribed only on the basis of a clinical assessment (Table 6.6). Vertical bitewing radiographs are of practical use in periodontitis affected patients. Panoramic oral radiographs, supplemented by a limited number of selected intraoral views, selected on the basis of the clinical findings and the appearance of the panoramic oral radiograph, can reach the "gold standard" with reduced radiation exposure.

BIBLIOGRAPHY

1. Akesson L, Rohlin M, Hakansson J, Hakansson H, Nasstrom K. Comparison between panoramic and posterior bitewing radiography in the diagnosis of periodontal bone loss. J Dent. 1989;17:266-71.
2. Allen KM, Hausmann E. Analytical methodology in quantitative digital subtraction radiography: analyses of the aluminum reference wedge. J Periodontol. 1996; 67:1317-21.
3. Caton J, Greenwell H, Mahanonda R, et al. Consensus report: dental plaque-induced gingival diseases. Ann Periodontl. 1999;4:18-9.

4. Dundar N, Ilgenli T, Kal BI, Boyacioglu H. The frequency of periodontal infrabony defects on panoramic radiographs of an adult population seeking dental care. Community Dent Health. 2008;25:226-30.
5. Highfield J. Diagnosis and classification of periodontal disease. Aust Dent J. 2009; 54(1 Suppl):S11–26.
6. *http://www.perio.org/index_pro.html.'* Accessed 12th December 2012.
7. Jenkins WM, Brocklebank LM, Winning SM, Wylupek M, Donaldson A, Strang RM. A comparison of two radiographic assessment protocols for patients with periodontal disease. Br Dent J. 2005;198:565-69; discussion 557; quiz 586.
8. Lai SM, Zee KY, Lai MK, Corbet EF. Clinical and radiographic investigation of the adjunctive effects of a low-power He-Ne laser in the treatment of moderate to advanced periodontal disease: a pilot study. Photomed Laser Surg. 2009;27: 287-93.
9. Lang N, Bartold PM, Cullinan M, et al. Consensus report: aggressive periodontitis. Ann Periodontl. 1999;4:53.
10. Lang N, Soskolne WA, Greenstein G, et al. Consensus report: abscesses of the periodontium. Ann Periodontol. 1999;4:83.
11. Lang N, Soskolne WA, Greenstein G, et al. Consensus report: necrotizing periodontal diseases. Ann Periodontol. 1999;4(1):78.
12. Li G, Engstrom PE, Nasstrom K, Lu ZY, Sanderink G, Welander U. Marginal bone levels measured in film and digital radiographs corrected for attenuation and visual response: an in vivo study. Dentomaxillofac Radiol. 2007;36:7-11.
13. Lindhe J, Ranney R, Lamster I, et al. Consensus report: chronic periodontitis. Ann Periodontl. 1999;4:38.
14. Pecoraro M, Azadivatan-le N, Janal M, Khocht A. Comparison of observer reliability in assessing alveolar bone height on direct digital and conventional radiographs. Dentomaxillofac Radiol. 2005;34:279-84.
15. Tugnait A, Hirschmann PN, Clerehugh V. Validation of a model to evaluate the role of radiographs in the diagnosis and treatment planning of periodontal diseases. J Dent. 2006;34:509-15.
16. Updegrave WJ. The paralleling extension-cone technique in intraoral dental radiography. Oral Surg Oral Med Oral Pathol. 1951;4:1250-61.

CHAPTER 7

DENTAL MATERIALS

Priyanka Jain

INTRODUCTION

The dental field is charged specifically with the conservation of oral health and with the diagnosis, prevention, and treatment of oral diseases, injuries, and deficiencies among general public. Dental materials used in the dental profession are indeed many, varied, and complex. This chapter deals with the composition, property, use, and manipulation of materials used in the dental profession.

Restorative dental materials are the metallic or nonmetallic materials used to restore diseased or damaged teeth to health and function. The corrosive nature of saliva, and the expansion and contraction of tooth structure with changes in temperature, and the stress brought to bear on the restoration by masticatory forces make great demands upon a restorative material. The stress brought to bear on the restoration by anterior region of the mouth, the materials must also be esthetically pleasing. Restorative materials, used when and where indicated, help to ensure the placement of a successful restoration and preservation of the tooth.

For many years the only available choices were metals. These are: (1) gold alloy or (2) a mixture or "amalgam" of mercury, silver and other metals. In the past few decades, other materials have been developed for restoring teeth. They are "tooth colored" rather than silver-colored or gold. They include composite resin, glass ionomer and porcelain materials. Dental fillings fall into two categories based on the method used to place them: They are: direct restorations and indirect restorations (Table 7.1).

Direct restorations are fillings placed immediately into a prepared cavity in a single visit. They include dental amalgam, glass ionomer, resin ionomer and most composite (resin) fillings. The dentist prepares the tooth, places the filling and adjusts it all during one appointment.

Indirect restorations may require two or more visits. They include inlays, onlays, veneers, crowns and bridges fabricated with gold, ceramics or composites. During the first visit, the dentist prepares the tooth and makes an impression of the area to be treated. The impression is sent to a dental laboratory, which creates the dental restoration (filling). The dentist cements the restoration to the prepared tooth in the next appointment.

Table 7.1 Dental materials

Direct restorative	*Indirect restorative*
Dental amalgam	*Impression materials* • Reversible hydrocolloid (Agar-Agar) • Irreversible hydrocolloid (Alginate)
Liners and bases • Thin film liners (solution liner and suspension liner) • Thick liner (cement liner)	*Cast metal restorations* • Noble metal alloys • Precious metal alloys • Low gold alloys • Gold substitute alloys • Base metal alloy
Dental adhesives	Dental cements
Pit and fissure sealants	Dental porcelain
Dental composites	Machined restorations
Glass ionomer cement	–
Direct filling gold	–

PHYSICAL PROPERTIES OF MATERIALS

- *Hardness:* Hardness is the measure of the resistance of a metal to indentation or scratching. It is an indication of the strength and wearability of an alloy or metal.
- *Ductility:* Ductility is the measure of the capacity of a metal to be stretched or drawn by a pulling or tensile force without fracturing. This property permits a metal to be drawn into a thin wire.
- *Malleability:* Malleability is the measure of the capacity of a metal to be extended in all directions by a compressive force, such as rolling or hammering. This property permits a metal to be shaped into a thin sheet or plate.
- *Flexibility and elasticity:* These terms differ in their technical definition but they are very closely related. Flexibility is the characteristic of a metal, which allows it to deform temporarily (Table 7.2). The elasticity of a metal is used when it returns to its original shape when the load or force is removed.
  - *Elastic deformation:* The reversible deformation of a material under load
  - *Plastic deformation:* The irreversible deformation of a material under load
  - *Creep:* It is the slow plastic deformation that occurs with the application of a static/dynamic force overtime.

Table 7.2 Properties of dental materials

The properties of dental materials can be classified as:
• Mechanical (strength) • Physical (thermal expansion) • Chemical (corrosion) • Biocompatibility (toxicity)

- *Fatigue:* Fatigue is the property of a metal to tire and to fracture after repeated stressing at loads below its proportional limit.
- *Strength:* Crushing strength is the amount of resistance of a material to fracture under compression.
- *Brittleness:* The fracturing of a material with little or no plastic deformation.
- *Stress:* Measure of force per unit cross-sectional area.
- *Strain:* The amount of deformation when a force is exerted.
- *Structure (crystalline or grain structure):* Metals are crystalline in nature and many of their physical properties depend largely upon the size and arrangement of their minute crystals called grains.
  - *Grain size:* The size of the grains in a solidified metal depends upon the number of nuclei of crystallization present and the rate of crystal growth. In the practical sense, the faster a molten is cooled to solidification, the greater will be the number of nuclei and the smaller will be the grain size. Generally speaking, small grains arranged in an orderly fashion give the most desirable properties.
  - *Grain shape:* The shape of the grains is also formed at the time of crystallization. If the metal is poured or forced into a mold before cooling, the grains will be in a flattened state. Metal formed by this method is known as cast metal. If the metal is shaped by rolling, bending, or twisting, the grains are elongated and the metal becomes a wrought wire.
- *Thermal conductivity:* Thermal conductivity is defined as the ability of a material to transmit heat or cold. A low thermal conductivity is desired in restorative materials used on the tooth, whereas a high thermal conductivity is desirable where the material covers soft tissue.
- *Thermal expansion:* Materials expand as the temperature rises and contract as it decreases.
- *Corrosion:* This is an electrochemical process which involves the movement of ions in an aqueous environment (saliva).
- *Wettability:* This is the ability of one material to flow across the surface of another.

METALLURGICAL TERMS

- *Cold working:* This is the process of changing the shape of a metal by rolling, pounding, bending, or twisting at normal room temperature.
- *Strain hardening:* This occurs when a metal becomes stiffer and harder because of continued or repeated application of a load or force. At this point, no further slippage of the atoms of the metal can occur without fracture.
- *Heat softening treatment (annealing):* This treatment is necessary in order to continue manipulating a metal after strain hardening to prevent it from fracturing. The process of annealing consists of heating the metal to the proper temperature (as indicated by the manufacturer's instructions) and cooling it rapidly by immersing in cold water. Annealing relieves stresses and strains caused by cold working and restores slipped atoms within the metal to their regular arrangement.
- *Heat hardening treatment (tempering):* This treatment is necessary to restore properties to metals that are decreased by annealing and cold working. Metals to be heat hardened should first be heat softened (annealed), so that all strain hardening is relieved and the hardening process can be properly controlled.

AMALGAM

An alloy is a solid mixture of two or more metals. It is possible to produce a material in which the desirable properties of each constituent are retained or even enhanced, while the less desirable properties are reduced or eliminated. With few exceptions, the metals used in dentistry are in fact alloys. A dental amalgam is a combination of mercury with a specially prepared silver alloy, which is used as a restorative material. Mercury is a silver-white, poisonous, metallic element that is liquid at room temperature (symbol Hg). Dental amalgams have commonly been called "silver fillings" because of their silver color when they are first placed. Today, amalgam is used most commonly in the back teeth. It is one of the oldest filling materials and has been used (and improved) for more than 150 years. Dental amalgam is the most thoroughly researched and tested filling material.

Components

Dental amalgam is a mix of approximately:
- Mercury (43–54%)
- Silver (67–74%)—imparts strength, durability, and color. It gives the alloy desirable setting expansion, decreases flow, and accelerates the setting time
- Copper (0–6%)—copper increases hardness, contributes to setting expansion, reduces flow, and decreases setting time

- Tin (25–27%)—tin makes amalgam easier to work, controls excessive setting expansion, and increases both flow and setting time
- Zinc increases workability, and unites with oxygen and other "impurities" to produce a clean amalgam
- Copper is added to decrease the gamma 2 phase (Table 7.3).

Setting Reaction

$Hg + AgSn \rightarrow Ag_2Hg_3 + Sn_{6\text{-}8}Hg$

There are mainly three methods of alloy formation:

1. *Lathe cut:* Ingots of solid alloy are turned on a lathe and homogenized. This is the oldest and the most traditional way of making an alloy.
2. *Spherical:* The particles are spray cooled and atomized in an inert environment. This results in better packaging and good mix on manipulation. This type of an alloy has greater strength.
3. *Dispersion:* This is a mixture of lathe cut and spherical types. It incorporates the properties of the spherical mix but also has a squeaky sound on condensation (Table 7.4).

Table 7.3 Properties of dental amalgam: Effects on the properties of amalgam restoration imparted by the components

Property		*Ingredient*		
	Silver	Tin	Copper	Zinc
Strength	Increases			
Durability	Increases			
Hardness			Increases	
Expansion	Increases	Decreases	Increases	
Flow	Decreases	Increases	Decreases	
Color	Imparts			
Setting time	Decreases	Increases	Decreases	
Workability		Increases		Increases
Cleanliness				Increases

Table 7.4 Dental amalgam

Phases in the setting reaction of amalgam		
Gamma	$Hg+AgSn$	Strongest phase
Gamma 1	Ag_2Hg_3	Intermediate
Gamma 2	$Sn_{6\text{-}8}Hg$	Weakest phase
Eta phase (Cu is added)	Cu_6Sn_5	

Abbreviations: Sn, Tin; Ag, Silver; Hg, Mercury; Cu, Copper

Properties of Amalgam

The most important physical properties of amalgam are:

- *Flow and creep:* The lower the creep value of an amalgam, the better the marginal integrity of the restoration. Alloys with high copper content usually have lower creep values than the conventional silver-tin alloys
- *Dimensional change:* An amalgam can expand or contract depending upon its usage. Dimensional change can be minimized by proper usage of alloy and mercury
- *Strength:* Sufficient strength to resist fracture is an important requirement for any restorative material. The strength of an amalgam is determined primarily by the composition of the alloy, the amount of residual mercury remaining after condensation, and the degree of porosity in the amalgam restoration
- No adhesion to enamel or dentin
- Double the thermal *expansion of the tooth.*

Advantages

- Strong, durable and stands up to biting force
- Can be placed in one visit
- The least expensive filling material
- Self-sealing with minimal-to-no shrinkage and resists leakage (leakage occurs when a filling does not completely seal, permitting food and bacteria to "leak in" and promote new decay behind or beneath the filling)
- Resistance to further decay is high
- Frequency of repair and replacement is low
- Amalgam may also be used in a wet environment, at times, especially important when treating small children or special needs patients.

Disadvantages

- Concerns about the low levels of mercury vapor released by amalgam
- Amalgam scraps (waste left over after repairing a cavity) contain mercury and require special handling to protect the environment
- Amalgam can darken overtime as it corrodes. This does not affect the function of the filling, but many people find it less attractive than tooth colored materials
- Placement of amalgam requires removal of some healthy tooth
- In rare cases, a localized, allergic reaction such as inflammation or rash may occur
- In larger amalgam fillings, the remaining tooth may weaken and fracture
- Because metal can conduct hot and cold temperatures, there may be a temporary sensitivity to hot and cold
- Contact with other metals may cause occasional, minute electrical flow.

Uses

- Used for restoring cavities in the posterior teeth with high occlusal loads
- May be used as core build up material for crowns.

> The durability of any dental restoration is influenced not only by the material, it is made from but also by the dentist's technique when placing the restoration. Other factors include the supporting materials used in the procedure and the patient's cooperation during the procedure. The length of time a restoration will last is dependent upon your dental hygiene, home care, diet and chewing habits.

Safety of Amalgam Restorations

Amalgam restorations do not constitute a hazard to patients. However, dental personnel may invite a health hazard, if exposed to concentrated mercurial vapors over an extended period of time. Mercury hygiene precautions should be used. Safety concerns due to mercury release should be taken into account while treating pregnant women, patient with multiple sclerosis or with CNS problems. Amalgam separators within the suction apparatus will help minimize the amount of amalgam entering the water supply and thus the food chain.

Mercury Hygiene Precautions

All cuts and abrasions on the skin must be covered when handling amalgam or mercury. All dental personnel must wash hands and arms thoroughly after coming in contact with amalgam operations. Capsules must be checked for general condition and seal. Cracked capsules or those in poor condition should be discarded. All dental personnel must wear masks when removing amalgam restorations. A water coolant must be used to reduce and minimize the dispersion of particles during removal of amalgam restorations. Handling amalgam with bare hands must be avoided.

Old amalgam and mercury must be stored under fresh, clean fixer solution in strong, closed containers in a cool, fireproof area. Disposable paper, cloths, and rubber items that are mercury or amalgam contaminated must be deposited into bag-lined, covered containers after use. Bag and contents must be disposed of daily. Waste amalgam should be stored in a solution and sent to a recognized waste disposal company for recycling. Amalgam mixing equipment, as well as mercury, must be kept away from any source of heat. Amalgamators must be kept inside closed containers as much as possible and cleaned at least once a week. There must be no carpeting in the part of the dental clinics where mercury or amalgam is used.

LINERS AND BASES

Dental cements are generally low strength materials prepared by mixing a powder with a liquid (Table 7.5). These cements vary in their chemical composition, properties, and uses. Dental cements have lower heat conductivity than most metallic restorative materials. However, they have the disadvantages of relatively low strength, varying degrees of solubility in mouth fluids, and setting shrinkage. As a group, they are more natural in appearance and are easier and faster to use. Although they are widely used in restorative dentistry, dental cements are considered to be among the least permanent of restorative materials. Types of cement used in dentistry are zinc phosphate cement, calcium hydroxide, polycarboxylate cement, glass ionomer cement, and zinc oxide eugenol.

Zinc Phosphate Cement

Clinical Uses

Zinc phosphate cement is used both as an intermediate base and as a cementing medium. As an intermediate base, a thick mix of zinc phosphate cement is used beneath a permanent metallic restoration. This layer of cement protects the pulp from sudden temperature changes that may be transmitted by the metallic restoration.

Table 7.5 Liners and bases

Liners	*Bases*
They are thin layers of materials used to provide a thermal barrier to protect the dentine	These are used to provide a strong structural lining and give thermal, mechanical and chemical protection to the dentine
Thickness: Liners can be: • Thin film liners (1–50 µm) can be divided into solution liners (varnishes, 2–5 µm) and suspension liners (20–25 µm) • Thick film liners (0.2–1 mm) are mainly used for thermal and pulpal protection and are also known as cement liners	The thickness is typically 1–2 mm
Liners are most importantly used with metallic restorations that are not well bonded to the tooth structure	Bases are mainly used to supplement mechanical support for the restoration
Examples of liners are: • Calcium hydroxide • Zinc oxide eugenol • Traditional glass ionomer	Examples of bases are: • Zinc phosphate cement • Zinc polycarboxylate cement • Glass ionomer

As a cementing medium, zinc phosphate cement is used to permanently cement crowns, inlays, and fixed partial dentures upon the remaining tooth structure. It is also used to hold splints, orthodontic appliances, and other appliances in place. This cement is used to cement facings to fixed partial dentures and certain types of artificial teeth to artificial denture bases. A creamy mix of cement is used to seat the restoration or appliance completely into place. The cementing medium does not cement two objects together. Instead, the cement holds the objects together by mechanical interlocking, filling the space between the irregularities of the tooth preparation and the cemented restoration. It is also used as a temporary restorative material.

Chemical Composition

The cement consists of a powder and a liquid:

Powder: The primary ingredients of zinc phosphate cement powder are zinc oxide and 10% magnesium oxide.

Liquid: The liquid used with the powder is phosphoric acid and water in the ratio of two parts acid to one part water. The solution may also contain aluminum phosphate and zinc phosphate. The water content of the liquid is critical as the water gain hastens setting; water loss lengthens setting time.

Advantages
- Inconspicuous appearance
- Speed and ease of usage
- Sufficient flow to form a thin layer for the cementing of closely adapted crowns, fixed partial dentures, and inlays
- Low thermal conductivity beneath a metallic restoration.

Disadvantages
- Low crushing strength
- Slight solubility in mouth fluids
- Opaque material not suitable for visible surfaces
- No adhesion to the tooth structure
- Can exhibit variable degree of pulpal effects, hence, if using in vital teeth, a lining is required.

Strength

The ratio of powder to liquid increases the strength of phosphate cements to a certain point. For this reason, the dental specialist must use as thick a mix as practical for the work being performed.

Setting Reactions

The chemical reaction that takes place between the powder and liquid of phosphate cement produces heat (exothermic set). The amount of heat produced depends upon the rate of reaction, the size of the mix, and the amount of heat extracted by the mixing slab. The less powder used in ratio to the liquid, the longer the cement will take to harden. Generally, for increased strength, decreased shrinkage, and resistance to solubility, it is advisable to blend as much powder as possible to reach the desired consistencies.

The setting time of zinc phosphate cement is normally between 5 and 9 minutes.

- Lower the temperature of the glass mixing slab (use a cool glass slab)
- Blend the powder slowly
- Mix the powder over a large area of the cool slab.

The Completed Mix

When a mix is ready for use, it should be similar to the consistency of melted ice cream or liquid glue (adhesive rubber). When the spatula is placed on the slab and the spatula is raised to one inch, the mix will cling to the spatula in a thin thread (peak) for one or two seconds, before it breaks and then gradually spreads.

Precautions

While using zinc phosphate, the clinician should try to prevent loss or gain of moisture in liquid cement by keeping bottles tightly closed. Dispense the liquid in drops only when ready to mix and use a cool, dry glass slab (65°–75° F). Always try to use the same brand of powder and liquid and add increments of powder slowly. Try to use the maximum amount of powder to obtain the desired consistency.

Zinc Polycarboxylate Cement

Clinical Uses

The primary use of polycarboxylate cement is as a cementing medium of cast alloy and porcelain restorations. In addition, it can be used as a cavity liner, as a base under metallic restorations, or as a temporary restorative material. Polycarboxylate cement is used in the same way as zinc phosphate cement, both as an intermediate base and as a cementing medium. It can also be used as a temporary restorative material.

Chemical Composition

The cement consists of powder and liquid:

Powder: The composition of polycarboxylate cement powder may vary slightly depending on the manufacturers. It generally contains zinc oxide, 1–5% magnesium oxide, 10–40% aluminum oxide and other reinforcing fillers. A small percentage of fluoride may be included.

Liquid: Polycarboxylate cement liquid is approximately a 40% aqueous solution of polyacrylic acid copolymer with other organic acids such as itaconic acid. Due to its high molecular weight, the solution is rather thick (viscous).

Properties

The advantages and disadvantages of polycarboxylate cement are identical to those of zinc phosphate cement with one exception. Polycarboxylate cement has lower compressive strength.

Setting Reaction

Unlike zinc phosphate cement, the setting reaction of polycarboxylate cement produces little heat. This has made it a material of choice. Manipulation is simpler, and trauma due to thermal shock to the pulp is reduced. The rate of setting is affected by the powder-liquid ratio, the reactivity of the zinc oxide, the particle size, the presence of additives, and the molecular weight and concentration of the polyacrylic acid. The strength can be increased by additives such as alumina and fluoride. The zinc oxide reacts with the polyacrylic acid forming a cross-linked structure of zinc polyacrylate. The set cement consists of residual zinc oxide bonded together by a gel-like matrix.

The Completed Mix

The correct cementing mix is more viscous than zinc phosphate cement. Because of its composition, the cementing mix flows adequately under pressure.

Precautions

While using, make sure that the interior of restorations and tooth surfaces are free of saliva. The mix should be used while it is still glossy. The powder and liquid should be stored in air tight containers under cool conditions as loss of moisture from the liquid will lead to thickening.

Glass Ionomer Cement

This is a polyalkeonate cement developed in the 1960s at the laboratory of a government chemist. Glass ionomers are tooth-colored materials made of a mixture of acrylic acids with fine glass powders that are used to fill cavities, particularly those on the root surfaces of teeth (Table 7.6). They are primarily used for small fillings in areas that need not withstand heavy chewing pressure.

Table 7.6 Various types of glass ionomer cements

Glass ionomer material	*Uses*	*Compositions*
Traditional	Liners, bases and cements	Smaller powder particle size
Metal modified	Filling materials, bases and core build up materials	• Miracle mix: With amalgam alloy admixed with cement • Cermet: This is a ceramic metal glass
Light cured	Liners and bases	• HEMA may be added to the liquid compositions • Polymers in the liquid may be modified with acrylic functional groups • Powder particles mixed with aluminosilicate glass
Hybrid (resin modified)	Cements, restorative filling materials and core build up materials	• HEMA added to the liquid component • Polymers added to the powder components

Clinical Uses

The primary use of glass ionomer cement is for permanent cementing of inlays, crowns, bridges, and/or orthodontic band/brackets. In addition, it can be used as a cavity liner and as a base. Glass ionomer cement is used in the same way as zinc phosphate cement, both as an intermediate base and as a cementing medium.

- Cervical abrasions and erosion cavities
- Deciduous tooth restoration
- Fissure sealing
- Root surface caries
- Sandwich restorations with composite resins.

Chemical Composition

The cement consists of a powder and a liquid.

- *Powder:* It generally contains fused ion-leachable aluminosilicate glass (the glass is mainly silicon dioxide, aluminum oxide and calcium fluoride) with dry polyacrylic/itaconic acid (polyalkeonic), tartaric acid (to improve the handling characteristics) and water.
- *Liquid:* Glass ionomer cement liquid consists of an aqueous solution containing an accelerator (a chemical accelerator shortens the setting time).

Properties

Glass ionomer cement is free from phosphoric acid and has very low solubility. It adheres chemically to enamel and dentin and, readily, to wet tooth structure, leaving minimal film thickness. It is well tolerated by the pulp and remains rigid under a load, exhibiting no creep. Glass ionomer possesses high compressive strength. It releases fluoride ions to tooth structure. It is simple to proportion, mix, apply, and clean up and is biocompatible.

Advantages
- Tooth-colored so the filling looks more natural
- May contain fluoride that may help prevent further decay
- Minimal amount of tooth structure removed
- Low incidence of localized allergic reaction
- Usually completed in a single visit.

Disadvantages
- It is hard and brittle
- It is susceptible to erosion in the first few minutes of placement
- There is an increase in the surface roughness of the material in the mouth over a period of time
- Low translucency
- Low abrasion wear resistance
- Low resistance to fracture. Use is limited to small areas of decay on non-biting surfaces of teeth
- Moderate cost, similar to composite (costs more than amalgam)
- May get dislodged at times
- In rare cases, a localized allergic reaction such as inflammation or rash may occur.

Setting Reaction

For glass ionomer cement as for other dental cements, the working time is reduced, if a higher powder to liquid ratio has been used. Higher temperature shortens working time and lower temperature extends working time. Glass ionomer cement should always have a glossy appearance. When the surface becomes dull, the setting reaction has started, and the mix should be discarded. Exceeding the working time will result in loss of adhesion to enamel and dentin. The setting reaction is an acid-base reaction between glass and polyalkeonic acid. There are three stages of the set:
1. *Dissolution phase:* There is initial cross linking of the polyacid chains.
2. *Gelation phase:* There is further cross linking which may take up to 24 hours. During this time, the physical properties improve.
3. *Maturation phase:* This takes place over weeks and months and involves further cross linking of the polyacid chains.

The Completed Mix

The right consistency is obtained when the material breaks away from the spatula when it is raised one-half inch from the glass slab.

Precautions

It is advisable not to insert glass ionomer cement as a ball of material into deep cavities or where the dentin is thin or where there is danger of pulpal involvement. In these cases, set in place a calcium hydroxide liner before inserting the glass ionomer cement. All enamel, dentin, and metal surfaces must be clean and dry before use of glass ionomer cement. Do not overfill the crown but brush a thin coat of glass ionomer cement on the internal crown surface and abutments. Bottles of liquid or powder should be tightly closed after use to prevent moisture contamination of the powder and evaporation of the liquid.

Resin-Ionomer Cement

Resin-ionomer cement is a mixture of glass and resin polymer and organic acid that hardens with exposure to a blue light used in the dental office. It is tooth colored but more translucent than glass ionomer cement. It is most often used for small fillings, cementing metal/porcelain metal crowns and liners. They are most commonly used in fillings on nonchewing surfaces and fillings in primary teeth.

Advantages

- Very good esthetics
- May provide some help against decay because it releases fluoride
- Minimal amount of tooth needs to be removed and it bonds well to both the enamel and the dentin beneath the enamel
- Good for nonbiting surfaces
- May be used for short-term primary teeth restorations
- May hold up better than glass ionomer but not as well as composite
- Good resistance to leakage
- Material has low incidence of producing tooth sensitivity
- Usually completed in one dental visit.

Disadvantages

- Cost is very similar to composite resin (which costs more than amalgam)
- Limited use because it is not recommended to restore the biting surfaces of adults
- Wears faster than composite and amalgam.

Cermets

These were developed to overcome the wear resistance of glass ionomers and were thus added with metal. They are composed of fused alumino silicate glass with sintered gold/silver. The setting reaction is similar to glass ionomer. It has higher wear resistance as compared to traditional glass ionomer and has very little marginal leakage. It is also hydrolytically more stable. The disadvantages include poor esthetics, and less fluoride release than glass ionomer. Cermets may be used in class V cavities, for the restoration of primary molar teeth, as core builds up materials and as intermediate filling materials in cases of endodontics.

Resin Modified Glass Ionomer

These materials contain both a composite and glass ionomer. The materials sets by light cure/chemical cure. The components include methacrylate resin, a polyacid, an ion leachable glass, water and HEMA (hydroxyethyl methacrylate). The setting reaction is similar to traditional glass ionomer as in acid-base reaction. They have improved wear resistance, fracture toughness and esthetics than glass ionomers. They adhere to the tooth structure but release less fluoride ions than glass ionomers.

Modified Composites and Compomer (Acid Modified Composite)

In these materials, the filler is replaced by an ion leachable alumino-silicate glass with no acid-base chemical reaction. On the other hand, in compomers, though the resin has acidic components to generate an acid-base chemical reaction, but is still set by resin polymerization. This may release more fluoride. Their uses and properties are same as resin modified.

Zinc Oxide Eugenol

This material is used for many dental purposes ranging from temporary restorative material to pulp capping. The material is composed of a powder that is basically zinc oxide and a liquid that is called eugenol.

Chemical Composition

The powder contains zinc oxide (70–100%), magnesium oxide, fillers, hydrogenated resins (to increase strength) and zinc acetate to hasten the set. The liquid contains eugenol, olive oil and acetic acid. Eugenol is usually derived from oil of cloves. It is an obtundent (pain-relieving agent) and is a clear liquid that gradually changes to amber when exposed to light.

Physical Properties

Zinc oxide (ZnO) is a weak and a bland material with no adhesion to the tooth structure. The set mix is accelerated by moisture. This material relieves pain, makes tissue less sensitive to pain, is slightly antiseptic, and is low in thermal conductivity. It provides a good marginal seal when placed in tooth cavities. The crushing strength (compression strength) of pure zinc oxide and eugenol is low in comparison to other cements. The addition of hydrogenated resin increases the crushing strength.

Clinical Uses

- *Treatment restoration:* The most frequent use of zinc oxide and eugenol is as a treatment restoration. It helps to prevent pulpal irritation when set in place for treatment of fractured teeth, lost restorations, advanced caries, or pulpitis. This dental material also exerts a palliative effect on the pulp
- *Temporary luting cement:* Zinc oxide and eugenol is used as a temporary cementing medium for crowns, inlays, and fixed partial dentures. These fixed appliances may later be permanently cemented with zinc phosphate cement
- *Pulp capping:* This material is used in pulp capping for near and direct exposures of the pulp, but this use is declining. Calcium hydroxide is now preferred for pulp capping
- Lining material
- Temporary restorative material
- Impression material in edentulous patients
- *Surgical packing or dressing:* This material is used as a surgical packing or dressing after certain periodontal surgical procedures. An example of this is the surgical dressing applied and adapted over the gingival area after a gingivectomy. This dressing protects the area and makes the tissue less sensitive.

Ethoxy Benzoic Acid (EBA)

This particular cement is based on zinc oxide eugenol to which orthoethoxy benzoic acid is added. A resin is also added to the composition for strength such as polystyrene. Its main use is as an intermediate restorative material. It can also be used for the retrograde sealing in endodontic surgeries.

Calcium Hydroxide

Calcium hydroxide is used in operative procedures such as pulp capping (protection for an exposed or nearly exposed pulp). It is available in premixed commercial preparations ready for immediate use. Because of its low compressive/crushing strength, calcium hydroxide alone is not used as an intermediate base. It is usually covered with zinc phosphate cement or zinc oxide and eugenol cement. Dycal, a commercial preparation, is an example of calcium hydroxide.

This material may be used as setting/nonsetting according to the clinical situation. It is alkaline in nature with a pH of 9–10. When used as a lining material, it sets with salicylic acid/light cure set. It forms a calcific bridge and thus protects the pulp.

Clinical Uses

- Indirect/direct pulp capping
- As nonsetting calcium hydroxide, it can be used as an endodontic intracanal dressing
- Root canal sealer
- Root perforations and resorption (as nonsetting material)
- Apexification (nonsetting material).

DENTAL ADHESIVES

Adhesion is a process of solid and/or liquid interaction of one material with another at a single interface (Table 7.7). Adhesion can be classified as:

- *Chemical:* This is the molecular attraction which occurs due to the bonds (ionic, covalent and metallic) formed across the interface
- *Mechanical/Micromechanical:* This is the result of an interface which involves undercuts and surface irregularities
- *Physical:* This involves the van der Waals forces and is relatively weak in nature.

The agents producing the adhesive joints are known as bonding agents (Table 7.8). The adhesive systems today can generally be placed into one of four categories: three-step total-etch systems (4th generation), two-step total-etch systems (5th generation), two-step self-etching systems (6th generation), and one-step or "all in one" self-etching systems (7th generation). Each system contains an acidic conditioner/component, a dentin primer, and a bonding resin.

Table 7.7 Dental adhesives

Ideal requirements of a bonding agent
• High bond strength • Thin film thickness • Fluoride releasing • User-friendly • Stable • Suitable for both moist and dry environments

Table 7.8 Evolution of bonding agents

Generation	*Comments*
First generation (1950s)	They were based on silane coupling agents model. The success rate was low due to high polymerization shrinkage. They did not recommend dentin etching and relied on the adhesion to smear layer
Second generation (1960s)	Similar concepts to first generation agents
Third generation (1980s)	They introduced the acid-etching concept of the dentin and a separate primer to increase the bond strength. There was marginal leakage
Fourth generation (1990s)	It forms a hybrid layer of collagen and resin by penetrating both the etched surface and the decalcified dentinal tubules. It is very technique sensitive and required multiple steps and bottles (three stages- etchant/primer/bonding resin)
Fifth generation (mid 1990s)	This combined the primer and the adhesive in one bottle while maintaining the high bond strength (two stages- etchant/combined primer and bonding resin)
Sixth generation (latter part of 1990s and early 2000s)	They are also called the self-etching primers. The separate acid-etching step was eliminated
Seventh generation (late 2002s)	These are the all-in-one systems. They combine etch, prime and bond in one single system and is user friendly. These can be used for enamel bonding, dentin bonding, amalgam bonding or composite to metal bonding

Acid Etch Technique

Cavities requiring added retention (to hold firmly) are treated with an acid etching technique. The enamel adjacent to the margins of the preparation is slightly decalcified with a phosphoric acid solution. This etched enamel enhances the mechanical retention. The acid is left on the cut tooth structure for only 15–20 seconds. The area is then flushed with water to remove the decalcified material. Etched tooth structure will have a chalky appearance.

Enamel Bonding Systems

These consist of an unfilled liquid acrylic monomer and are based on the total etch procedure where the bonding agent is applied to both the enamel and the dentin. These are made from resins combined with diluents to lower the viscosity (Bis-GMA + TEGDMA). Types of etchants used for these systems may be strong acids (37% phosphoric acid used for 15 seconds) or weak acids (2.5% nitric acid or 17% maleic acid for 30–60 seconds).

Dentin Bonding Systems

These systems involve an unfilled, liquid acrylic monomer which is placed onto an acid conditioned and primed dentin surface. They consist of:

- *Etchant/Conditioner*—phosphoric acid (to remove the smear layer)
- *Primer*—HEMA (to increase the surface energy)
- *Bonding resin*—Bis-GMA.

Amalgam Bonding Systems

These systems are used to bond amalgam to the tooth structure, amalgam to amalgam, and/or amalgam to other metals. 4-META (4-methyloxyethyl trimellitate anhydride) is used as, it has both hydrophobic and hydrophilic ends required for optimal bonding.

> *Note*
> For cast metal restoration bonding/porcelain bonding, it is recommended to use solvent based adhesives.

RESINS

Due to its esthetic properties, resin can be used for the reproduction of lost tooth structure. These materials are often referred to as direct-filling resins. There are two types of direct filling resins. The older type is an unfilled polymethyl methacrylate. Such a resin is often referred to as an acrylic resin. The newer type is the composite resin.

Composite Resins

Composite resins are the most commonly used material for all permanent anterior restorations. These resins make excellent restorative materials because of their good resistance to wear and their excellent esthetics. Composite is a mixture of acrylic resin and powdered glass-like particles that produces, a tooth-colored filling. This type of material may be self-hardening or may be hardened by exposure to blue light (Table 7.9).

Chemical Composition

Composite resins are composed of universal paste with filler and resin. Fillers used may be quartz, silica, borosilicate glass. Filler decreases the curing shrinkage and the thermal expansion of the material. Barium glass is used for radio-opacity. Filler loading is >60% by volume for posterior use and <60% by volume for anterior use. The resin component is based on bis-phenol A and glycidyl methacrylate (Bis-GMA). These help in decreasing

Table 7.9 Composite resins

Types of composites	
Coarse	Large filler particles with good wear resistance. They have poor esthetics and are difficult to polish
Microfill	Smaller filler particles (less than 1 μm) results in better esthetics. They have poor wear resistance but are easier to polish
Hybrid	This combines the coarse and the microfill particle to improve esthetics
Flowable composites	–

the shrinkage. Other resins which may be used are tri-ethylene glycol dimethacrylate or TEGDMA (as Bis-GMA may be viscous).

Properties
- Composite resins have excellent esthetic properties
- Composite resins have good resistance to wear because of the filler
- They also have an acceptable compressive and tensile strength comparable to the tooth
- Polymerization shrinkage.

Dental composites set by the formation of polymer chains. In a two paste system (base and catalyst), the reaction between the tertiary amine and peroxide results in the set of the material. In case of a visible light cure (470 nm wavelength), the material sets by the use of light reacting with 1, 2 diketone (e.g. camphorquinone) and a tertiary amine.

Direct Composites
Microfill, hybrid and flowable, all three may be used as direct composites. Microfill may be used for Class 111 and Class V cavities and small Class 1 cavities. Flowable may be used for repair of marginal defects or as a liner. Hybrid composite is used mainly for core build up and large Class 1 and Class 2 cavities.

Indirect Composites
These require two clinical visits. They have better esthetics. They are mainly used for composite veneers.

Advantages
- Good esthetics
- Often permits preservation of the tooth structure
- Low-risk of leakage, if bonded only to enamel
- Does not corrode.

Disadvantages

- This type of filling can break and wear out more easily than metal fillings, especially in areas of heavy biting force. Therefore, composite fillings may need to be replaced more often than metal fillings
- They cannot be used in all situations
- Composite generally is more expensive than amalgam
- May require more than one visit for inlays, veneers and crowns
- May wear faster than natural dental enamel
- Polymerization shrinkage
- Light cured materials have a limited depth of cure.

PIT AND FISSURE SEALANTS

Pit and fissure sealants are similar to the unfilled resin portion of acid etch composite filling materials. This is used as a prophylactic seal of occlusal pits and fissures. The purpose is to prevent carious destruction of tooth structure. The sealant is used when there is a deep occlusal pit or fossa or a lingual pit, when there is an intact occlusal surface with a carious or restored contralateral tooth surface, and where there is high carious activity, poor oral hygiene, or newly erupted posterior teeth.

CAVITY LINING VARNISH

Cavity lining varnish is used as a seal under an otherwise unbased restoration. It is composed of resins dissolved in a volatile thinner. It is used extensively to seal dentin tubules and thus isolate the pulp of the tooth from the acidity of zinc phosphate cement. In some cases, it is used to help prevent marginal leakage around restorations. This is available as a liquid in a container, usually together with a bottle of thinner. The bottle of varnish should be kept tightly sealed when not in use. If the varnish gets too thick, thinner is added to restore the original consistency.

INTERMEDIATE RESTORATIVE MATERIAL

Intermediate restorative material (IRM) is zinc oxide and eugenol cement that has been reinforced for increased strength. It is used as an intermediate base beneath a metallic restoration and also as a temporary restoration.

DIRECT FILLING GOLD

Gold, the most noble of metals, seldom tarnishes or corrodes in the oral cavity. Gold is frequently used in combination with other metals to produce alloys that can be used to fabricate various types of dental restorations where metal is indicated. The basic types of gold alloys used in dentistry are casting gold, gold solder, wrought gold and gold plate. The principal metals used in combination with gold to form the alloys are silver, copper, platinum, palladium, and zinc. Gold foil is a restorative material used in the pure state. It is used most often on facial surfaces, proximal surfaces of anterior teeth, and occlusal surfaces of posterior teeth. Its chief disadvantages are color, high thermal conductivity, and difficulty in manipulation. Gold foil is available in either adhesive or nonadhesive form. To prevent pellets of adhesive foil from sticking together before use, their surfaces are treated with moisture or gas residues. When ready for use, the moisture and gas residues are vaporized by heating.

INDIRECT RESTORATIVE MATERIALS

Impression Materials

An impression is a negative reproduction of a given area of the oral cavity. The area reproduced may be composed of either hard or soft tissues or both.

Classification of Impression Materials

- *Rigid*
  - Impression plaster
  - Impression compound
  - Zinc oxide eugenol
- *Elastic*
  - *Hydrocolloids*
    - Reversible-Agar-Agar
    - Irreversible-Alginate
  - *Elastomers*
    - Polysulphides (rubber-base)
    - Silicones
    - Polyethers.

Rigid Impression Materials

These materials have limited use for dentulous patients as they are solids and hence, incapable of being removed directly from the undercut areas. Plaster of Paris is used for pouring casts, making matrices for prosthodontic restorations, for attaching casts to articulators, and general use in the dental laboratory where strength is not important. It contains 4% potassium sulphate and 0.4% borax (retards the set).

Impression compound has poor accuracy and distorts easily. They are of two types:

1. *Type 1:* Low fusing used for primary impressions.
2. *Type 2:* High fusing used for peripheral adaptation of impression trays.

Elastic Impression Materials

Properties

These exhibit poor dimensional stability due to:

- *Syneresis:* When an impression made of this material is removed from the mouth into the air at room temperature, the surface contracts by giving off water to the air. This process is called syneresis and causes the outer layer of the impression to shrink and become distorted
- *Imbibition:* If the impression is placed in water, it will expand (take up water). This process is called imbibition. Unfortunately, the expansion caused by imbibition will not restore an impression to its original dimensions
- *Expansion after shrinkage:* The expansion does not equal the shrinkage either in volume or direction. Therefore, any attempt to restore an impression after syneresis has occurred will result in a distorted cast oxide.

Agar-Agar

The agar-type hydrocolloids are thermoplastic, elastic materials. They are called reversible hydrocolloids because they are softened by heating, hardened by cooling, and used repeatedly. In the hardened state, they are flexible and elastic. The basic component of these hydrocolloids is agar-agar, a product extracted from certain types of seaweed. The exact composition of the material varies with different manufacturers. Most preparations contain about 80 percent water, 15 percent agar-agar, and 5 percent chemicals and inert substances. It has largely been superseded by impression materials.

Alginate

An alginate is a salt of alginic acid (an extract from seaweed). Alginate-type hydrocolloids gel by chemical action. Once the gelation process begins, it is irreversible.

The components are a soluble alginate (either potassium alginate or sodium alginate) and a reactor (calcium sulfate), which causes the alginate to gel. The material also contains a retarder (sodium or potassium sulfate, oxalate, or carbonate) to prevent gelation from occurring too rapidly. A fluoride is usually added to prevent retardation of the setting time of the casts. The remainder of the material is composed of fillers that increase the strength and stiffness of the gel.

Elastomers

Synthetic rubber base impression materials are flexible, rubber-like, and sufficiently elastic to return to their original shape after slight distortion. They are used for making impressions of areas containing undercuts, especially for crowns, inlays, and removable and fixed partial dentures. There are two types of rubber base impression materials. Type one has a synthetic rubber base of silicone. Type two has a synthetic rubber base of polysulfide. Both types are polymeric compounds. These compounds are composed of molecules of the same elements in the same proportions but differing in size. The compound containing small, simple molecules is called monomer. The compound containing large complex molecules in which the atoms are joined in chains or rings is called a polymer. Because of their different molecular structure, the compounds have different physical properties. The chemical process by which the molecules of monomer are combined to form polymer is called polymerization.

Both the silicone and polysulfide bases are liquids. They are mixed with liquid chemical reactors which polymerize them. Inert substances or plasticizers are added to make paste of a consistency that will remain in an impression tray, until polymerization has taken place.

Polyether: The catalyst is usually an aromatic sulphonate ester. It is used for crown and bridge impressions and implant impressions. It is rigid and is difficult to remove from the undercuts.

Polysulphides: This contains a prepolymer, an ether link and a plasticizer. It has a noxious odor and stains clothes. It is used for crown and bridge impressions, implant impressions and for multiple preparations and the setting reaction is accelerated by moisture.

Addition Silicones: This is based on dimethylsiloxane and polymerizes by the addition to an unsaturated end group. It is high accuracy and is dimensionally stable but not as strong as other elastomers.

CAST METAL RESTORATIONS

Gold Casting Alloy

Restorations made with gold foil do not exhibit as much overall strength and resilience as do restorations made with gold alloys (Table 7.10). Casting gold alloy is used in the fabrication of various types and classes of restorations. It is alloyed and made into ingots suitable for melting and casting into molds for the restorations. It is biocompatible with good corrosion resistance.

Fineness, Carat and Weighing

The amount of gold in a gold alloy may be rated in terms of fineness or carat. Fineness is determined by the parts per thousand of pure gold contained in the alloy. In terms of fineness, pure gold is 1,000 fine, and an alloy with three-fourths pure gold is 750 fine. In the carat system of rating, the carat refers to the parts of gold determined by dividing the substance into 24 units

Table 7.10 Different types of alloys

Noble metal alloys	*Precious metal alloys*	*Gold alloys*	*Base metal alloys*
They are resistant to corrosion. These are based on gold, platinum, palladium, rhodium and iridium	These contain metals of high value and include all the noble metals and silver	These are precious metal alloys that do not contain gold. Example is silver-palladium	These alloys are formulated with 18–28% chromium

and then counting the number of units of gold. Thus, a 24-carat substance would be pure gold and a 12-carat alloy would be one-half gold.

Annealing and Tempering

Through the use of controlled heat and rate of cooling, gold alloys can be annealed (softened) or tempered (hardened). Gold alloys are hardened by slow cooling. Rapid cooling from a high temperature will soften a gold alloy. Rapid cooling is done by quenching the heated gold alloy in tap water.

Types of Casting Gold Alloys

- Type I—For inlays not subjected to stress
- Type II—For inlays and onlays work
- Type III—For onlays, full crowns, three-quarter crowns, and retainers
- Type IV—Used for crowns, bridges and removable partial dentures.

Chemical Composition

Main components are gold and copper. Copper causes the solution hardening and causes the gold to be red in color. Silver is added to counteract the color of copper. Palladium provides hardness and platinum elevates the melting temperature of gold. Zinc is added to act as a scavenger.

White Gold

Casting gold alloys can be whitened (white gold) by adding palladium, platinum, or silver. This may be used for crowns and abutments requiring great strength and hardness.

Nickel and Cobalt-Chromium Alloys

Nickel or cobalt-chrome alloys are mixtures of nickel and chromium. They are a dark silver metal color and are used for crowns and fixed bridges and most partial denture frameworks. Cobalt-chromium alloys contain 40–60% cobalt, 25–35% chromium with small amounts of nickel to improve the ductility. The alloy is corrosion resistant and less expensive than gold. It is strong and hard but less flexible than gold and does not bond to porcelain. Its main clinical use is for partial dentures and clasps. On the other side, nickel-chromium alloys contain 70–80% nickel, 15–20% chromium and some trace metals. The alloy bonds to porcelain and can be cast accurately. The disadvantage is that it is not as strong as cobalt-chromium. Its main use is for crowns and bridges (Table 7.11).

Table 7.11 Indirect restorative materials

Factors	*All-porcelain (ceramic)*	*Porcelain fused to metal*	*Gold alloys*	*Base metal alloys*
Description	Porcelain, ceramic and glass like fillings and crowns	Porcelain is fused to an underlying metal structure to provide strength to the restoration	Alloy of gold, copper and other metals resulting in a strong and effective restoration	Alloys of non-noble metals resulting in high strength restorations
Uses	Inlays, onlays, crowns and veneers	Crowns and fixed bridges	Inlays, onlays, crowns and fixed bridges	Crowns, fixed bridges and partial dentures
Strength and durability	Brittle material, may fracture under heavy biting loads	Strong and durable	High strength and fracture resistance	High strength and fracture resistance
Bio-compatibility	Well tolerated	Well tolerated but some individuals may have allergic sensitivity to base metals	Well tolerated	Well tolerated but some individuals may have allergic sensitivity to base metals
Esthetics	Color and translucency mimic a natural tooth	Porcelain may mimic the natural tooth but the metal limits the translucency	No esthetic value	No esthetic value

Advantages

- Good resistance to further decay, if the restoration fits well
- Excellent durability; does not fracture under stress
- Does not corrode in the mouth
- Minimal amount of tooth needs to be removed.

Disadvantages

- Is not tooth colored; alloy is a dark silver metal color
- Conducts heat and cold; may irritate sensitive teeth
- Can be abrasive to opposing teeth
- High cost; requires at least two office visits and laboratory services
- Wear to opposing teeth.

DENTAL PORCELAIN (CERAMICS)

Porcelains are inorganic salts that fuse when heated. Dental porcelain is manufactured as a powder. When it is heated to a very high temperature in a special oven, it fuses into a homogeneous mass. The heating process is called baking. Upon cooling, the mass is hard and dense. The material is made in a variety of shades to closely match most tooth colors. Baked porcelain has a translucency similar to that of dental enamel, so that porcelain crowns, pontics, and inlays of highly pleasing appearance can be made. Ingredients of porcelain include feldspar, kaolin, silica (in the form of quartz), materials which act as fluxes to lower the fusion point, metallic oxide, and binders (Table 7.12).

Table 7.12 Types of porcelain (based on strength)

Type	*Comments*
Aluminous porcelain	Strong and hard but opaque. Used mainly as a core porcelain
Sintered alumina cores	High flexural strength and improved translucency
Injection moulded	Excellent strength, acceptable esthetics but poor accuracy at the margins
Computer-aided design and computer-aided manufacturing(CAD and CAM)	Marginal fit may pose a problem
Leucite reinforced	Good strength and esthetics

Porcelains are classified into high-fusing, medium-fusing, and low-fusing groups, depending upon the temperature at which fusion takes place:

- *High-fusing porcelains:* High-fusing porcelains fuse at 2400° F. They are used for the fabrication of full porcelain crowns (jacket crowns). Kaolin is used as a binder
- *Medium-fusing porcelains:* Medium-fusing porcelains fuse between 2,000° and 2,400° F. They are used in the fabrication of inlays, crowns, facings, and pontics (a pontic is the portion of a fixed partial denture, which replaces a missing tooth)
- *Low-fusing porcelains:* Low-fusing porcelains fuse between 1,600° and 2,000° F. They are used primarily to correct or modify the contours of previously baked high- or medium-fusing porcelain restorations.

Advantages

- Tooth-colored with excellent translucency; the color looks similar to natural tooth enamel
- Very little tooth is removed when used as a veneer
- Good resistance to further decay
- Resists leakage because of precise shaping and fitting.

Disadvantages

- Material is brittle and is prone to cracking under biting force
- Requires a minimum of two appointments to complete
- High cost, similar to gold.

PORCELAIN FUSED TO METAL

This type of porcelain is a glass-like material that is "enameled" on top of metal shells. It is tooth-colored and is used for crowns and fixed bridges.

Advantages

- Good resistance to further decay, if the restoration fits well
- Very durable, due to metal substructure
- The material does not cause tooth sensitivity
- Resists leakage because it can be shaped for a very accurate fit.

Disadvantages

- More tooth must be removed (than for porcelain) for the metal substructure
- Higher cost because it requires at least two office visits and laboratory services.

MACHINED RESTORATIONS

There are two methods of machining dental restorations:

1. Copy milling
2. Computer aided design/Computer aided machining (CAD/CAM) milling.

Copy milling uses an impression of the desired form as a guide for the milling machine. Composite and ceramic materials are mainly used. The choice of the material also depends on the type of restoration and the margins required. CAD (Computer aided design)/CAM (Computer aided machining) uses digital information about the cavity preparation and the type and pattern of the restoration. The CEREC (Ceramic Reconstruction) was the first CAD/CAM system used in dentistry. CAD/CAM restorations are mainly fabricated from ceramics. Examples of some CAD/CAM systems currently used in dentistry are *CEREC*-used for inlays, onlays and veneers, *DentiCAD*-used for inlays, onlays and crowns and bridges, *CICERO (Computer integrated crown reconstruction)*-used for porcelain fused to metal crowns, *ProCera*-used for copy milling restorations and porcelain fused to metal restorations and *CELAY* (used for copy-milled composite/ceramic inlays, onlays or veneers).

DENTAL CEMENTS

These are based on reactions between acidic liquids and powders to produce salts. Since most of the cements have been discussed under liners and bases, just a brief mention would be given here to recapitulate. Dental cements are most often used as luting indirect restorations but may also be used as bases (Table 7.13). Zinc phosphate cements have the potential to irritate the pulp. Hence, while using this product, the dentin should be protected with cavity varnish.

MISCELLANEOUS

Root Canal Filling Materials

Root canal filling materials consist of tapered gutta-percha in standard sizes that match the size of the files used. The points are cemented in place with root canal sealer that is usually a zinc oxide and eugenol preparation, calcium hydroxide based or a glass ionomer based. Root canal filling materials are used to fill previously prepared root canals.

Gutta-Percha Points

Gutta-percha points are made from the refined, coagulated, milky exudate of trees in the Malay Peninsula. Gutta-percha is pink or gray in color. It is softened (at 65°C) by heat and is easily molded. When cool, gutta-percha

Table 7.13 Dental cements

Type	*Composition*
Zinc oxide eugenol • Unmodified • Reinforced • ZOE-EBA	Powder consists of ZnO, polymer, resins and aluminum oxide. Liquid consists of eugenol
Zinc phosphate	Powder is mainly ZnO and the liquid component consists of phosphoric acid
Zinc polycarboxylate	Powder is ZnO and the liquid part is polyacrylic acid
Calcium hydroxide	Powder is $Ca(OH)_2$ with phenolic esters as the liquid component
Glass ionomer (conventional)	Powder is F1-Al silicate glass and polyacrylic acid as the liquid
Glass ionomer (light-cured)	Powder is F1-Al silicate glass with polyacrylic acid monomers as the liquid part
Glass ionomer (resin-modified/hybrid)	Powder is F1-Al silicate glass and resin and the liquid is polyacrylic acid monomers

Abbreviations: ZnO, Zinc oxide eugenol; $Ca(OH)_2$, Calcium hydroxide; F1-Al, Fluoroalumino

maintains its shape. It is 60% crystalline and 40% amorphous at room temperature and melts at 100°C. Gutta-percha points are used as a root canal filling material.

Advantages

- They have a high thermal expansion
- They do not shrink unless used with solvent
- They are radiopaque, conduct heat poorly, and are easy to remove from the root canal
- They may be kept sterile in antiseptic solution, are impervious to moisture, and are bacteriostatic.

Disadvantages

They shrink when used with a solvent.

Polishing Materials

Tin Oxide: Tin oxide is used in polishing teeth and metal restorations. It is a fine, white powder that is made into a paste by adding water or glycerin.

Pumice: Pumice is used as an abrasive and polishing agent for acrylic resins, amalgams, and gold. It consists mainly of complex silicates of aluminum, potassium, and sodium. Two grades—flour of pumice and coarse pumice—are listed in the Federal Supply Catalog.

Chalk (Whiting): Chalk is used for polishing acrylic resins and metals. It is composed primarily of calcium carbonate.

Tripoli: Tripoli is usually used for polishing gold and other metals. It is made from certain porous rocks.

Waxes

Many different waxes are used in dentistry. The composition, form, and color of each wax is designed to facilitate its use and to produce the best possible results. The discussion in this chapter is limited to aspects of clinical interest.

Inlay Wax

Inlay wax is used to prepare patterns. These patterns are reproduced in gold or other material in the fabrication of inlays, crowns, and fixed and removable partial dentures. Inlay wax is sometimes called casting wax. The wax should harden at body temperature but soften at a temperature low enough to permit it to be manipulated in a plastic state in the mouth without injury to pulp or oral tissues. Its color should contrast with the colors of teeth and oral tissues to facilitate carving, except that ivory wax is used to avoid risk of color contamination when porcelain or acrylic restorations are constructed. Inlay wax is available in blue, green, ivory, or deep purple sticks, in preformed shapes for partial dentures, and in solidly packed cans. It is hard at room temperatures and breaks if bent sharply. This wax remains hard at mouth temperature and may be carved either in or out of the mouth. It is softened with dry heat or by immersion in warm water until pliable.

Baseplate Wax

Baseplate wax is used mainly for making occlusion rims and for holding artificial teeth to baseplates during the fabrication of dentures. Baseplate wax is composed mainly of beeswax , paraffin, and coloring matters, which are mixed together, cast into blocks, and rolled into sheets. The sheets are red or pink, 3 inches wide and 6 inches long. Baseplate wax is relatively hard and slightly brittle at room temperature but becomes soft and pliable when heated. Baseplate wax must be capable of holding porcelain or acrylic teeth in position both at normal room temperature and at mouth temperature. There are two types of baseplate wax, hard and medium. The hard type is suitable for use in warm temperatures but tends to crack and flake at low temperatures. The medium type is suitable for use at low temperatures but flows excessively at high temperatures.

Sticky Wax

Sticky wax has many uses in a dental clinic and dental laboratory. It holds broken pieces of a denture together, assembles components of fixed partial dentures and wrought partial dentures in preparation for soldering. Sticky wax becomes sticky when melted and has the property of adhering to the surfaces of various materials. It is composed of beeswax, paraffin, and resins. It is usually supplied as hexagonal sticks of various colors, often orange or purple. It is brittle at room temperature and assumes a thick liquid consistency when heated.

Disclosing Wax

Disclosing wax is used to determine unequal pressure points in a denture that may cause discomfort to the patient. These points are located by painting the wax on the tissue side of the denture base and holding the denture in place under pressure in the mouth. The wax flows away from the points needing relief. Disclosing wax is sometimes known as pressure indicator paste.

Boxing Wax/Carding Wax

Boxing wax is used to form a box around impressions of the mouth when making a cast (model). This limits the flow of either plaster of Paris or artificial stone gypsum material. Boxing wax is usually issued in red strips measuring 1 1/2 inches wide, 12 inches long, and 1/8 inch thick. It is soft and pliable enough at room temperature to be formed into a desired shape without heating. For further softening, a strip of wax can be passed through an open flame.

Low-fusing Impression Wax

Low-fusing impression wax is a wax that is especially compounded so that when subjected to controlled pressure, it will flow to some extent in the mouth. Low-fusing impression wax is often used in relining or rebasing complete and partial dentures. Because it is easily distorted, impressions must be handled with care.

SAFETY AND EFFICACY

Dental products such as acrylics, resins and polymer materials used in restorative dentistry represent a major advance in dentistry. Although these products may act as allergens, we should not forget that every technology, no matter how beneficial, can exert a negative impact on some members of the population. The reality of public health will always involve balancing maximum benefit and minimum harm to the public health and well-being. Some guideline or protocols should be followed to help combat the hazardous effects of materials used in dentistry.

Dental personnel should be familiar with the major signs and symptoms of allergic reactions, including anaphylaxis, should an allergic emergency arise during a consultation. Previous allergic status of patients and personnel should be noted. Dental personnel should always keep records of dental materials used. If allergic reaction occurs, backtracking is necessary in order to identify the specific allergen. Local exhaust ventilation systems can significantly reduce the peak concentration of acrylate vapor in the breathing zone of dental technicians. Nitrile, vinyl, or 4 H gloves should be used by the dental practitioner, if acrylate or latex sensitivity is suspected. If sensitivity is suspected, inform the patient about possible clinical tests to determine origin of allergy, e.g. acrylate patch testing. Delayed sensitivity may be prevalent in certain cases. Be aware of cross-sensitivity towards coloring agents of dentures. It is always helpful to create a latex-free environment for personnel and patients with latex sensitivity.

BIBLIOGRAPHY

1. Eley BM. The future of dental amalgam: a review of the literature. British Dental Association, London; 1998.
2. Lonnroth EC, Shahnavaz H. Use of polymer materials in dental clinics. Swed Dent J. 1997;(21):149-50.
3. McCabe JF, Walls AWG. Applied Dental materials, 8th edn. Blackwell Science, oxford; 1998.
4. Reiss B, Walther W. Clinical long-term results and 10-year Kaplan-Meier analysis of CERE C restorations. Int J Comput Dent. 2000;3(1):9-23.
5. Reiss B, Walther W. Ereignisanalyse und klinische Langzeitergebnisse mit CEREC-Keramikinlays. Dtsch ahnarztl Z. 1998;53(1):65-68. In German.
6. Ritter RG. Where are we and where are we going? Adhesive Update; PennWell Pub Co; 2007.
7. Van Meerbeek B, Inoue S, Pedigao J, et al. In Fundamentals of Operative Dentistry, 2nd edn. Carol Stream, Ill: Quintessence Publishing; 2001.pp.194-214.
8. Van Noort R. Introduction to Dental Materials, 2nd edn. Mosby, Edinburgh; 2002.

CHAPTER **8**

NONCARIOUS TOOTH SURFACE LOSS

Balaram Naik, Priyanka Jain

INTRODUCTION

Noncarious tooth surface loss can be defined as the loss of dental hard tissue due to causes not attributed to bacterial action on fermentable carbohydrates. Noncarious tooth surface loss (NCTSL) is a process occurring throughout life, but it can become a problem affecting function and esthetics and often causing pain. It is also referred to as nonbacterial tooth surface loss or tooth wear. Different forms of chronic destructive processes other than caries affecting the teeth and leading to an irreversible loss of tooth structure from the external surface can be described. They are referred to as abrasion, demastication, attrition, abfraction, resorption and erosion. These processes can be viewed as physiological and/or pathological. Noncarious loss of dental hard tissue is hardly ever caused by one of the above processes alone. Tooth wear in any one individual is therefore, likely to be multifactorial.

Tooth wear was and is considered a normal physiologic process as some degree of tooth wear is essential for efficient functioning of the teeth. This is also considered important in establishing unhindered guidance during mastication. But if the rate of wear challenges, the viability of teeth tooth surface loss is considered to be pathologic.

FACTORS PRECIPITATING TOOTH WEAR

The loss of tooth wear is commonly termed as attrition, abrasion, erosion and abfraction. Often, tooth wear is a complex combination of any of the two problems mentioned above. Knowledge of the etiology is very important in preventing occurrence of further lesions and halting the progression of those already present. Noncarious lesions may have a multifactorial etiology and may not be related to any one factor. A combination of erosion, abrasion and abfraction may operate in the initiation and progression of these lesions.

- *Congenital abnormalities:* Amelogenesis and dentinogenesis imperfecta may cause regressive changes in teeth and extensive tooth wear can result from normal function.
- *Increase in the life expectancy of an individual:* This may be attributed to the increased functional demand on the teeth, longer exposure to erosive foods as the diet pattern changes, and increased use of medication which may affect the tooth wear (by their acidic nature).
- *Quantitative and qualitative reduction in salivary flow:* The quantity and quality of saliva may also have a role in the development of noncarious lesions. Drugs and conditions which reduce salivary flow may accelerate the loss of tooth structure in the cervical region. Reasons for the link between salivary dysfunction and tooth wear may be due to the:
  - Reduced clearance of dietary acids
  - Reduced pH of saliva
  - Reduced buffering capacity of saliva which prevents the dietary acids from being neutralized
  - Softening of tooth structure leading to accelerated wear from normal wear and tear under occlusal forces.
- *Loss of teeth increases the demands on the remaining teeth.*
- *Diet:* Dietary changes have resulted in the diets being less abrasive. Excessive consumption of erosive beverages and foods has had a potentiating effect on the increased prevalence of NCTSL. Implicated foods in this category can be fizzy drinks (pH 2.2–3.8), fruit juices (pH 3.0–4.0), wines (pH 3.2–4.8), cider and beer (pH 3.5–4.0) and citrus fruits.
- *Parafunctional habits:* Habits like bruxism, object biting, etc. increase the masticatory load on the teeth by nearly 700 times, as compared to the normal masticatory load. The force used is considerably greater than during normal mastication. Patients with parafunctional habits may present clinically as having wear in nonfunctional cusps, prominent masseters and tenderness of muscles of mastication.
- *Intrinsic acid:* The pH of the gastric acid is 1–2. This causes tooth wear due to gastric regurgitation, vomiting, etc. which are described later in the chapter. This type of a wear classically presents as a lingual/palatal erosive defect.
- *Abrasive restorative materials:* Unglazed porcelain can accelerate tooth wear (Mahalick JA et al, 1971).
- *Abrasive dentifrices and hard brushing in horizontal strokes.*
- *Defective enamel and dentine deposition and maturation.*
- *Instrument biting, needles, etc.*

TYPES OF WEAR

The excessive differential wears of teeth and restorative materials have significant deleterious effects on the biologic, functional, and esthetic condition of the masticatory system. The loss by physical wear of tooth substance or restorative material caused by direct tooth contact between the occluding or proximal surfaces is known as *attrition*. A similar loss caused by physical factors other than direct tooth contact, namely exogenous material being forced over the tooth and restoration surfaces, is known as *abrasion*. The loss of tooth substance or restorative material caused by nonbacterial chemical action is usually known as *erosion*. Erosion is not directly associated with physical wear or dental caries, although all of these processes may coexist to varying extents. Acids weaken the tooth or restoration surfaces, allowing other wear processes to occur more easily. The hydroxyapatite crystals of tooth substance and the matrices of conventional GICs are particularly susceptible to acid degradation. Tensile forces induced by occlusal loads may also result in the microfracture of cervical enamel on the facial and lingual tooth surfaces, a process described as *abfraction*.

The presence of an intervening medium or slurry between the moving opposing surfaces is known as three body wear. This occurs typically during the "open phase" of mastication, and the degree of wear present is determined partly by the hardness, shape, and size of the particles in the slurry. The direct contact of teeth and restorative materials moving without an intervening medium is known as two-body wear. This is observed with tooth grinding, or bruxism especially, where the opposing occlusal surfaces show close fitting matching facets on mandibular excursion. The production of microfine fragments of tooth and restorative materials converts this process to three-body wear.

Physiologic tooth wear results in a slow, progressive loss of tooth substance. Initially, this process manifests as a flattening of the occlusal cusp tips and incisal edge mammelons. The proximal surfaces also flatten and increase in area. Continued wear leads to the exposure of softer dentin and potentially an acceleration of the wear rate. However, as the facet area increases, there is a substantial reduction in pressure and a slowing of the wear process. The anisotropic nature of tooth substance adds further variability to this wear process. The clinical significance of the extent and rate of tooth wear varies with age, but wear can be regarded as pathologic when the biologic, functional, and esthetic condition of the masticatory system is effectively compromised.

Restoration Wear

The different structure and physical properties of tooth substance and dental restorative materials eventually result in their differential wear, even in the same oral environment. Gold (high-noble metal) alloy restorations have a long history of satisfactory clinical performance and are said to be "kind" to opposing tooth substance and restorative materials, wearing at approximately the same rate as enamel, depending on the type of alloy used. Base-metal (nonnoble metal) nickel-chromium alloy restorations are more economic and mechanically stiffer alternatives to type III gold alloys, with a lower wear rate. However, base-metal restorations are also harder and more difficult to adjust and polish, and they may wear the opposing teeth more than gold alloys. Rough porcelain surfaces can cause substantial wear of opposing teeth and other restorations. This is also the case with resin-bonded all-ceramic restorations. Porcelain is wear resistant, but the surfaces of the material must remain smoothly glazed or highly polished to reduce damage to opposing teeth and restorations.

Amalgam alloy restorations are wear resistant, largely because of their ability to adapt through smearing from deformation under load. Resin composite materials show higher wear rates than amalgam alloys when placed as large posterior restorations. Conventional GIC and resin-modified GIC (RM-GIC) materials are unsuitable as long-term restorations in high-stress situations. The occlusal wear resistance of an RM-GIC can be improved by combining its usage with a resin composite.

The roughness of surface of restorative materials has been regarded as both the consequence of restoration wear and the cause of antagonistic tooth and restoration wear.

Clinical Implications

The wear of restorative materials should be matched to that of normal tooth wear; otherwise, the occlusion may be destabilized leading to various other problems. Excessive wear of both restorative materials and opposing teeth may occur from incorrect selection of materials for the particular clinical situation. In general dental practice, most restoration failures occur because of caries, fracture, and debonding, or discoloration and marginal deterioration.

Patient factors that might enhance the extent and rate of tooth and restoration wear include heavy biting forces and parafunctional habits, incorrect tooth brushing/dentifrices, abrasive and acidic diets, regurgitation, reduced salivary flow and altered composition, defective tooth structure, and reduced posterior tooth support. Careful monitoring of the extent and rate of tooth and restoration wear should be part of routine dental treatment management.

TOOTH WEAR

The average rate of enamel occlusal contact area wear varies widely, but it has been reported as approximately 30–40 μm per year in the molar region. However, many factors will influence the rate and extent of enamel wear.

Types of Tooth Wear

Attrition

The term attrition is derived from the Latin verb *uttrrrre, uttrilti, crttrituiii,* describing the action of rubbing against something. The clinical term dental attrition is used to describe the physiological wearing away of dental hard tissue as a result of tooth-to-tooth contact with no foreign substance intervening. Such contact occurs while grinding the teeth, e.g. during swallowing, speech, and the resulting wear involves the occlusal and incisal surfaces of teeth. Proximal surfaces may also be worn away by attrition during mastication. Clinically, this loss of substance leads to the formation of facets.

Attrition is associated with occlusal function and maybe exaggerated by habits or parafunctional activity like bruxism. This type of tooth wear is significant in populations with high abrasive diets. This is an age related process and can vary from individual to individual.

Causes of Attrition

- Parafunctional habits like bruxism
- Marked misalignment or malocclusion
- Highly abrasive diet
- Loss of posterior teeth
- Constant chewing like betel nut or tobacco
- Occupational habits like putting nails or pins in mouth
- Physiological like in canine guidance.

Clinical Features of Attrition

- Flat cusp tips
- Polished facets on enamel surfaces
- Wear on nonfunctional cusps
- The upper and lower incisal edges are shortened and at one level
- Mostly seen in anterior teeth when posteriors are lost
- Erosion potentiates attrition (Demastication)
- Occasional full loss of enamel resulting in the exposure of dentine with heavy staining
- Exposed dentine will wear at the same rate as enamel
- Attrition may be generalized or localized. If it is localized, it is usually pathological caused by restoration or bad habits.

In extreme cases, the teeth may be worn down to the level of the gingiva. Attrition ranges from part of the enamel being worn away in the early stages to full thickness of the enamel wearing away in the advanced stages of attrition. The process of attrition is slow. Secondary dentine is laid down in response and this is rarely associated with pain. Men show a greater degree of attrition than women.

ABRASION

Abrasion, derived from the Latin verb *abradere, nhrasi, ahrasum* (to scrape off), describes the wearing away of a substance or structure through mechanical processes, such as grinding, rubbing or scraping. The clinical term dental abrasion is used to describe the pathological wearing away of dental hard tissue through abnormal mechanical processes involving foreign objects or substances repeatedly introduced in the mouth and contacting the teeth like pins, tooth brushing, etc. (Table 8.1). It usually occurs on the exposed root surfaces after gingival recession has exposed the cementum. Sometimes, it may be seen on the incisal or interproximal surfaces of the teeth. The buccal cervical areas are the sites for predilection. Furthermore, canines and premolars are the most affected teeth due to their position in the arch where they receive most attention during cleaning.

Depending on the etiology, the pattern of wear can be diffuse or localized. Based on the clinical observation of the frequent coincidence of smooth-surface and/or cervical abrasion and extensive oral hygiene, the latter has been incriminated to be a main etiological factor in dental abrasion. Both patient related and material related factors influence the prevalence of abrasion. Abrasion on proximal tooth surfaces may be caused by extensive use of interdental cleaning devices such as tooth picks or interdental brushes, especially when they are inserted along with toothpaste or toothpowder. Occupational abrasion, i.e. excessive tooth wear due to any professional cause such as abrasive dust at the work place, holding nails between the teeth, biting thread, etc. are only rarely seen today.

Table 8.1 Causes of abrasion

Patient related factors	*Material related factors*
Frequency of brushing	Use of an abrasive dentifrice (whitening agents). The enamel and dentine is worn away to produce a V shaped notch at the neck of the tooth. Areas most affected are the labial and the buccal surfaces of the canines and the premolars
Time spent on brushing. Longer than 1 to 3 minutes can lead to abrasion lesions	Stiffness and end rounding of the bristles
Incorrect or aggressive use of a tooth brush	pH and amount of dentifrice used
Improper brushing technique. Cross technique creates a V shaped notch and cross and horizontal technique increases the chances of cervical abrasion	Tuft design of the brush
Use of a hard tooth brush	Flexibility and length of the toothbrush grip
Habits like biting finger nails or opening bobby pins using teeth	–
Arch where brushing is begun. Most commonly the cervical thirds of the posterior teeth in the upper left quadrant in a right handed individual are affected	–

Clinical Features of Abrasion

- Common in the left quadrant of a right handed individual
- Common on the facial surfaces of the teeth
- Canine and the 1st premolars are the most commonly affected teeth
- Notched, wedge shaped or V shaped lesions
- Margins are sharp and well defined
- Smooth surfaces may show scratches
- Worn, shiny yellow/brown areas at the cervical margins
- Worn notches on the incisal surfaces of anterior teeth.

ABFRACTION

This is used to describe a special form of wedge-shaped defect at the cemento-enamel junction (CEJ) of a tooth. Such lesions observed on a single tooth are hypothesized to be the result of eccentrically applied occlusal forces leading to tooth flexure rather than the result of abrasion alone. According to the tooth flexure theory masticatory or parafunctional forces in areas of malocclusion may expose one or several teeth to strong tensile, compressive or shearing stress with the resultant weakening of the cervical tooth structure. These forces are focused on the CEJ where they provoke microfractures in enamel and dentin. The microfractures are thought to propagate with time, perpendicular to the long axis of the stressed teeth, until enamel and dentin break away, as there is progressive disruption of the hydroxylapatite crystals leading to dentin exposure. Abfraction has been used to describe the cervical abrasive lesions.

Causes of Abfraction

- Excessive occlusal stresses which cause the tooth to flex and small enamel flecks to break off inducing these abrasive lesions
- Parafunctional habits like bruxism and clenching of teeth.

Clinical Features of Abfraction

- These are wedge shaped lesions with sharp angles occurring at the facial surfaces of teeth
- Enamel surfaces are rough in the initial stages but may show groves in the later stages
- May be seen in a single tooth
- Subgingival location is also possible.

They can also be found on the occlusal surfaces presenting as circular areas. These lesions can occur with occlusion alone or can be associated with tooth brush erosion. They are often misdiagnosed as tooth brush abrasion, but they differ as their angles are much sharper. They are common in individuals with poor teeth alignment and can be associated with anterior open bite, abnormal tongue movements and occlusal restorations that change the cuspal movements.

DEMASTICATION

Demastication is mainly derived from the Latin verb *mandere. mundi, mansum* (to chew). This describes the wearing away of tooth substance during the mastication of food with the bolus intervening between opposing teeth. Wear is thus influenced by the abrasiveness of the food. Demastication is normally a physiological process affecting primarily the occlusal and incisal surfaces, but may be termed pathological when it occurs due to improper food consumption such as betel nut. This type of wear can also be looked upon as a combination of abrasion and attrition.

RESORPTION

Resorption, derived from the Latin verb *resorberc'* (to suck back), describes the process of biological degradation and assimilation of substances or structures previously produced by the body. The clinical terms dental resorption, root resorption, tooth resorption describe the biological removal of dental hard tissue by cementoclastic, dentinoclastic and ameloclastic activity. This can be either a physiological process, as in the case of root resorption of deciduous teeth, or a pathological process, such as resorption owing to trauma, cysts or neoplasms. Resorption cannot be omitted from the list of noncarious destructive processes.

EROSION

Erosion, derived from the Latin verb *erotlere, erosi* (to gnaw, to corrode), describes the process of gradual destruction of a surface usually by electrolytic or chemical processes. The clinical term dental erosion is used to describe the physical result of a pathologic, chronic, localized, painless loss of dental hard tissue chemically etched away from the tooth surface by acid without bacterial involvement. The acids demineralize the enamel by binding to the calcium and removing it from the enamel. The acids responsible for erosion are not products of the intraoral flora; they stem from dietary, occupational or intrinsic sources. This is a noncarious pathological loss of tooth structure and plaque is not involved in this process.

Erosion can be classified as based on:

- Etiology
- Clinical severity
- Activity of progression
- Localization of erosion.

Classification Based on Etiology

Tooth erosion can be termed extrinsic, intrinsic, or idiopathic. *Extrinsic erosion* is the result of exogenous acids such as industrial acids, or acidic water of swimming pools. Another reason may be the oral administration of medicaments such as iron tonics. Dietary acids, however, undoubtedly are the principal causative factor for extrinsic tooth erosion. Habitual consumption of highly acidic, low pH carbonated drinks, or concentrated fruit juices often lead to erosion. A diet high in acidic food and drinks can cause tooth wear. The lower the pH of a particular food item, the more acidic it is. Any food or drink with a pH lower than 5 may cause tooth wear and sensitivity (Table 8.2).

These lesions appear as generalized to moderate and affect the cervical and buccal surfaces of the upper teeth and the occlusal surfaces of the lower teeth. Factors affecting the erosion severity are the method of consumption (straw is better than direct), frequency of ingestion (reduce citrus fruit juices), forms of acids (Vitamin C is better than tablets), and the amount of time acid is in contact with the teeth (chew quickly). Extrinsic erosive lesions appear as a wide shallow lesion affecting the labial and the palatal surfaces of the upper teeth. They have an etched like appearance. These appear in either the upper or lower anterior teeth.

Intrinsic erosion is the result of endogenous acid. This is gastric acid contacting the teeth during recurrent vomiting, regurgitation or reflux. Eating disorders of psychosomatic origin, such as nervous vomiting, anorexia nervosa or bulimia are often the cause of regurgitation or vomiting which is self-induced. This is characterized by voluntary or involuntary regurgitation and rechewing of partially digested food that is either reswallowed or expelled. This regurgitation appears effortless, and does not involve retching or nausea. Involuntary regurgitation (regurgitation erosion) can occur as a result of gastrointestinal complications like hiatus hernia, chronic alcoholism or as a consequence of pregnancy. Voluntary regurgitation is

Table 8.2 The pH of common foods and drinks

Food	*pH*
Milk	6.9
Tap water	6.0
Cheese	5.9
Coffee	5.0
Beer	4.5
Orange juice	3.5
Apple juice	3.4
Pickles	3.2
Common soft drinks	2.7
Red wine	2.5
Lemon juice	2.2
Vinegar	2.0

associated with an underlying psychological problem. *Anorexia nervosa* is the aversion of food resulting from complex interaction of biological, social, individual, & family factors, leading to severe weight loss. It manifests as extreme aversion of food, behavior directed toward weight loss and intense fear of gaining weight (Table 8.3).

Bulimia nervosa is the over-eating followed by inappropriate compensatory behavior and manifests as having the irreversible urge to over eat, morbid fear of becoming fat and avoidance of all these by vomiting. Chronic regurgitation, be it of somatic or of psychosomatic origin, often leads to a typical distribution of erosion within the dental arches and on the teeth. This is known as *Permolysis.* Perimolysis affects the maxillary and mandibular teeth in different ways. While affecting the palatal and occlusal surfaces of all teeth in the maxilla, the erosion remains confined to the buccal and occlusal surfaces of premolars and molars only in the mandible. The buccal surfaces of the maxilla are not affected by the acid, as they are protected by the neutralizing effect of the saliva. The lingual surfaces of the mandibular teeth are covered by the tongue and are also spared from the acid. The restorations remain intact and stand proud.

Clinical Features of Bulimia Nervosa and Anorexia Patients with Erosive Lesions

- Permolysis is seen in patients with bulimia nervosa and is characterized by erosive lesions localized to the palatal aspects of maxillary teeth
- Raised restorations
- Caries
- Xerostomia caused by vomit induced dehydration or drugs such as diuretics, appetite suppressants and antidepressants
- Wide shallow lesions.

Preventive Measures for Bulimia Nervosa: The first step is medical consultation: tackle the problem with care. The individual may not admit to the unattractive aspect of a psychological illness. Advise to rinse the mouth with sodium bicarbonate or magnesium hydroxide to change the saliva

Table 8.3 Differences between bulimia nervosa and anorexia nervosa

Bulimia nervosa	*Anorexia nervosa*
F>M 10:1	20:1
Age 25 years and up	16 years
10% below body weight	15% below body weight
Extrovert	Introvert
Can't be identified	Very thin looking
Mortality 0.3%	4–20%

to alkaline and use of a neutral pH sodium fluoride dentifrice. Also, it is advisable to eat cheese or milk after vomiting or use xylitol chewing gum.

Signs of Erosive Lesions

- They are broad, shallow or saucer shaped lesions
- Their margins are not well-defined
- Prevalence and size increases with age
- Females are more susceptible than males
- Progression of erosion is faster in the maxillary teeth
- Sensitive teeth
- Teeth appear yellow due to the darker tissue showing through the thinning tooth enamel
- Teeth appearing glazed and smooth due to the tooth surface being worn away
- Sensitive teeth
- Proud restorations
- Teeth appearing to become shorter.

Classification According to Clinical Severity

Erosive lesions can be classified as (Eccles 1979).

Class 1: Superficial lesion involving enamel only.

Class 2: Localized lesion, less than 1/3 of the tooth surface involving dentin.

Class 3: Generalized lesion, more than 1/3 of the tooth surface involving dentine. This can be further classified as according to the site.

- Facial
- Palatal or lingual
- Incisal or occlusal
- Severe and multisurfaces are involved.

Classification According to Pathogenic Activity

Actively progressing erosion (manifest erosion) is clinically diagnosed by its enamel border zones. These are thin where they meet the exposed dentin. In the scanning electron microscope (SEM), they show a honeycomb enamel prism pattern, resembling acid etched enamel. Latent or inactive erosions have prominent thick enamel borders and are no longer subject to further decalcification.

To minimize the risk of dental erosion, individual should:

- Eat a well-balanced diet, and reduce the amount of acidic and sugary foods and drinks. Try to limit snacking
- Eat foods that act as a buffer by neutralizing saliva pH more quickly (e.g. dairy products contain a protein called casein which protects teeth from acid)

- Avoid holding or 'swishing' acidic drinks around the mouth, as this increases the likelihood of tooth decay and tooth wear
- When drinking, use a straw whenever possible, as this minimizes exposure of the drink to your teeth
- Chew sugar free gum to stimulate saliva flow and wash acids away
- Drink plenty of water frequently throughout the day, especially if exercising. If available, drink fluoridated water
- Avoid caffeinated beverages, as caffeine causes dehydration
- Do not brush immediately after eating or drinking acidic or sugary foods or drinks, as tooth enamel will be softened and could be 'brushed off'.

Effects of Tooth Surface Loss

- *Tooth sensitivity:* Exposure of dentin in the cervical area may result in dentin hypersensitivity (Tables 8.4 and 8.5).

Table 8.4 Occlusal problems

Clinical signs and features of noncarious tooth surface loss and occlusal problems
• Tooth mobility
• Open contacts
• Tilted or drifted teeth
• Atypical occlusal wear
• Over-erupted teeth
• Cross bites, deep bites and open bites
• Fewer number of occluding teeth.

Table 8.5 Causes of tooth wear

Etiology of noncarious cervical lesions		
Erosion	**Abrasion**	**Abfraction**
Extrinsic erosion • Dietary acids (citrus fruits, carbonated drinks) • Environmental erosion (battery manufacturers, metal plating) *Intrinsic erosion* • Gastric disorders (ulcers, hiatus hernia, alcoholism) • Chronic vomiting • Pregnancy	*Tooth brushing* • Over vigorous brushing • Use of a hard brush • Improper brushing *Abnormal habits* • Biting a pipe stem • Nail biting • Opening bobby pins	*Excessive occlusal stresses* • Parafunctional habits • Bruxism • Clenching

- *Compromised esthetics:* Loss of tooth structure in the cervical region of teeth may produce an unaesthetic appearance especially in the anterior region (Table 8.6).
- *Risk of tooth fracture:* Deep, wedge-shaped lesions in the cervical area of teeth can increase the risk for tooth fracture due to lowered strength at this critical region.
- *Pulpal damage:* Deep cervical lesions are also likely to result in irreversible pulpitis and pulpal death.
- *Caries:* Noncarious cervical lesions also favor plaque accumulation which would eventually lead to the development of caries.
- *Poor periodontal health:* The gingival may be irritated and inflamed due to noncarious cervical lesion.

DIAGNOSIS

This involves the need to identify the factors causing tooth wear. This is done to preserve the remaining dentition and improve the long term prognosis of any treatment already completed.

Aids to Diagnosis: An initial comprehensive examination is performed which includes a thorough and detailed medical and dental history including occupation, social history and dietary analysis. Questions

Table 8.6 Clinical features

Clinical features of noncervical carious lesions			
	Erosion	**Abrasion**	**Abfraction**
Location	Facial/Lingual	Facial	Facial
Shape	Broad, shallow/ saucer shaped	Notched, Wedge-shaped or V-shaped	Wedge-shaped
Margins	Ill-defined	Sharp and well-defined	Sharp
Enamel surface	Smooth and polished	Smooth but may show scratches	Initial stage—rough Later stage—may show grooves
Teeth affected	Multiple teeth affected, usually lingual surfaces of maxillary molars	Multiple teeth affected, usually facial surfaces of maxillary left canine to molar regions in right handed individuals and vice-versa	May be evident even in a single tooth

regarding diet, lifestyle, medications, stress, brushing habits and consumption of juices and soft drinks can help in the diagnosis. Note down any history of intrinsic or extrinsic erosion. The dentist must try to identify digestive problems like anorexia, gastric regurgitation, etc., by a diet diary. This proves useful in detecting excessive consumption of citrus fruits, carbonated drinks, vitamin C tablets, vinegar, natural yoghurt, etc., which are the common cause of dietary erosion. The dentist must also question the patient about abnormal habits like clenching, grinding, etc., which may be factors responsible for abfraction. Radiographs and other special tests like saliva test, pulpal sensitivity tests, etc., are then carried out according to the requirement. Radiographs may prove useful in identifying changes like altered lamina dura and periodontal space, evidence of hypercementosis, resorption, and pulpal calcifications. The muscles of mastication should also be examined.

A classification of the tooth wear should be made from the clinical observations, habits and history, as all this information is required to determine the risk factors and educate the patients to help minimize the long term damage. Tooth wear has to be diagnosed as to physiological or pathological. If the wear has compromised esthetics, is causing tooth sensitivity, responsible for the reduction in facial height and occlusal vertical dimension, then tooth wear is considered pathological and needs treatment. A period of monitoring is essential to decide on the most appropriate treatment. This monitoring can be accomplished by photographic records, dated study models, teeth measurements, impression of splint and comparison of changes over three months and tooth wear indices. Erosive tooth wear from a clinical observation is a surface phenomenon occurring on areas accessible for visual view. Diagnosis is therefore, a visual approach and should be compared with different tooth wear indices.

MEASUREMENTS OF WEAR

Numerous direct and indirect clinical assessment methods have been used to measure tooth and restoration wear. Direct clinical methods include the US Public Health Service (USPHS)-Ryge criteria. The rating scale intervals used by the USPHS-Ryge method detects the wear at the margins of restorations as coarse and is unable to detect early changes. Therefore, they are unreliable for measuring restoration wear.

Indirect clinical methods include the use of somewhat less subjective, semiquantitative methods for measuring margin wear from replicas made of the restorations. These methods are reasonably accurate for ranking relatively fast-wearing restorative materials.

However, these research methods are not of much practical relevance to the dental practitioner who might need to monitor the wear rates of teeth and restorations. Instead, it is recommended that changes in wear are best observed by the careful comparison of serial casts.

The most common method to record changes on teeth resulting from wear has been the use of indices. The most frequently reported index is the Smith and Knight Tooth Wear Index [1984], which classifies tooth wear on a 5-point scale at 4 sites per tooth (Table 8.7). The index records wear or depth changes into dentine with 3 grades, whereas changes to enamel, which can be equally widespread, are notified as a single grade. The difficulty with most indices is that wear on enamel is normally given a single score, which under-represents the damage to enamel particularly, if the surface lesion is widespread.

Basic Erosive Wear Examination

0 No erosive wear
1 Initial loss of surface texture
2 Distinct defect, hard tissue <50% of the surface area
3 Hard tissue loss >50% of the surface area
2/3rd dentine involved

Table 8.7 Tooth wear index by Smith and Knight

Score	*Surface*	*Characteristics*
0	B/L/O/I	No loss of enamel surface characteristic
	C	No loss of contour
1	B/L/O/I	Loss of enamel surface characteristic
	C	Minimal loss of contour
2	B/L/O	Loss of enamel exposing dentine for less than one-third of the surface
	I	Loss of enamel just exposing dentine
	C	Defect less than 1mm deep
3	B/L/O	Loss of enamel exposing dentine for more than one-third of the surface
	I	Loss of enamel and substantial loss of dentine
	C	Defect less than 1–2 mm deep
4	B/L/O	Complete loss of enamel, or pulp exposure, or exposure of secondary dentine
	I	Pulp exposure or exposure of secondary dentine
	C	Defect more than 2 mm deep, or pulp exposure, or exposure of secondary dentine

Abbreviations: B, Buccal; L, Lingual; O, Occlusal; I, Incisal; C, Cervical

TREATMENT

Treatment options for noncarious tooth wear includes:

- Dentin desensitization
- Restorative treatment
- Removable and fixed prosthesis
- Endodontic therapy
- Periodontal therapy.

Preventive and Initial Management

Before any definitive restorative treatment is undertaken, plaque-induced dental disease such as caries and periodontal disease should be controlled. The long term success of rehabilitation is dependent on good oral hygiene and its regular maintenance. Efforts should be made to eliminate or control the etiological factors. The strategies in the initial management of these cases also include psychosocial support, medical referrals, habit intervention, reduction in consumption of erosive beverages, using a straw and soft mouth guards to protect teeth during gastric regurgitation with the addition of fluoride gel.

Dentin Desensitization

This is a viable treatment option for those situations where minimal amount of dentin is exposed (less than 1 mm) and the patient experiences hypersensitivity. This may be managed by any of the methods suggested for dentin desensitization such as fluoride varnishes, dentin-bonding agents or use of desensitizing tooth pastes.

Restorative Management

Restorations are deemed necessary, when the lesions show considerable loss of enamel and dentin, esthetics is compromised, or the lesions are deep affecting the strength of the tooth and pulpal integrity. Caries beginning in the cervical lesion with significant sensitivity of the exposed dentin also require restorative management.

Class V noncarious lesions may be restored with any of the permanent restorative materials presently available. Of these materials, amalgam, direct gold, cast gold inlays and ceramic inlays are no longer preferred, as they require some amount of cavity preparation to make the restoration retentive. Currently, composite resins and glass ionomer cements are more popular in restoring noncarious cervical lesions primarily because they are adhesive and do not require any extensive cavity preparations (Table 8.8).

Table 8.8 Comparison of materials in the treatment of NCTSL

	Advantages	*Disadvantages*
Composite resins	• Superior esthetics • Excellent polishability • High bond strength with good abrasion resistance	• Technique sensitive • Polymerization shrinkage
Glass ionomer	• Adhesion to tooth structure • Biocompatible and release fluoride • Coefficient of thermal expansion similar to tooth structure	• Less esthetic • Brittle and sensitive to moisture • Contamination

Tooth wear can be classified as physiological or pathological, but no universally accepted guidelines are available to differentiate the two entities, the same loss of tooth substance may be regarded as physiological in an elderly person, but pathological in young one. Clinical indications for restorative management can be:

- *Biological:* Where the loss of tooth substance could lead to irregular tooth surfaces which may enhance plaque retention, there is evidence of pulpal exposure and weakening of tooth structure.
- *Functional:* Where the loss of tooth substance cannot be compensated by continuous eruption, and there is reduced masticatory efficiency because of occlusal wear.
- *Esthetic:* This treatment is required in cases, where the loss of tooth substance is esthetically unacceptable to the patient.

A systematic treatment approach should be used to manage characteristic worn out dentitions involving different tooth surfaces and degree of severity. The worn out dentition can be classified according to location as:

- Localized anterior tooth wear
- Localized posterior tooth wear
- Generalized tooth wear.

Localized Tooth Wear

When erosion is the primary etiological factor and the palatal surfaces of the upper anterior teeth are most commonly involved in tooth wear, less frequently the posterior teeth may also be affected in a localized manner. Adhesive techniques with minimal tooth preparation should be employed in these cases. It is difficult to construct a crown on a shortened tooth without clinical crown lengthening surgery or subgingival placement of the crown margin. As a result of compensatory tooth eruption and alveolar bone growth, several methods are used to create interocclusal space needed for the management of localized tooth wear before the placement of the final restoration. These includes:

- Fixed or removable anterior bite planes (Dahl appliance)
- Tooth preparation at existing intercuspal position
- Occlusal adjustment
- In addition to these methods, provisional or permanent restorations can be placed at increased OVD. These supraoccluding appliances are used as "Individual Dahl appliances".

Removable and Fixed Prosthesis

Challenges in the management include lack of vertical space due to dento-alveolar compensation mechanisms and excessive loading of restorations. Primary aim in treatment should be to prevent/reduce the causes and replace what is lost. The use of removable prosthesis can be broadly divided into two categories:

Conformative Approach

In these, the appearance of the worn teeth is acceptable to the patient. Therefore, the management should be directed at trying to prevent progression of the tooth surface loss. Partial dentures are provided to ensure there is adequate occlusal support. The new restorations are placed conforming to the existing occlusal vertical dimension and intercuspal position. This means that the restorations are easier to make and the patient needs to make minimal adaptation to them.

The conformative approach is usually the more convenient method of treatment for single crowns or simple bridges. The maintenance in these cases is usually the least demanding, because the degree of intervention necessary is limited and simple. The conformative approach is usually the more convenient method of treatment for single crowns or simple bridges. This will consist of regular reviews, and very often the provision of a soft, vacuum formed, night mouth guard to protect the remaining teeth. The use of a night mouth guard is inadvisable for patients with gastric acid reflux, as they may reflux silently in a supine position during sleep.

Reorganized Approach

The appearance is unacceptable to the individual. In such circumstances, treatment options can be divided broadly into tooth reduction and the provision of overdentures, treatment combining removable prostheses and adhesive techniques and treatment combining fixed and removable prostheses. This approach is required, when the vertical dimension or intercuspal position must be altered significantly or when multiple units are needed. In cases of tooth wear, the vertical dimension often needs to be increased and a new occlusal relationship has to be defined/created to correct the mandibular posture and articulate the crowns.

Treatment with Tooth Reduction and Overdentures

In cases of severe tooth wear, the most appropriate treatment is to reduce the worn teeth further and restore the missing crowns with an overdenture. But it is important to consider the consequence of retention of overdenture abutments upon the success of the removable prosthesis. The retention of the overdenture abutments reduces the space for the artificial teeth and base. This increases the likelihood of fatigue fracture, particularly in those individuals who have a tooth clenching or grinding habit. Therefore, it is worth considering the use of porcelain teeth on the denture, as they have a high abrasion resistance and will therefore, resist wear and help to maintain the occlusal vertical dimension. However, porcelain teeth may crack and, if left rough following occlusal adjustment, will wear down natural teeth. In addition, attaching porcelain teeth to the denture can be particularly difficult, if there is limited space available, as the means of mechanical retention may be ground away. An alternative would be to replace the occlusal surfaces of conventional resin teeth with cast gold alloy restorations.

Treatment with Combination of Adhesive Techniques and Removable Prostheses

The main aim should be to protect the remaining natural tooth substance from further wear in lateral excursive movements and also to protect the restorations on the incisor teeth from unwanted occlusal loading.

Endodontic Therapy

When cervical tooth loss is extensive resulting is pulpal involvement, endodontic therapy is necessary followed by post placement and full coverage restoration in the form of a crown.

Periodontal Therapy

This is required when noncarious cervical lesions are associated with considerable gingival recession and mucogingival defects. The treatment options include root coverage procedures using free gingival grafts or connective tissue grafts, root coverage using nongrafting procedures like rotational and coronally advanced flaps or guided tissue regeneration.

PREVENTION

Causes of tooth surface loss must be understood to adopt appropriate preventive measures. Abrasive effects of aggressive tooth brushing can be minimized with education, but can be difficult to change specially with in-built memory. Advise patients to modify their brushing techniques and recommend the use of soft brushes and less abrasive toothpastes. Other abrasive habits may also be changed like nail biting, holding objects like pins, pipes, etc., in the mouth. Erosive effects may require change in dietary intake to minimize acidic drinks/food. Some chronic cases may require medical referral. Milder cases can be controlled with self-medication and diet control. In patients with gastric regurgitation, a sodium bicarbonate mouth-rinse should be prescribed to neutralize the effect of the acid. Patients must be advised not to brush their teeth immediately after acid intake or regurgitation but to rinse their mouth carefully. Such patients may also benefit from a fluoride mouth rinse. Erosion can also be exacerbated by a reduction in salivary flow. Chewing gum (Xylitol) may help in boosting the flow of saliva. Bruxism and attrition may be prevented with the help of occlusal splints and stress management. For suspected anorectics and bulimics, psychiatric consultation is required.

Monitoring of all preventive measures needs to be performed even, if no restorative treatment is performed to ensure long term success and maintenance for patients suffering from tooth surface loss.

DENTIN HYPERSENSITIVITY

The lifestyle and behaviors in the present world including the oral self-care habits of today's dental patients pose a number of challenges that may contribute to increased dentin hypersensitivity. It is through greater awareness and knowledge of the risk factors that we may more effectively manage dentin hypersensitivity for the dental patient. In the early 1980s, dentin hypersensitivity was described as an enigma because it was frequently encountered yet poorly understood. Before we begin discussing the etiology of dentin hypersensitivity, risk factors, and prevention strategies, it is important to fully understand the definition of dentin hypersensitivity.

Dentine sensitivity (DS) or dentinal hypersensitivity (DH) is one of the most commonly encountered clinical problems. Dentin hypersensitivity is a common condition of transient tooth pain caused by a variety of exogenous stimuli. The exogenous stimuli include thermal (cold), tactile (touch), or osmotic changes (sweets or drying the surface). The response to a stimulus varies from person to person due to differences in pain tolerance, environmental factors, and emotional state. The primary underlying clinical cause for dentin hypersensitivity is exposed dentinal tubules. The only hypersensitivity not associated with this etiology is the transient spontaneously resolving hypersensitivity associated with the dental bleaching process.

Dentin hypersensitivity is a condition characterized by short, sharp pain arising from exposed dentin in response to stimuli typically thermal, evaporative, tactile, osmotic or chemical and which cannot be ascribed to any other form of dental defect or pathology (Holland et al, 1997).

The phenomenon of dentin hypersensitivity is characterized predominantly by erosion, which both exposes dentin and initiates the lesions. Dentin hypersensitivity occurs when dentin becomes exposed and tubules are open at the dentin surface. Gingival recession is the primary way dentin is exposed in the cervical region of the tooth. Once the root is exposed, the protective layer of cementum is easily removed, resulting in open dentin tubules. Other causes of the typically short and sharp pain may include caries, chipped teeth, fractured or faulty restorations, specific restorative materials and cracked tooth syndrome. It is important to rule out any other possible etiology before proceeding with specific management of dentin hypersensitivity (Table 8.9).

Prevalence and Epidemiology

Dentinal hypersensitivity (DH) is a painful clinical condition with an incidence ranging from 4 to 74%. The variations in the reports may be because of difference in populations and different methods of investigations. Age is broad, spanning from early teenage to more than 70 years. (Fischer, et al, 1992), however, peak incidence is between 20–40 years. This may be due to the development of secondary or sclerotic dentin. A slightly higher incidence of DH is reported in females than in males. Buccal aspect of cervical area is the commonly affected site. Sites of predilection in descending order are canines and first premolars, incisors and second premolars, molars.

Pathogenesis

Dentinal hypersensitivity (DH) develops in two phases:

1. *Lesion localization:* Lesion localization occurs by loss of protective covering over the dentin, thereby exposing it to external environment. It includes loss of enamel via attrition, abrasion, erosion or abfraction. Another cause for lesion localization is gingival recession which can be due to toothbrush abrasion, pocket reduction surgery, tooth preparation for crown, excessive flossing or secondary to periodontal diseases.
2. *Lesion initiation:* As stated earlier, not all exposed dentine is sensitive. For DH to occur, the lesion localization has to be initiated. It occurs after the protective covering of smear layer is removed, leading to exposure

Table 8.9 Conditions resembling dentinal hypersensitivity

Conditions where sensitivity is identical to that experienced with dentinal sensitivity
• Chipped or fractured teeth • Caries • Marginal leakage of restorations • Cracked cusps of teeth

and opening of dentinal tubules. Dentin is naturally sensitive owing to its close structural and functional relationship with the dental pulp. Normally, the dentin is well protected, so sensitivity does not present an issue. It is a calcified tissue of the body usually covered by enamel on the crown and cementum on the root surface and is similar in composition to bone.

Dentin consists of microscopic channels called dentinal tubules which radiate outward through the dentin from the pulp to the exterior cementum or enamel border. It gives a honeycomb appearance under the microscope. As a result, dentin has a degree of permeability which can increase the sensation of pain. The diameters of the tubules also play an important part in determining the intensity of the sensitivity. If the larger tubules are exposed, then there is more pain as compared to if more tubules are exposed which causes more sensitivity. Dentin is thought to be covered by a smear layer, forming a smear plug or natural "bandage" that blocks stimuli. Conversely, removal of these occluding materials can also frequently occur as a result of physical or chemical agents that open the dentinal tubules.

Etiological and Predisposing Factors

There are potentially numerous and varied etiological and predisposing factors that collectively place the patient at risk for dentine hypersensitivity. No single primary cause can be identified. These include gingival recession, tooth wear, lifestyle behaviors, oral self-care habits, and the pH of the oral environment which may be related to dietary as well as xerostomia like conditions. By definition, dentine hypersensitivity may arise as a result of loss of enamel and/or root surface denudation due to gingival recession with exposure of underlying dentine. Enamel loss as a part of tooth wear may result from attrition, abrasion, abfraction or erosion. As tooth wear has already been discussed in the text, we will concentrate on other factors.

Gingival recession and subsequent root surface exposure results in a more rapid and extensive exposure of dentinal tubules because the cementum layer overlying the root surface is thin and is easily removed. Gingival recession can be caused by a variety of factors. Tooth brushing has long been implicated in gingival recession on buccal surfaces.

Common Reasons for Gingival Recession Includes

- Inadequate attached gingiva
- Prominent roots
- Toothbrush abrasion
- Periodontal surgery
- Oral habits resulting in gingival laceration like tooth picking or eating hard foods
- Excessive tooth cleaning and flossing

- Gingival loss secondary to specific diseases like anug
- Periodontitis
- Herpetic gingiva-stomatitis
- Crown preparation
- Aging.

Diet sensitivity: This is associated with a low pH of the food, such as fresh tomatoes, orange juice, cola drinks.

Restorative sensitivity: This is usually triggered following placement of a restoration for several possible reasons like during setting, inadequate moisture control during composite placement or improper etching of the tooth resulting in microleakage, incorrect preparation of glass ionomer or zinc phosphate cements, general pulpal insult from cavity preparation technique, thermal or occlusal causes; galvanic reaction to dissimilar metals.

Medication sensitivity: This can occur as some medications may result in a dry mouth like antihistamines thereby, compromising the protective effects of saliva and aggravating diet-related trauma or proliferating plaque. This further leads to an increase in erosive lesions.

Bleaching sensitivity: This is associated with carbamide peroxide vital tooth bleaching and thought to be due to the by-products of 10 percent carbamide peroxide (3 percent hydrogen peroxide and 7 percent urea) readily passing through the enamel and dentine into the pulp in a matter of minutes. Sensitivity can be caused by all other forms of bleaching (in-office, with or without light activation, and over-the-counter) and depends on peroxide concentration.

Mechanism of Action

Many theories have been proposed to understand the mechanism of dentinal hypersensitivity.

- Direct innervation theory
- Odontoblast receptor theory
- Transducer theory
- Gate control theory/vibration theory
- Fluid movement/hydrodynamic theory.

Direct Dentine Innervation Theory

The dentin contains nerve endings that respond when it is stimulated. No evidence has been found for nerves in the outer-dentin, which is most sensitive. Direct mechanical stimulation of these nerves will initiate an action potential. There are many shortcomings of this theory. There is lack of evidence that outer dentin, which is usually the most sensitive part, is innervated. Developmental studies have shown that the plexus of Rashkow and intratubular nerves do not establish themselves, until the tooth has erupted; yet, newly erupted tooth is sensitive.

Odontoblast Receptor Theory

This theory proposes that odontoblasts receive and pass on impulses and that when they are touched cause the sensation of pain. The drawback in this theory is that, odontoblasts are matrix forming cells and thus are not considered to be excitable cells. No synapses have been demonstrated between odontoblasts and nerve terminals. This is not the most likely theory, as there are no synapses between the odontoblasts and Nerve Plexus of Rashkow (synapses-junctions between neurons where chemicals transmit the impulse).

Transducer Theory

This theory of dentinal sensation takes into consideration the synaptic relationship between the terminal sensory nerve endings and odontoblastic process. If a true synapse were present between these two elements to facilitate the transmission of dentinal sensations, then a neural transmitting substance such as acetylcholine could be expected, but there is no direct evidence of its presence.

Gate Control Theory

When the dentin is irritated, for example, by cavity preparation, then all the pulpal nerves become activated from these vibrations. The larger myelinated fibers may accommodate these sensations but the smaller C-fibers may tend to be maintained and not adjust to the stimulus. Thus, as the low-intensity pain gates from the larger fibers are closed, the high-intensity "pain gates" from the smaller fibers are enhanced. However, the gate theory does little to explain, how pain responses from the dentin are transmitted and perceived by the nerve endings of the pulp.

Fluid Movement/Hydrodynamic Theory

This was first proposed by Brannstrom. This mechanism explains that dentin sensitivity involves movement of fluid through the dentinal tubules. This is based on Brännström's hydrodynamic theory that stimuli create a pressure change or disturbance within the fluid that fills the dentinal tubules. The movement of the fluid backwards and forwards, on stimulation by temperature or touch or sweet, within the open tubules gives the sensation of pain. This is then transmitted to the A-delta nerve fibers. Heat, cold, air, and pressure can cause this rapid movement of fluid in open dentin tubules. The hydrodynamic hypothesis explains, why pain is produced by thermal change, mechanical probing, hypotonic solutions and dehydration. This theory answers more questions like:

- Hot/cold caused expansion/contraction causing the fluid to flow
- Salt/sweet causes osmotic pressure, flows towards the concentrate
- Tactile/electrical (touch) causes contraction of the fluid.

Clinical Features

Not all areas of exposed dentin are sensitive and hypersensitive surfaces can vary in their sensitivity to different stimuli. As like any other clinical condition, an accurate diagnosis is important before starting the management of DH. DH has features which are similar to other conditions like caries, fractured or chipped enamel/dentine, pain due to reversible pulpitis, and post dental bleaching sensitivity. Diagnosis of DH starts with a thorough clinical history and examination. The other causes of dental pain should be excluded before a definite diagnosis of DH is made.

Pain is the only consistent symptom of dentin hypersensitivity. The severity or degree of pain can be quantified either according to categorical scale (i.e., slight, moderate or severe pain) or using a visual analogue scale (VAS) (for example 0–100). To elicit a pain response for examination and diagnosis purposes, the dentist can use a probe or jet of air. The patient's own evaluation of the severity of his or her sensitivity should also be recorded.

An important clinical feature of dentinal hypersensitivity, gingival recession occurs in descending order of canines and premolars followed by incisors and second premolars and finally molars with the majority of sites being buccal and cervical. They are more common on the left than on the right sides of the mouth and also possess an inverse relationship with plaque scores.

EVALUATION STRATEGIES

Both chronic and acute pain related to dentin hypersensitivity can be particularly challenging for our dental patient. Acute pain often causes anxiety and may lead to avoidance of dental treatment. Often patients will not schedule an appointment specifically to address their sensitivity. It is unlikely that the topic will even be discussed without some form of prompting by the dentist. It is our responsibility to initiate the discussion and also to evaluate the level of sensitivity the patient is experiencing. Dentin hypersensitivity is mainly evaluated on the individual patient's response to the stimulus.

Stimuli can be grouped into five categories, namely:

1. Mechanical (tactile) stimuli—explorer, constant pressure probe, scaling procedures.
2. Electrical stimulation—electrical pulp testers, cold air blast.
3. Chemical (osmotic) stimuli—hypertonic solutions. For example, sodium chloride, glucose, and calcium chloride.

4. Thermal stimuli—cold water testing, heat, ethyl chloride, ice stick.
5. Evaporative stimuli—cold air blast.

There are a number of questions we may employ in order to obtain further information regarding dentin hypersensitivity. The following questions are suggested to initiate the discussion of dentin hypersensitivity and to evaluate the intensity of pain:

- Which tooth or teeth is/are sensitive and on which aspect?
- On a scale from 1 to 10, how much does it hurt, with 10 being the most painful?
- How long does the pain last?
- Can the pain be characterized as sharp, dull, shooting, throbbing, persistent, constant, pressure, burning, intermittent?
- Does it hurt when you bite down (pressure)?
- Does the discomfort linger or stop immediately after a stimulus such as cold water is removed?
- On a scale from 1 to 10, how much does the pain impact your daily life?
- Is the pain stimulated by certain foods: Sweet? Sour? Acidic?
- Does sensitivity result from hot or cold food or beverages?
- Does discomfort stop immediately upon removal of the painful stimuli, such as cold food or beverage?
- How effectively are you managing the stress in your life?

Subjective Evaluation Techniques

There are a number of ways to evaluate the degree of hypersensitivity.

- Using a *verbal rating scale* and the use of a short, intermittent "air blast" to quantify the subjective level of pain as follows (Gilliam and Newman 1993) (Table 8.10).
- *Visual analogue scale (VAS)* is a line 10 cm in length, the extreme of the line representing the limits of pain, a patient might experience from external stimulus. No pain at one end and most severe pain at the other end. Patients are asked to place a mark on the 10 cm line which indicates the intensity of their current level of sensitivity or discomfort following application of stimuli. VAS can give only a one-dimensional assessment of pain and as such cannot distinguish between the sensory, intensity and affective aspects of pain.

Table 8.10 Verbal rating scale

0	No discomfort/pain; no discomfort/pain but aware of stimulus
1	Mild discomfort/pain—described as mild discomfort during but not following the air blast
2	Marked discomfort/pain—described as definitive discomfort during the air blast
3	Marked discomfort/pain lasting more than 10 seconds following exposure to air

There are a number of predisposing factors that individually or collectively place the patient at risk for dentin hypersensitivity. These include gingival recession, tooth wear, lifestyle behaviors, oral self-care habits, and the pH of the oral environment which may be related to dietary as well as xerostomia like conditions.

The assessment and evaluative phase should include the careful identification and elimination of any predisposing factors affecting the pH of the oral environment. The pH of the oral environment is the single most contributory factor to hypersensitive cervical and occlusal surfaces. This is due to both exogenous and endogenous contributing factors. Any food substance with a critical pH value of less than 5.5 can become an erosive agent and demineralize the tooth structure. Erosion of the dentin appears to bring about a rapid loss of the smear layer and the opening of dentinal tubules. Foods and beverages with a low pH readily remove the smear layer after a few minutes of exposure. A dietary history may be obtained from the patient in order to identify predisposing acidic factors in the diet.

Whitening agents may also induce dentin hypersensitivity. Endogenous or internal contributory factors may include regurgitation associated with gastroesophageal reflux disease or eating disorders, both of which are capable of lowering the pH of the oral environment rapidly and significantly. Xerostomia as a result of the vast array of prescription medications can severely diminish the saliva's ability to buffer the oral environment. Oral self-care habits can add another dimension which can be particularly destructive in combination with lowered oral pH. The combination of erosion and abrasion can exacerbate dentin hypersensitivity quickly.

MANAGEMENT OF DENTINE HYPERSENSITIVITY

When a patient presents with what appears to be sensitive dentin, the initial diagnosis should eliminate any possible reasons such as decay, cracked tooth, or irreversible pulpitis that may mimic dentin hypersensitivity. The next appropriate step, once the problem has been identified as dentin hypersensitivity, is to identify the reason for the exposed dentinal tubules and to see if the etiology process causing the hypersensitivity can be eliminated. The greatest clinical implication of dentine hypersensitivity is, how the condition may be prevented either from occurring or recurring, and this can only be debated by considering the probable etiologic factors.

Grossman has stated—The best treatment for hypersensitivity lies in its prevention.

Management Strategy

- Take a detailed clinical and dietary history
- Differentially diagnose the condition from other dental pain conditions
- Identify and manage etiological and predisposing factors

- In case of mild-to-moderate sensitivity, advice at home desensitizing therapy
- If there is no relief or in case of severe sensitivity, initiate in-office treatment
- In extreme cases, if patient does not respond to the therapy and there are individual teeth exhibiting the symptoms, then endodontic therapy can be initiated
- A regular review should be made with an emphasis on prevention of the condition.

Clinical Management

Often dentin hypersensitivity abates without treatment. This is probably related to the fact that dentin permeability can decrease spontaneously. This may be probably due to the:

- Natural process contributing by the formation of reparative dentin
- Obturation of the tubules by the formation of mineral deposits (dentinal sclerosis)
- Calculus formation on the surface of the dentin.

Treatments can be self-administered by the patient at home or to be applied by a dental professional in the dental office. At home, methods are simpler and may be used to treat several teeth at one time. In office, treatments are more complex and generally target DH localized to one or a few teeth. There are essentially two basic approaches to the treatment of dentin hypersensitivity namely *direct inhibition of sensory nerve activity and tubule occlusion.*

To occlude the dentinal tubules, ingredients that may be used include oxalate compounds, strontium chloride, hydroxyethyl methacrylate (HEMA), and fluorides. Compounds not associated with fluoride compounds that may be used to treat sensitivity include calcium phosphate compounds, calcium hydroxide, amorphous calcium phosphate, casein phosphopeptide-amorphous calcium phosphate (CPP-ACP) and calcium sodium phosphosilicate. Recent advances include remineralizing the tooth structure by increasing salivary calcium and phosphate levels, increasing the salivary pH, and stimulating the formation of calcium phosphate or hydroxyapatite. Calcium phosphate compounds occlude the tubules by forming a calcium phosphate precipitate, while, calcium hydroxide occludes the dentin formation. Products that interfere with the transmission of the nerve impulse work by raising the extracellular potassium ion concentrations and affecting polarization.

At-Home Treatments

Mild, generalized dentinal hypersensitivity can usually be managed well with at home treatment. At-home treatments for sensitivity relief are cost-effective, safe, noninvasive and simple to use. These at home treatments come in a variety of applications including dentifrices, gels, or rinses and are incorporated into the daily oral home care regimen.

Treatments Interfering with Neural Transmission

The "at home" desensitizing agents include toothpastes, mouthwashes and chewing gums. Majority of the toothpastes contain potassium salts (potassium nitrate, potassium chloride or potassium citrate, sodium fluoride, strontium chloride, dibasic sodium citrate, formaldehyde, sodium mono-fluorphosphate and stannous fluoride). The most popular ingredient that affect neural transmission is 5% potassium nitrate, the concentration recognized by the FDA for this ingredient.

Potassium ions work by penetrating the length of the dentinal tubule and block the repolarization of the myelinated A-fibers. This increase in extracellular potassium allows for the large enough concentration to depolarize the nerve fibers and does not allow repolarization to occur. As a result, neural transmission will not occur following exposure to the stimulus and the patient will have no sensation of sensitivity or pain.

Toothpastes containing potassium nitrate and fluorides have been shown to reduce post-bleaching sensitivity. The desensitizing toothpastes should be used with the help of a toothbrush with soft bristles. For the treatment to be effective, frequent and regular application is needed. A significant reduction in hypersensitivity may be observed by using them for two weeks twice daily. Dentists should educate patients on how to use dentifrices and monitor their tooth brushing techniques. Rinsing with water immediately after tooth brushing may cause the active agent to be diluted and cleared from the mouth and thus, reduce the efficacy. Therefore, patients should be advised accordingly.

Along with the desensitizing toothpastes, mouthwashes and chewing gums containing potassium nitrate, sodium fluoride or potassium citrate are also recommended.

Strontium Chloride: Strontium chloride is contained in some toothpaste. Strontium combines with phosphate in the dentinal fluid and exchanges for calcium in the hydroxyapatite of the dentinal tubule walls. This may produce strontium phosphate crystals and dentinal tubules closure. Strontium may also stimulate the formation of dentin.

Self-care Strategies: Oral self-care can influence the degree of dentin hypersensitivity. Patients who brush excessively or use undue pressure while brushing should be instructed on proper tooth brushing techniques to avoid gingival recession. Tooth brushing (with variations to be considered such as filament stiffness; end rounding; and tooth brushing force, duration, and frequency) has long since been associated with gingival recession and has been considered relevant. Also, repeated brushing, immediately following the intake of a low pH food or beverage, can further exacerbate the dissolution of both the enamel and dentin. Wear of enamel and dentin can dramatically increase, if tooth brushing follows an erosive challenge. It is for this reason that the patient should avoid tooth brushing for a minimum of 30–60 minutes or longer after consuming acidic foods or drinks to reduce the co-effects of acids and abrasion.

Treatments for Tubule Occlusion

One of the main active ingredients used in this manner is fluoride. When fluoride is applied to exposed dentin, they decrease the permeability of the dentin and block the dentinal tubules. Long-term relief will require the continued use of the product. Calcium and phosphate precipitates formed following use of dentifrices containing calcium and phosphate technologies have also been found to relieve hypersensitivity.

Desensitizing Agents

Grossman listed the requirements for an ideal dentine desensitizing agent as:

- Rapidly acting with long-term effects
- Non-irritant to pulp, painless and easy to apply
- Should not stain the tooth.

These agents are applied over the open end of dentinal tubules. The options can be periodontal surgery/grafting in extreme cases, composite/glass ionomer restorations placement, or crown placement, dentine bonding agents that form a chemical bond with the dentine locking into the tubules and resins and adhesives. The results of "at-home" desensitizing therapy should be reviewed after every 3–4 weeks. If there is no relief in DH, "in-office" therapy should be initiated (Table 8.11).

In-Office Treatment

Stimulation of Secondary Dentine/Desensitizing Agents: In-office, desensitizing procedures help by the stimulation of secondary dentine formation.

Table 8.11 Treatment options

Reversible	*Nonreversible*
Desensitizing toothpastes	Glass ionomer
Fluoride gels, rinses and varnishes	Filled/unfilled resins
Oxalates of ferric, potassium or aluminum	Periodontal flaps/grafts
	Endodontic therapy
	Extraction

For this high concentration of fluoride, a varnish can be used. Fluoride irritates the dentine sufficiently for it to lay down a secondary layer and therefore, protect the tooth from further stimuli. Fluoride achieves this by occluding the tubules. Treatment options includes:

- Mouthwashes daily 0.05% and weekly 0.2% solutions
- High fluoride toothpastes-Duraphat 2800, 5000
- Varnishes-Duraphat 22,000 ppm
- Gels-0.04% stannous fluoride.

Other materials used in desensitization of dentine are calcium phosphates, oxalates (act by reducing the dentinal permeability and occluding dentinal tubules like copal varnish), adhesive materials like fluoride varnishes, sealants and primers (act by forming a hybrid layer like GLUMA), bio-glass (used in dentistry to fill the osseous defects during periodontal surgery and helps in promoting infiltration and remineralization of dentinal tubules like Nova Min technology) and Portland cement.

OTHER PROCEDURES

Iontophoresis: This procedure uses electricity to enhance diffusion of ions into the tissues. This is used in conjunction with fluoride pastes or solutions.

Lasers: The Nd:YAG laser has been used experimentally in dentistry, since 1970s. Recently systems have become available which are tailored specifically for dental surgery using fiber optic delivery to a hand piece. The tool was effective in reducing dentin hypersensitivity to cold stimuli. Although, the mechanism of laser action has yet to be confirmed, it would appear that obturation of the dentinal tubules may be the most logical hypothesis. It has been found to produce quick response with few side effects. It is also simple and fast to administer.

Pro-Argin Technology in Toothpastes: The active ingredients argin, calcium carbonate, hydroxyapatite and sodium monofluorophosphate bind to the tooth surface. This arginine complex then encourages a calcium rich mineral layer into the exposed and open dentinal tubules. This acts as an effective plug and is acid resistant but needs to be applied twice daily.

Future therapies for dentine hypersensitivity

Gene therapy in the future may include treatment of sensory nerves to dental restorative procedures, as well as surgical and nonsurgical debridement that elicits its dentin hypersensitivity. One such method may include blocking the increased production of nerve growth factor (NGF) by pulpal fibroblasts near the lesion thought to contribute to tooth hypersensitivity after restorative procedures.

CONCLUSION

Although wear is usually slowly progressive, the extent and rate can be exacerbated by many patient factors.

Tooth wear is an increasing problem, and many persons now wish to retain their natural dentitions for a lifetime.

However, oral rehabilitation is often necessary because of the extensive "wear and tear" that has occurred over many years. The selection of appropriate materials to minimize further tooth and restoration wear is an important consideration during treatment planning. The wear can be enhanced by adverse parafunctional, tooth brushing/dentifrice, and dietary habits; regurgitation; reduced salivary flow; defective tooth structure; and lack of posterior tooth support.

Dentinal hypersensitivity is a problem that plagues many dental patients. When a patient presents with dentinal hypersensitivity symptoms, they should be examined and informed of the multiple treatment options that may be necessary to eliminate the problem. The patient should be responsible for the decision making process, since some of their daily habits may be contributing to the problem and if not changed, the condition will persist. With the acquired knowledge of the role that causative factors play in localizing and initiating dentin hypersensitivity, prevention strategies may now be included in the dental care plan. Active management will involve a combination of chairside and oral self-care therapies. Although dentin hypersensitivity is not the enigma it once was, there is still much to learn about the condition itself, the management of risk, and prevention behaviors. Our profession is strategically positioned to not only evaluate but also to educate to improve the comfort and quality of life for our patients.

BIBLIOGRAPHY

1. Addy M, Hunter ML. Can tooth brushing damage your health? Effects on oral and dental tissues. Int Dent J. 2003;53(Suppl 3):177-86.
2. Ailor JE Jr. Managing incomplete tooth fractures. J Am Dent Assoc. 2000;131: 1158-74.
3. Available at: http://www.jada. info/cgi/content/full/136/1/71.
4. Dahl Bl, Carlson GE, Ekfeldt A. Occlusal wear of teeth and restorative materials. A review of classification, etiology, mechanisms of wear, and some aspects of restorative procedures. Acta Odontol Scand. 1993;51:299-311.
5. Dugmore CR, Rock WP. A multifactorial analysis of factors associated with dental erosion. Brit Dent J. 2004;196(5):283-6.
6. Eccles JD. Tooth surface loss from abrasion, attrition and erosion. Dent Update. 1982;9:373-81.
7. Idle M. The differential diagnosis of sensitive teeth. Dent Update. 1998;25:462-6.
8. Imfeld T. Dental erosion. Definition, classification and links. Eur J Oral Sci. 1996; 104:151-5.

9. Levitch LC, Bader JD, Sugars DA, et al. Noncarious cervical lesions. J Dent. 1994;22:195-207.
10. Mandel L. Dental erosion due to wine consumption. J Am Dent Assoc. 2005;136(1):71-5.
11. Orchardson R, Gillam DG. Managing dentinal hypersensitivity. J Am Dent Assoc. 2006;137:990-8.
12. Walters PA. Dentinal hypersensitivity: A review. J Contemp Dent Pract. 2005;2(6): 107-17.
13. Zipkin I, McClure FJ. Salivary citrate and dental erosion. J Dent Rest. 1949;28: 613-26.

CHAPTER 9

TREATMENT OF DISCOLORED TEETH

Balaram Naik, Priyanka Jain

INTRODUCTION

One of the most frequent reasons for seeking dental treatment is discolored anterior teeth. Even people having teeth with normal color often request to have them whiter. Over a period of time, individuals may experience loss of tooth structure due to caries, erosion, abrasion or attrition.

Discolorations are not confined to any surface/part of the tooth but may be located on any part like the outer surface of the tooth structure. While some discolorations may be caused by stain taken up by the enamel or dentin, others may occur during tooth development and result in an alteration of the light transmitting properties of the tooth structures. These may be caused by multiple factors like medications, genetic defects, diseases, trauma, caries, normal aging processes, etc. The prevention and treatment of these conditions is clinically and esthetically desirable. Traditional treatment and prevention options have included fluoride and chemotherapeutics to help prevent tooth structure loss, and abrasives and hydrogen peroxide to treat tooth discoloration and staining. Recently introduced calcium and phosphate technologies have increased the treatment options available.

DISCOLORATIONS

These can be classified as intrinsic, extrinsic or internalized.

Intrinsic Discolorations

Intrinsic discoloration can be defined as discoloration which is incorporated into the structure of either enamel or dentine and which cannot be removed by prophylaxis with toothpaste or pumice. This can be a significant cosmetic, and in some instances, functional, problem. Loss of vitality secondary to trauma or infection frequently results in tooth discoloration which is not responsive to conventional endodontic therapy. Fluorosis, tetracycline

Table 9.1 Causes of intrinsic discolorations

Vital teeth	*Local causes*	*Systemic causes*
Within enamel	• Caries • Idiopathic • Injury/infection of the primary predecessor • Internal resorption • Enamel cracks • White spots due to failure of enamel to calcify properly resulting in decalcified white spots • Enamel hypoplasia	• Amelogenesis imperfecta, drugs like tetracycline • Fluorosis, systemic illnesses during tooth formation
Within dentine	• Caries • Internal resorption • Metallic restorative materials • Necrotic pulp tissue • Root canal filling materials • Secondary caries around existing restorations • Aging	• Congenital porphyria • Dentinogenesis imperfecta • Hemolytic disease of the newborn (bilirubin) • Drug induced (tetracycline, ciprofloxacin)
Nonvital teeth	• Infected or degeneration of the pulp due to trauma • Deep caries or irritation from restorative procedures	

staining, localized/chronological hypoplasia, and both amelogenesis and dentinogenesis imperfecta can all produce a cosmetically unsatisfactory problem. Intrinsic staining starts from inside the tooth and results from stain penetrating into the dentin from the surface of the tooth. Trauma to teeth may also result in nonvitality and a gradual graying and blackening of the crown of the tooth.

Causes for the intrinsic discolorations can be divided into two groups, systemic and local causes (Table 9.1). Systemic causes may further be separated into genetic defects or drug induced. The developing dentition can be affected of a number of metabolic diseases and systemic factors (Table 9.2). Teeth with vital/nonvital pulps as well as endodontically treated teeth may be affected.

Tetracycline Stains

Tetracycline has the ability to cause staining of both primary and permanent dentitions during odontogenesis. The mechanism to explain the staining by tetracycline is its ability to form a complex with calcium ions, i.e. chelation. Tetracycline chelates with calcium ions to form a stable tetracycline

Table 9.2 Etiology of intrinsic discolorations (Plotino et al, 2008)

Pre-eruptive causes	*Posteruptive causes*
• Medications (tetracycline)	• Pulpal necrosis
• Metabolism (fluorosis)	• Intrapulpal hemorrhage
• Genetics (hyperbilirubinemia, amelogenesis imperfect, cystic fibrosis of the pancreas)	• Residual pulp tissue after endodontic treatment
• Dental trauma	• Endodontic materials (medications/irrigant, root canal sealer)
	• Filling materials
	• Root resorption
	• Aging process

calcium ortophosphate complex. These complexes are deposited into bone and teeth. Dentine is more susceptible to staining than enamel. Tooth discoloration may be yellow, yellow-brown, brown, dark gray, or blue in color, depending on the type of tetracycline, dosage, duration of intake, and patient's age at the time of administration. Discoloration is usually bilateral, affecting multiple teeth in both arches. Deposition of the tetracycline may be continuous or laid down in stripes depending on whether the ingestion was continuous or interrupted. This type of discoloration is permanent since dentine and enamel cannot be remodeled. The staining may also vary, from yellow or gray to brown with or without banding, brown, dark gray, or blue, depending on all the factors already mentioned.

Chlortetracycline causes for example a gray-brown discoloration, whereas tetracycline, dimethyl chlortetracycline and oxytetracycline give a yellow discoloration. Oxytetracycline is the least discoloring. The affected teeth tend to be yellow on eruption and after exposure to light, the fluorescent yellow staining changes to nonfluorescent brown color with time. The severity of the staining is related to the time of the administration, dose, frequency, duration of administration and the stage of odontogenesis (the primary teeth begin the calcification stage at about the end of the fourth month of gestation and ends at 11–14 months of age).

The calcification of the permanent dentition begins after birth and can therefore not be affected by prenatal administration of tetracycline. The permanent teeth continue their calcification until 8 years of age, except for the third molars. Therefore, tetracycline should be avoided for pregnant women during the second and third trimester of pregnancy and for children up to the age of eight. Tetracycline discoloration is classified according to the extent, degree and location of the staining (Table 9.3).

Table 9.3 Tetracycline staining classification

Severity	*Comments*
First degree (mild)	Varies from yellow to gray with no banding and occurs uniformly throughout the crown
Second degree (moderate)	Yellow-brown to dark gray staining with no banding
Third degree (severe)	Blue gray or black with significant horizontal banding across the tooth. This predominates in the cervical region

Fluorosis

The ingestion of fluorides is particularly important in infants as dental fluorosis can originate during the tooth development. Fluoride is highly reactive and reacts rapidly with mineralizing tissues. Fluoride gradually gets be incorporated into the crystal lattice structure in the form of fluorhydroxyapatite, and is then stored in bones and teeth. Ingestion of excessive amounts of fluoride during tooth formation may produce a defect in mineralized structures, particularly in the enamel matrix, causing hypoplasia. The severity and degree of subsequent staining generally depend on the degree of hypoplasia and is directly related to the amount of fluoride ingested during odontogenesis.

The teeth are not discolored on eruption, but their surface is porous and gradually absorbs colored chemicals present in the oral cavity. Discoloration is usually bilateral, affecting multiple teeth in both arches. It presents as various degrees of intermittent white spotting, chalky or opaque areas, yellow or brown discoloration, and, in severe cases, surface pitting of the enamel (Table 9.4). Posteruptive, this chalky white enamel may change to more severe forms of fluorosis depending on the degree of hypo mineralization as a result of posteruptive mechanical damage such as mastication, attrition and abrasion. Since the discoloration is in the porous enamel, such teeth can be bleached externally.

Enamel Hypoplasia

Enamel hypoplasia (EH) is a condition of deficient amelogenesis, resulting from an injury to the formative cells, the ameloblasts. A consequence of this is less quantity of enamel formation than normal. Hypoplasia of primary teeth is rarely as severe as in the permanent teeth. Enamel hypoplasia may be localized or generalized. Trauma and localized infections in the primary dentitions are the most common reasons of EH. Turner's hypoplasia is a common term for EH where an apical localized infection in the deciduous dentition causes disturbances of the normal amelogenesis. Generalized EH may be the result of any disturbance caused by fetal or maternal conditions

Table 9.4 Causes of discolorations

Discoloration	*Cause*
White	Fluorosis
Light yellow	Fluorosis, aging, tetracycline (Type 1)
Dark yellow (moderate stain)	Aging, tetracycline (Type 2)
Brown (dark stain)	Fluorosis, tetracycline (Type 1 and 2), endodontic therapy
Bluish gray (severe stain)	Tetracycline stain or endodontic therapy
Black	Caries, fluorosis, amalgam stain

such as maternal vitamin D deficiency, rubella infection, or drug intake during pregnancy.

Clinical Presentation of EH

The defects of EH on the tooth surface appear as thin, or pitted, single or multiple, shallow or deep, or scattered. The pits and grooves are exposed to extrinsic staining of the enamel. The thickness of the enamel is reduced, and may be translucent or opaque. Another interesting developmental dental defect in this context is molar-incisor hypomineralization, MIH, which has a different clinical appearance, (MIH) presents as demarcated opacities, resulting from incomplete mineralization and is a defect, in the permanent first molars and incisors. Demarcated opacities have a clear and distinct boundary to the near areas of normal enamel. They vary from white, yellow to brown in color, and do not always appear symmetrically. The number of affected teeth also varies. EH and MIH can be difficult to differentiate diagnostically if the affected molars have a posteruptive breakdown caused by caries or trauma from masticatory forces. EH and MIH can occur together, especially at a histological level. Enamel *hypocalcification* is a distinct brownish or whitish area, commonly found on the facial aspect of affected crowns. The enamel is well formed with an intact surface. Enamel *hypoplasia* differs from hypocalcification in that the enamel is defective and porous. This condition may be hereditary, as in amelogenesis imperfecta, or a result of environmental factors such as infections, tumors, or trauma.

Extrinsic Discolorations

These are stains which are located on the outer surface of the teeth and can easily be removed. In young patients, stains of almost any color can be found and are usually more prominent in the cervical areas of the teeth. These may be related to poor oral hygiene, existing restorations, bleeding gums, plaque accumulation, eating habits or the presence of chromogenic bacteria or fungi. Smoking can result in severe and stubborn staining, while tea, coffee

Table 9.5 Factors in tooth discoloration

Intrinsic	*Extrinsic*
Aging	Age changes of the tooth
Trauma	Surface defects
Enamel cracks	Tobacco
Medications	Red wine, coffee and tea
Structure and the thickness of the hard tissue	Level of oral hygiene
Systemic conditions and metabolic diseases	Chlorhexidine gluconate mouth rinse

and red wine are common culprits associated with surface staining. In older patients, staining is more likely on the areas adjacent to the gingival tissues (Table 9.5).

Causes for Extrinsic Staining

These may be classified into metallic or nonmetallic. Metallic may be due to occupational exposure to metallic salts or to medicines containing metal salts for example, characteristic black staining of teeth in people using iron supplements, mouth rinses containing copper salts resulting in green colored staining. Nonmetallic satins are those which are adapted into the tooth surface, for example deposits such as plaque/acquired pellicle. When the extrinsic stain is incorporated within the tooth substance during the dental development, it is known as *internalized discoloration.*

MANAGEMENT OF DISCOLORATIONS

The justification of the treatment is very important. Mild discolorations may be left untreated or treated conservatively as no restorative material is as good as the natural, healthy tooth structure.

The treatment of choice is dependent on the diagnosis. In many cases of discoloration there is a hierarchy of treatment options. These should be pursued in a logical order until a satisfactory cosmetic outcome is achieved. Pretreatment photographs, shade taking and sensibility tests are recommended in all cases.

History

A careful, detailed history is essential for the accurate diagnosis of intrinsic tooth discoloration, as the choice of treatment is greatly influenced by the etiology. Specifically details of childhood illness and any drugs taken, dental history including infections relating to primary teeth, trauma to the primary and permanent teeth and fluoride history should all be included in the history.

Clinical Examination

A standard extraoral examination and full mouth intraoral examination should be undertaken, with special emphasis on the presence and/or absence of both primary and permanent teeth. If possible, the extent of discoloration should be identified with respect to the depth of affected enamel or dentine.

TREATMENT OPTIONS FOR DISCOLORED TEETH

- Microabrasion and macroabrasion
- Dentifrice use for stain removal and prevention in extrinsic discolorations
- Bleaching
- Composite resin restorations
- Porcelain veneers.

MICROABRASION AND MACROABRASION

Microabrasion

This is a combination of chemical and mechanical technique where a microscopic layer of the enamel is eroded and abraded away. This was introduced in 1984 by McCloskey. This technique works well with single line or patch types of enamel opacities, and the improvement is long-term. It involves the softening and removal of both enamel and the surface defect through hydrochloric acid (HCL) 18% mixed with pumice, in a special geared-down handpiece under rubber dam isolation. This technique does result in the physical removal of the tooth structure and, therefore, is indicated only for stains or enamel defects that do not extend beyond a few tenths of a millimeter in depth. If the defect or discoloration still remains after treatment with microabrasion or macroabrasion, a restorative alternative is suggested and indicated.

There are two main microabrading techniques for discolored or hypoplastic teeth:

1. The hydrochloric acid/pumice technique which requires very careful isolation of the affected teeth.
2. The phosphoric acid/pumice technique.

These techniques are simple to perform and the depth of enamel removed in 10 applications is approximately 100 μm. (0.1 mm). Microabrasion can be used for discolorations caused by fluorosis, postorthodontic demineralization, localized hypoplasia due to infection or trauma, and idiopathic hypoplasia where the discoloration is limited to the outer enamel layer. This technique is not effective in improving the appearance of multi-line and diffuse types of opacities.

Technique

After the teeth are isolated with a rubber dam, abrasive paste mixed with 18% hydrochloric acid is rubbed on the surface of the enamel using a hand applicator for 5–10 minutes with intermittent washing. At the end of the treatment, after thorough washing with copious water, the teeth are dried and 0.2% sodium fluoride liquid is applied in order to enhance remineralization. The patients are instructed not to rinse for one hour. This procedure is repeated after two weeks. The appearance of the teeth after microabrasion continues to improve for approximately one month.

Macroabrasion

This is an alternative technique for the removal of localized superficial white spots and other surface stains or defects. This technique utilizes a 12 fluted composite finishing bur or micron finishing diamond in a high speed hand-piece to remove the defect. Care must be taken to use light intermittent pressure and to carefully monitor the removal of the tooth structure in order to avoid irreversible damage to the tooth. Following removal of the defect or upon termination of any further removal of tooth structure, a 30 fluted composite finishing bur is used to remove any striations or roughness created. Final polishing should be accomplished with an abrasive rubber point (Table 9.6).

STAIN REMOVAL AND PREVENTION BY THE USE OF DENTIFRICE

Surfactants contained in dentifrices and rinses, such as sodium lauryl sulfate, help lift and remove stain from the tooth surface. A dentifrice should ideally contain sufficient cleaning power to remove and help prevent staining without being so abrasive that it results in loss of tooth structure.

Table 9.6 Differences between microabrasion and macroabrasion

Microabrasion	*Macroabrasion*
• Ensures better control of the removal of the tooth structure	• High speed instrumentation. Therefore, it is technique sensitive to the operator's ability
• Recommended over macroabrasion for the treatment of superficial defects	• This is faster and does not require the use of a rubber dam
	• Defect removal is easier

Increasingly, abrasives with fine, rounded particles have been used in modern-day dentifrices, to gently remove stain and simultaneously help impart a polish that gives the appearance of whiter teeth. Typical agents include calcium phosphate, calcium carbonate and sodium bicarbonate. *Sodium Bicarbonate* (baking soda) functions as both a mechanical and a chemical cleaning agent. Mechanical cleaning relies on abrasives. The recent introduction of the calcium and the phosphate technology—*amorphous calcium phosphate* (ACP) has the potential for both esthetic and preventive benefits from dentifrices. Two other calcium and phosphate technologies include Novamin® and casein phosphopeptide—amorphous calcium phosphate (CPP-ACP). These release calcium and phosphate for remineralization.

BLEACHING

Bleaching is the lightening of the color of a tooth through the application of a chemical agent to oxidize the organic pigmentation in the tooth. Bleaching can be done for both vital and nonvital teeth. Many different bleaching agents are available today; the ones most commonly used are hydrogen peroxide, sodium perborate, and carbamide peroxide. Hydrogen peroxide and carbamide peroxide are mainly indicated for extracoronal bleaching, whereas sodium perborate is used for intracoronal bleaching.

Hydrogen Peroxide

Various concentrations are available, but 30–35% stabilized aqueous solutions (Superoxol) are the most common. Gel forms containing 35% hydrogen peroxide are also available which are activated by a composite curing light. Hydrogen peroxide is caustic and can burn tissues on contact, releasing toxic free radicals, perhydroxyl anions, or both. Therefore, high-concentration solutions of hydrogen peroxide must be handled with care.

Sodium Perborate

This is available in a powdered form or as commercial preparations. Sodium perborate is stable when dry. It occurs in the form of sodium mono, tri or tetrahydrate. In the presence of acid, warm air, or water, however, it decomposes to form sodium metaborate, hydrogen peroxide, and nascent oxygen. Commonly used sodium perborate preparations are alkaline, and their pH depends on the amount of hydrogen peroxide released and the residual sodium metaborate. Sodium perborate is more easily controlled and safer than concentrated hydrogen peroxide solutions. Therefore, it should be the material of choice in most intracoronal bleaching procedures.

Carbamide Peroxide

Ten percent carbamide peroxide was introduced and commercially made available in 1989. This agent, also known as urea hydrogen peroxide, is available in the concentration range of 3–45%. 10% carbamide peroxide breaks down into urea, ammonia, carbon dioxide, and approximately 3.5% hydrogen peroxide. Bleaching preparations containing carbamide peroxide usually include glycerine or propylene glycol, sodium stannate, phosphoric or citric acid, and flavor additives. In some preparations, carbopol, a water-soluble polyacrylic acid polymer, is added as a thickening agent. Carbopol improves the shelf life and also extends the bleaching potential of the gel. Carbamide peroxide-based preparations have been associated with various degrees of damage to the teeth and surrounding mucosa.

Bleaching Mechanism

Bleaching gels usually contain either carbamide peroxide ($CH_6N_2O_3$), hydrogen peroxide (H_2O_2) or nonhydrogen peroxide chemicals. 10% gel of carbamide peroxide breaks down to 3.35% hydrogen peroxide (H_2O_2) and 6,65% urea (CH_4N_2O) (Table 9.7). Urea further decomposes into CO_2 and ammonia. High pH of the ammonia facilitates the bleaching process. Hydrogen peroxide is an oxidizing agent and breaks down to produce unstable free radicals. These unstable free radicals attack organic pigmented molecules in the spaces between the inorganic salts in tooth enamel resulting in smaller, less heavily pigmented constituents. These smaller molecules reflect less light, thus creating "whitening effect". Most bleaching procedures use hydrogen peroxide because it is unstable and decomposes into oxygen and water. The mechanisms of nonhydrogen peroxide containing materials are that the moist tooth structure and the gel interact and activate the gel. The oxidation-reduction reaction that occurs during bleaching is known as a redox reaction.

Bleaching Techniques for Vital Teeth

The fundamental bleaching approaches can be described as dentist supervised night guard bleaching (Matrix Bleaching), in-office or power bleaching (calcific metamorphosis) and bleaching systems which are available over the counter (Table 9.8).

Table 9.7 Bleaching mechanism

Na perborate → Na metaborate + H_2O_2 and releases O^+
When mixed with the superoxol solution (H_2O_2), it breaks down into
Na perborate + Superoxol → Na metaborate + H_2O_2 + active O_2 (which oxidizes and discolors the stain slowly)

Table 9.8 Constituents of the bleaching gel for vital bleaching techniques

Constituent	*Role*
Carbamide peroxide	–
Hydrogen peroxide	–
Thickening agent (carbopol)	• Enhances viscosity and delays the breakdown on contact with saliva
Urea	• Stabilizes the solution
Vehicle (glycerin, glycol, dentifrice)	• Glycerin enhances viscosity and ease of manipulation
Surfactant	• This is the wetting agent and allows H_2O_2 to diffuse into the tooth
Pigment dispersers	• Keeps the pigments in suspension
Preservatives (phosphoric acid, citric acid and sodium stannate)	• Provides durability and stability
Flavoring agents	–

Night Guard Bleaching

This process involves the daily use and placement of carbamide peroxide gel into a custom fitted tray of either the upper or lower arch at night. The night guard is made from a model of the patient's teeth. Instructions typically call for twice daily treatments of about 30 minutes to 2 hours a day for 2 to 6 weeks, depending on the color of the teeth at the start of treatment. There are 2 basic regimes for the application of the whitening solution. One is sleeping with the night guard filled with the bleaching material at night and second is wearing the loaded night guard during the day while changing the solution every 2 hours not exceeding 12 hours (Table 9.9).

At-home tray bleaching requires a number of steps to achieve success, which include accurate study casts that need to be trimmed to allow for a vacuum-down, thin, flexible mouth guard to be fabricated. The mouth guard can be trimmed to be scalloped (for the higher concentrations of bleaching peroxides) or with a 0.5–1 mm extension from the free gingival margin. The patient should be instructed on how to place the bleaching gel in the trays and how to remove any excess gel after insertion.

Advantages include lower cost to patient and minimal in-office chair time. The major disadvantage is that significant patient compliance is necessary for optimal results, longer treatment time is required and there is an unknown potential for the soft tissue changes with excessively extended uses.

This technique is indicated for mild, and moderate fluorosis as an adjunct to microabrasion. It has been shown to be effective for lightening primary teeth discolored by trauma, lightening tetracycline-stained teeth,

Table 9.9 Indications and contraindications for mouth guard vital bleaching

Indications	*Contraindications*
• Superficial enamel discolorations	• Severe enamel loss
• Mild yellow discolorations	• Hypersensitive teeth
• Brown fluorosis discolorations	• Presence of caries
• Age-related discolorations	• Defective coronal restorations
	• Allergy to bleaching gels
	• Bruxism

and lightening teeth stained by nicotine and can be used before and after restorations to harmonize shades of the restorative materials in the mouth. It will not, however, change the color of roots of teeth, and this should be taken into consideration in the patient's treatment plan.

One arch should be bleached at a time, beginning with the maxillary arch. This permits the untreated mandibular arch to serve as a constant standard for comparison. Also, by doing so, it reduces the potential for occlusal problems which could potentially occur if the thickness of two mouth guards were interposed simultaneously.

Examples of products for night-time use include:

- Opalescence PF (Ultradent Products), containing 10%, 15%, and 20% carbamide peroxide
- Nupro White Gold (Dentsply Professional), containing 10% and 15% carbamide peroxide
- Nite White Turbo (Discus Dental), containing 6% hydrogen peroxide.

In-Office Bleaching

This technique generally uses high levels of bleaching agents (e.g. 25%–35% hydrogen-peroxide-containing products) for shorter periods. This technique involves the external application of hydrogen peroxide to the surface of the tooth followed by activation with a heat source. The dental practitioner has the choice to use one of the light enhanced bleaching techniques, laser-activated bleach or merely paint-on bleaching gel or solution. The light system is based on a plasma arc high-intensity photopolymerization device (Table 9.10).

This technique is mainly indicated for mild tetracycline staining without any obvious banding, mild fluorosis, and single teeth with sclerosed pulp chambers and root canals. The in-office treatment can result in significant bleaching after only one treatment visit but may require multiple treatment appointments for optimum whitening. The main advantage of using this

Table 9.10 Indications and contraindications for thermo/photo extracoronal bleaching

Indications	*Contraindications*
• Light enamel discolorations	• Severe dark discolorations
• Mild tetracycline discolorations	• Severe enamel loss
• Endemic fluorosis discolorations	• Proximity of pulp horns
• Age-related discolorations	• Hypersensitive teeth
	• Presence of caries
	• Large/poor coronal restorations

technique is that while using very caustic chemicals, it is totally under the dentist's control, the soft tissue is protected and this has the potential for bleaching teeth more rapidly. Disadvantage can be related to the unpredictable outcome of the treatment.

Combination Bleaching Treatment

This treatment option involves application (in the office) of a high-concentration hydrogen-peroxide agent followed by a professionally dispensed and supervised product for at-home use for 5 days, often followed by an additional chairside application. Compared with in-office stand-alone treatment, combination treatments take less time, require fewer office visits, and is cost effective for the patients. The major disadvantage is the need for in-office chair time. Also, combination treatment is not a one-time treatment, which is preferred by most patients.

Light-Activated Bleaching Treatment

The mechanism of treatment involves application in the office of a high-concentration hydrogen-peroxide agent, which is then "activated" by plasma arc, light-emitting diodes, argon lasers, and metal halide and xenon-halogen light sources. The theory behind the treatment is that light or heat will speed the breakdown of the hydrogen peroxide and thus lighten the teeth more rapidly. The advantage is that the procedure is less time-consuming while producing faster results.

Over-the-Counter Bleaching Systems

Such products typically contain low levels of bleaching agent (e.g. 3–6% hydrogen peroxide), which are self-applied to the teeth via gum shields, strips, or paint-on product formats. These typically require twice-per-day application for up to 2 weeks. Bleaching strips use 6.5% hydrogen peroxide and the paint-on brush application uses 18% carbamide peroxide as the bleaching agent. These methods are excellent for maintaining already bleached teeth and are a good option for patients who cannot afford the professionally prescribed products or for patients who do not have time for multiple office visits.

Laser-Activated Bleaching

This technique uses lasers for extracoronal bleaching. Two types of lasers may be employed: the argon laser that emits a visible blue light and a carbon-dioxide laser that emits invisible infrared light. These lasers can be targeted to stain molecules and, with the use of a catalyst, rapidly decompose hydrogen peroxide to oxygen and water. The catalyst/peroxide combination may be damaging; therefore, exposed soft tissues, eyes, and clothing should be protected. Combination of both lasers can effectively reduce intrinsic stains in the dentin. It is easy to use and is best for removal of initial dark stains, such as those caused by tetracycline.

Side Effects of Bleaching: The most commonly reported side effect during a bleaching treatment is *tooth sensitivity*. Carbamide peroxide decomposes to hydrogen peroxide and urea. Hydrogen peroxide further decomposes to water and oxygen and the urea breaks down to ammonia and carbon dioxide. These by-products pass through the dentinal tubules reaching the pulp, thus causing reversible pulpitis resulting in tooth sensitivity. If the bleaching products contain glycerin as one of the ingredients, then that can cause dehydration during the bleaching treatment as glycerin absorbs water. This can contribute to the tooth sensitivity.

The sensitivity related to tooth bleaching is generally mild and transient and occurs early in the treatment. The sensitivity decreases as treatment continues with cessation shortly after the treatment ends. Recommended treatment for the sensitivity includes treatment with fluoride gel or a potassium nitrate toothpaste in the tray for 10 to 30 minutes before use of the bleaching agent, treatment of the teeth with a desensitizing agent after treatment, and reduction of the number of applications by requiring fewer applications per day. In addition to this, use of potassium nitrate plus fluoride toothpaste 2 weeks before bleaching and during the bleaching treatment will also help. These agents can also adversely affect the color of various restorative materials, with glass ionomer exhibiting the greatest color change.

Dental Hard Tissue Damage: Hydrogen peroxide can cause morphologic and structural changes in enamel, dentin, and cementum. These changes may cause dental hard tissues to be more susceptible to degradation and to secondary caries formation.

Mucosal Damage: Caustic bleaching agents if come in contact with the oral mucosa may cause peroxide-induced tissue damage. Ulceration and sloughing of the mucosa are caused by oxygen gas bubbles in the tissue. Generally, the mucosa appears white but does not become necrotic or leave scar tissue. The associated burning sensation is extremely uncomfortable for the patient. Treatment is by extensive water rinses until the whiteness is reduced. In more severe cases, a topical anesthetic, limited movements, and good oral hygiene aid healing. Application of protective cream or catalase can prevent most of these complications.

Bleaching of Nonvital Teeth

This technique is indicated for endodontically treated teeth which have become discolored due to the deposition of the blood degradation products in the dentinal tubules. The presence of a well-adapted and condensed root canal filling is mandatory for this procedure. A successful outcome of the treatment depends on the etiology, correct diagnosis, and proper selection of the bleaching technique (Table 9.11).

There are three different options/ways for bleaching endodontically treated teeth:

1. Walking bleach (out of the office technique)
2. In-office technique
3. The inside/outside technique.

Walking Bleach Technique was first described by Spasser. Commonly used agents are:

- Superoxol (30% H_2O_2 by wt. and 100% by vol. in pure distilled H_2O)
- Sodium perborate + H_2O
- Sodium perborate + H_2O_2
- Sodium perborate + 10% carbamide peroxide.

Predominantly, the technique utilizes sodium perborate mixed with either water or hydrogen peroxide and filled into the access cavity. Bleaching

Table 9.11 Indications and contraindications for bleaching endodontically treated teeth

Indications	*Contraindications*
• Discolorations of pulp chamber	• Superficial enamel discolorations
• Dentin discolorations	• Defective enamel formation
• Discolorations not amenable to extracoronal bleaching	• Severe dentin loss
	• Presence of caries
	• Discolored composites

success depends on the application duration of the agent. The bleaching mixture is very active for 24 hours, after which very little potential for damage to the tissue remains. The mixture maybe changed every 3 to 5 days and usually 1–3 treatments are required for the optimal result. If sodium perborate is used alone, then it should be changed bi-weekly.

An application of calcium hydroxide is recommended after the bleaching process. This helps to diminish the oxygen inhibition of the polymerization of the definitive post obturation filling and to counteract the increased permeability of the dentin caused by the bleaching agent.

Inside/Outside Bleaching Technique

This was first described by Settembrini et al. and was later modified (Liebenberg 1997). This is a modified walking bleach technique using 10% carbamide peroxide. As the name implies, the idea is to apply bleaching agent on the external and the internal surfaces of the tooth. The access cavity remains open during the entire treatment process. One advantage of this technique is that a low concentration of bleaching gel is sufficient to obtain the desired effect. The technique success relies on patient compliance. This technique may be indicated where simultaneous bleaching of nonvital and vital teeth is possible and required. A disadvantage is the lack of bacterial control during bleaching. The microorganisms can colonize the dentin tubules, and the danger exists not only to the bleaching result but also to the long-term success of the endodontic treatment which may be compromised.

In-Office Bleaching Technique

This technique may also be used for nonvital teeth. This is historically a thermocatalytic technique which involves the placement of 30–35% hydrogen peroxide in the pulp chamber and activation of the oxidation process by placement of a heating instrument inside the pulp chamber. This may initiate a local inflammatory reaction attributable to the oxidizing agent combined with heating. Hence, the potential damage is external cervical root resorption caused by irritation to the cementum and periodontal ligament. Therefore, the preferred technique these days utilizes a 2 minute exposure to ultraviolet light on the labial surface of the tooth to be bleached. 30–35% hydrogen peroxide solution is placed in the pulp chamber on a cotton pellet. In both these techniques, it is imperative that sealing cement like polycarboxylate or light cured GIC is placed over the exposed root canal filling prior to the application of the bleaching agent.

Side Effects of Bleaching in Nonvital Teeth

External cervical root resorption probably caused by the oxidizing agent, particularly 30 to 35% hydrogen peroxide. Presumably, the irritating chemical diffuses via unprotected dentinal tubules and cementum defects and causes necrosis of the cementum, inflammation of the periodontal ligament, and, finally, root resorption. The process may be enhanced if heat is applied or in the presence of bacteria. Previous traumatic injury and age may act as predisposing factors.

Chemical burns and sloughing of the gingiva are caused by the caustic nature of hydrogen peroxide. When using such solutions, the soft tissues should always be protected with vaseline or orabase.

COMPOSITE RESIN RESTORATIONS

Composite resin offers a satisfactory alternative and may be used in child and adolescent patients. Resin can be used by either to camouflage/replace discrete localized areas of abnormal enamel or to cover the entire enamel surface (veneer). Composite resin restorations are indicated in cases of hypoplasia caused by moderate to severe fluorosis, localized hypoplasia not responsive to microabrasion, chronological hypoplasia, tetracycline staining, discoloration due to loss of vitality not responsive to nonvital bleaching, amelogenesis and dentinogenesis imperfecta, and idiopathic hypoplasia. Composite veneers may be placed directly on to the tooth surface or fabricated indirectly in the laboratory.

PORCELAIN VENEERS

Porcelain veneers are indicated for hypoplastic and discolored teeth in patients aged 16 years and over, when techniques such as microabrasion, nonvital bleaching and composite resins have failed to produce a satisfactory clinical result. The large size of the immature pulp chamber and pulp horns, and the immature gingival contour of the adolescent patient contraindicates the use of porcelain veneers.

CROWNS

These are indicated when the discoloration cannot be completely diminished, in cases of congenital discolorations, congenitally malformed teeth, when there is weakening of the tooth structure, in cases of heavily restored teeth and in patients contraindicated for bleaching.

CONCLUSION

Tooth discoloration is prevalent, and varies with age, habits and by individual patient. The treatment of tooth discoloration and its prevention have been central in dentistry for a number of decades. The typical result is a whiter appearance of the patients. This whiter appearance often leads to a heightened awareness of other problems with the dentition and a desire for further treatment. The dentist may play an active role in encouraging patients and educating them about choices for tooth whitening and in providing the best treatment option. Vital tooth bleaching, when administered correctly may prove to be a safe, conservative and effective esthetic procedure available to patients.

BIBLIOGRAPHY

1. Alaudin SS, Fontana M. Evaluation of NovaMin® as an adjunct to fluoride for caries remineralization. Novqamin Research Report. Available at: http://novamin.com/pdf/Evaluation_of_NovaMin_As_An_Adjunct_to_Fluoride.pdf. Accessed Jan 2013.
2. Bailey SJ, Swift EJ. Effects of home bleaching products on resin composites [abstract]. J Dent Res. 1991;70:570.
3. Bowles WH, Thompson LR. Vital bleaching: the effect of heat and hydrogen peroxide on pulpal enzymes. J Endod. 1986;12(3):108-12.
4. Bowles WH, Ugwuneri Z. Pulp chamber penetration by hydrogen peroxide following vital bleaching procedures. J Endod. 1987;13(8):375-7.
5. Fuss Z, Szajkis S, Tagger M. Tubular permeability to calcium hydroxide and to bleaching agents. J Endod. 1989;15(8):362-4.
6. Gokay O, Tuncbilek M, Ertan P. Penetration of the pulp chamber by carbamide peroxide bleaching agents on teeth restored with composite resin. J Oral Rehabil. 2000;27(5):428-31.
7. Haywood VB, Leech T, Heymann HO, et al. Nightguard vital bleaching: effects on enamel surface texture and diffusion. Quintessence Int. 1990;21:801-4.
8. Haywood VB, Leonard RH, Chauncy NF, et al. Effectiveness, side effects and long-term status of nightguard vital bleaching. J Am Dent Assoc. 1994;125(9):1219-26.
9. Leonard RH, Haywood VB, Phillips C. Risk factors for developing tooth sensitivity and gingival irritation associated with nightguard vital bleaching. Quintessence Int. 1997;28(8):527-34.
10. Miller WD. Experiments and observations on the wasting of tooth tissue variously described as erosion, abrasion, chemical abrasion, denudation, etc. Dent Cosmos. 1907;49:1-23, 109-124, 225-247.
11. Pohjola R, Browning WD, Hackman ST, et al. Sensitivity and tooth whitening agents. J Esthet Restor Dent. 2002;14(2):85-91.
12. Shen P, Cai F, Nowicki A, et al. Remineralization of enamel subsurface lesions by sugar-free chewing gum containing casein phosphopeptide-amorphous calcium phosphate. J Dent Res. 2001;80(12):458-96.
13. Tung MS, Eichmiller FC. Amorphous calcium phosphates for tooth mineralization. Comp Cont Educ Dent. 2004;25(9, Suppl. 1):9-13.
14. Wülknitz P. Cleaning power and abrasivity of European toothpastes. Adv Dent Res. 1997;11:576-9.

CHAPTER **10**

DRUG PRESCRIBING AND THERAPEUTICS

Balaram Naik, Priyanka Jain

INTRODUCTION

There are several types of medications that are used to manage a variety of diseases involving the oral cavity (mouth) that are part of good dental care. There are a number of different medications a dentist may prescribe, depending on the condition. Some medications are prescribed to fight certain oral diseases, some to prevent or treat infections, and others to control pain and relieve anxiety.

This chapter will deal with the most commonly used medications in dental care. The dose of the drugs and instructions on how to take them will differ from patient to patient, depending on what the drug is being used for, patient's age, weight and other considerations. Dosage should be appropriately reduced by age or body weight in children. Elderly people show exaggerated reactions to drugs, hence doses need to be modified as per the requirements. Polypharmacy is quite common in the elderly. Therefore, any possible interaction should be identified before prescribing.

DRUGS USED TO CONTROL PAIN

Pain, as defined by the *International Association for the Study of Pain*, is "an unpleasant sensory and emotional experience arising from actual or potential tissue damage or described in terms of such damage." It is often pain that brings the patient to the dental clinic. The two components of pain are *perception and reaction*. Perception is the physical component of pain and involves the message of pain that is carried through the nerves eventually to the cortex. Reaction is the psychological component of pain and involves the patient's emotional response to the pain. Although individuals are surprisingly uniform in their perception of pain, they vary greatly in their reaction to it. A decrease in the pain threshold (a greater reaction to pain) has been associated with emotional instability, anxiety, fatigue, youth, certain nationalities, women, and fear and apprehension. The pain threshold is raised by sleep, sympathy, activities, and analgesics.

Pain is a subjective phenomenon. The patient's self-report is the single most accurate and reliable indicator of the existence and intensity of pain and any resultant distress. Pain is whatever the experiencing person says it is and exists whenever he says it does. The most common types of odontogenic pain are characterized as acute pain, sharp and shooting pain, dull pain, etc. (Table 10.1). Characteristically, acute pain is accompanied by some recognizable evidence of tissue injury or inflammation, and it resolves spontaneously once the underlying cause (inflamed pulp, abscessed tooth, carious lesion) is definitively treated. Few underlying psychological or behavioral issues affect the dentist's choice of therapies, and, most commonly, a pharmacologic approach to pain management is most appropriate.

Dentists must be able to diagnose the source of pain and have strategies for its management. The '*3-D's*' principle—diagnosis, dental treatment and drugs may be used to manage pain. Most painful problems that require analgesics will be due to inflammation. Pain management drugs include nonopioid, nonnarcotic analgesics (e.g. nonsteroidal anti-inflammatory

Table 10.1 Painful conditions in the dental practice

Condition	*Comments*
Reversible pulpitis	Pain is poorly localized and is of short duration. Tooth is not tender to percussion and normal radiographic anatomy and features are seen
Irreversible pulpitis	Spontaneous pain lasting from few seconds to hours. Pain is exacerbated by hot/cold stimulus
Acute periapical periodontitis	Spontaneous pain aggravated by biting. Tooth is nonvital
Lateral periodontal abscess	Swollen/inflamed gingiva around the affected tooth, tender on percussion, is mobile and vital. Pain is continuous
Periodontitis	Localized dull pain, tooth is tender to percussion
Pericoronitis	Spontaneous pain aggravated by biting, visible signs of inflammation over the operculum. May be associated with fever
Cellulitis	Swelling sand tenderness of the affected part of the face with associated lymphadenopathy. Tooth is tender and associated with an abscess
Hypersensitivity	Sharp pain of short duration initiated by hot/cold or sweets
Cracked tooth	Pain is initiated by hot/cold, and aggravates on biting. This condition is difficult to diagnose
Acute necrotizing ulcerative gingivitis (ANUG)	Bleeding gums, soreness. Associated with halitosis and fever
Bacterial sialadenitis	Affected salivary gland is swollen and painful especially during eating

drugs, paracetamol, etc.) or opioids analgesics (i.e. narcotics) (Table 10.2). Nonsteroidal anti-inflammatory drugs (NSAIDs) provide excellent pain relief due to their anti-inflammatory and analgesic action. The most common NSAIDs are aspirin and ibuprofen. Paracetamol gives very effective analgesia but has little anti-inflammatory action. The opioids are powerful analgesics but have significant side effects and therefore they should be reserved for severe pain only. The most commonly used opioid is codeine, usually used in combination with paracetamol (Table 10.3).

Nonopioid analgesics act primarily at the peripheral nerve endings, although they also act centrally (Table 10.4). Opioids act within the central nervous system. Another difference between the opioids and the nonopioid analgesic agents is their mechanism of action. The action of the nonopioid analgesic agents is related to their ability to inhibit prostaglandin synthesis. The opioids affect the amount of pain by depressing the CNS (the reaction) (Flow chart 10.1).

NONSTEROIDAL ANTI-INFLAMMATORY DRUGS

Nonsteroidal anti-inflammatory drugs (NSAIDs) produce analgesic and anti-inflammatory actions by inhibition of cyclo-oxygenase, thereby reducing the synthesis of arachidonic acid metabolites such as prostaglandins

Table 10.2 Common drugs used in dentistry

Drugs	*Category*
Drugs used to control pain	• Nonopioid analgesics • Salicylates (Aspirin) • NSAIDs (Ibuprofen) • Acetaminophen (Paracetamol) • Opioid analgesics • Codeine • Morphine • Corticosteroids
Drugs used to treat infections	• Antibiotics/antimicrobials • Therapeutic • Prophylactic • Topical • Antiseptics • Antifungals • Antivirals
Drugs used to treat anxiety	• Benzodiazepines
Other drugs	• Topical anesthetics • Saliva substitutes

Table 10.3 Differences between nonopioid and opioid analgesics

Nonopioid	*Opioid*
Act peripherally and centrally	Act centrally
Inhibit the prostaglandin synthesis	Depress the central nervous system
Do not produce tolerance/physical dependence	Produce physical dependence
Have a ceiling effect to analgesia	No ceiling effect
Most effective when given before the procedure	Never used as a first-line therapy drug

Table 10.4 Nonopioid analgesics

Salicylates	*NSAIDs*	*Acetaminophen*
Aspirin	Ibuprofen	Tylenol/Paracetamol
Magnesium salicylate	Ketorolac	
Choline salicylate	Diflunisal	

Flow chart 10.1 Choice of analgesics

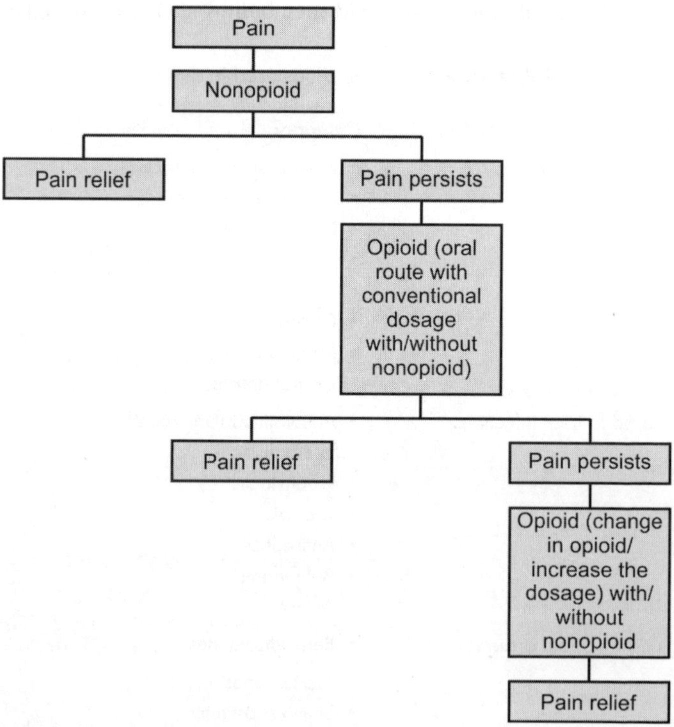

and thromboxanes. Prostaglandins play a key role in the development of pain and inflammation. They potentiate the pain producing action of various chemicals like bradykinin and 5-hydroxytryptamine by sensitizing the pain receptors. Many NSAIDs including ibuprofen, aspirin, diflunisal, mefenamic acid produce significant reductions in dental pain arising from surgical, periodontal, operative or endodontic procedures. Redness and swelling of the tissues is dependent on the vasodilation and the capillary permeability action of the prostaglandins. NSAIDs reduce these manifestations by inhibiting the prostaglandin synthesis.

Aspirin

Aspirin has been commercially available since 1899, and, until the late 1970s, no peripherally acting analgesics could claim greater efficacy. Aspirin, (the most prominent member of the salicylate group), derives its analgesic, antipyretic, and anti-inflammatory action from its ability to inhibit prostaglandin synthesis. Aspirin inhibits the enzyme cyclo-oxygenase (prostaglandin synthase) by acetylating a serine, which results in inhibition of the production of prostaglandins. A reduction in prostaglandins results in a reduction in painful perception. Many dental patients are advised to take aspirin before the painful stimuli is experienced, such as a "throbbing" pain caused by inflammation. Aspirin is typically used to relieve mild-to-moderate pain such as a headache or toothache.

The antipyretic properties of aspirin are best demonstrated in febrile patients. Normal subjects show no marked change in body temperature when therapeutic doses of aspirin are administered. It is difficult to separate the analgesic and anti-inflammatory effects of aspirin, since the vast majority of painful conditions have an inflammatory component.

The choice of the route of administration is via the oral method. It may be administered rectally when vomiting is present. Since, this route is more erratic and unpredictable it should only be used when the oral route is not feasible. An aspirin tablet should never be applied topically to the oral mucosa to treat a toothache. A painful ulceration may occur. It is not effective against intense pain because the analgesic potency of aspirin is weaker than that of the opioids. Apart from the effects mentioned above, aspirin also has an effect on the metabolism of the body. It reduces the blood sugar level in diabetics by raising the peripheral utilization of glucose, increases the basal metabolic rate, causes a reduction in the platelet adhesiveness, and causes an increase in the thyroid hormone when used for a long period of time. Aspirin is rapidly and almost completely absorbed from the stomach and small intestine, reaching its peak on an empty stomach in 30 minutes.

Adverse Effects

Aspirin has numerous side effects at therapeutic doses, most of which are more annoying than serious. The most commonly reported side effect is nausea. Certainly, many dental surgical procedures have the potential for causing nausea because of the swallowing of blood and debris, the use of sedative or anesthetic drugs, and the anxiety associated with dental surgery. However, aspirin can cause gastric irritation that leads to nausea and, occasionally, vomiting. In addition to the effects of aspirin on the gastric mucosa, aspirin causes local irritation directly while the tablet is disintegrating and in contact with the gastric tissues.

Aspirin significantly increases bleeding time by inhibiting the aggregation of platelets. Although the prolongation of clotting time is tolerated in healthy patients, the possibility exists that aspirin could promote postoperative hemorrhaging, especially if a clot has not fully formed.

Toxicity caused by aspirin overdose is common. Its symptoms and severity depend on dose. Chronic toxicity is characterized by tinnitus, nausea, vomiting, headache, and hyperventilation. Chronic toxicity usually only requires removal of the drug and eventual dose adjustment. Acute toxicity often requires respiratory support, gastric lavage, maintenance of electrolyte balance (e.g. potassium replacement if necessary), maintenance of plasma pH, and alkalinization of the urine by intravenous (IV) bicarbonate (Table 10.5).

Aspirin is contraindicated in a number of medical conditions. Serious internal bleeding can result from the ingestion of aspirin by a patient with an ulcer condition. It causes an increase in acid production and a reduction in mucin leading to erosive and ulcerative effects on the stomach and the duodenum. This leads to bleeding and perforation. In such cases, paracetamol can be given. Aspirin enhances the effect of warfarin leading to increased anticoagulant effect. This increases the blood loss from the GI tract. Hence, it should be avoided in patients undergoing anticoagulant therapy. Aspirin is not contraindicated in pregnancy, but it should be used with caution. In the third trimester, aspirin tends to prolong labor by inhibiting the synthesis of prostaglandins involved in initiating uterine contractions and can also cause bleeding at birth in both mother and the baby. Aspirin should also be avoided in children less than 16 years with influenza or chickenpox (varicella). There is epidemiologic data

Table 10.5 Contraindications to the use of aspirin

Disease	*Effect of aspirin*
Ulcer	Internal bleeding
Asthma	Asthmatic attack is initiated
Diabetes	May cause hyperglycemia/hypoglycemia in high doses
Influenza	Reye's syndrome in children
Hypocoagulation state	Excessive bleeding

indicating that aspirin usage during or shortly after these viral diseases increases the risk of developing *Reye's syndrome* (a fatty degeneration in the liver and kidney with an associated encephalopathy). Aspirin can also precipitate severe bronchospasms in known asthmatics. Therefore, caution should be used.

Dosage: 600–900 mg per 4–6 hours. Maximum dose is 4 gm daily.

Ibuprofen

The anti-inflammatory action is less than that of aspirin. Ibuprofen is readily absorbed after oral administration and peak blood levels occur about one to two hours after ingestion. Ibuprofen can be used in several different formulations. Gels provide faster absorption and therefore a quicker onset for meaningful analgesia that occurs about 25–30 minutes after ingestion. Another way of using is the mucoadhesive patch that permits intraoral delivery of ibuprofen. Paracetamol (1000 mg) when added to ibuprofen (600 mg) can be used to improve pain relief after endodontic treatment when compared with ibuprofen (600 mg) alone.

Adverse Effects

The adverse effects are similar to those produced by aspirin; however, they may vary in severity. Gastric irritation (nausea and abdominal pain) is usually the most troublesome adverse effect. Dizziness, gastrointestinal bleeding, fluid retention, and nephrotoxicity can also occur in some cases. Inhibition of platelet aggregation is transient and reversible. This analgesic should be avoided in most patients whose medical conditions contraindicate the use of aspirin. Of particular concern are patients with gastrointestinal ulcers, and coagulation defects. Ibuprofen occasionally causes xerostomia that may increase oral plaque and dental caries.

Dosage: Ibuprofen should be considered the drug of first choice for management of acute inflammatory pain. 200–800 mg every 4–6 hours is the recommended dose. The maximum dose should not exceed a total daily dose of 3200 mg. 400–600 mg of ibuprofen taken every six hours is very effective for treating moderate inflammatory pain. This is not recommended for children under 7 years of age. All NSAIDs should be used with caution in elderly patients.

Acetaminophen/Paracetamol

Paracetamol (also known as acetaminophen in some countries) acts primarily in the central nervous system. It has analgesic and antipyretic effects, but is a weak inhibitor of the cyclo-oxygenase system. Paracetamol readily crosses into the cerebrospinal fluid. Within the central nervous system (CNS) it works by inhibiting prostaglandin synthesis in the hypothalamus. At therapeutic doses it does not inhibit prostaglandin in the peripheral tissues so there is very little, if any anti-inflammatory action. Paracetamol is rapidly absorbed from the stomach and peak blood levels are reached within 30–60 minutes. It is nontoxic at therapeutic concentrations. Elimination half-life is about two hours. It is metabolized in the liver and the metabolites are excreted via the kidneys. It does not cause the same gastric irritation or the other complications associated with aspirin and other NSAIDs.

Adverse Effects

Since paracetamol is metabolized in the liver, patients with liver disease need to take care. Other patients who may have increased toxicity are those with a high alcohol intake and those taking enzyme-inducing drugs (e.g. antiepileptics and rifampicin). Paracetamol may cause prolongation of prothrombin time in patients taking anticoagulants and it can occasionally cause urticarial or erythematous skin rashes, or fever.

Dosage: 500 mg–1 gm orally 4–6 hourly. Maximum adult dose is 4 gm daily.

An overdose of paracetamol is defined as a single dose of more than 100 mg/kg of body weight. Overdose will produce hepatotoxicity (delayed hepatocellular necrosis), hypoglycemia and acute renal tubular necrosis. In adults, a dose of 7.5–15 mg/kg is considered potentially toxic. Symptoms occur 24–48 hours after ingestion.

Topical Analgesic

These are indicated in all painful oral conditions (burns, inflammation, ulcers, etc.) and are available as benzydamine hydrochloride (mouthwash), lignocaine rinse and lignocaine hydrochloride as spray.

OPIOID ANALGESICS (NARCOTICS)

Opioid analgesics are primarily employed for the relief of pain and consequently find widespread application in dentistry. Opioid analgesia occurs by activation of opioid receptors expressed on neurons in supraspinal sites, spinal sites and in peripheral tissue. In general, the opioid receptors are thought to inhibit neuronal activity. Opioids tend to produce variable responses in patients, with some patients reporting considerably greater analgesia than others, even after administration of identical doses. The variability in patient response forms the basis for recommendations that analgesics be prescribed based on patient report rather than on prior expectations of the clinician. This can be attributed to various factors like environmental (e.g. psychosocial status, secondary gain, etc.), pathophysiological (e.g. liver function, enzyme/receptor expression) and genetic factors. Opioids also possess therapeutically useful antitussive (cough suppressant) and constipating effects. Repeated use of opioids for control of pain can lead to analgesic tolerance (loss of analgesic effect), as well as physical and sometimes psychological dependence.

Fear of addiction on the part of both the practitioner and the patient is a common barrier to the effective use of opioid analgesics. Addiction refers to *psychological dependence*, a behavioral pattern of drug use marked by craving, drug-seeking behavior, and compulsive use that may interfere with the person's ability to function in society. *Physical dependence,* on the other hand, is a pharmacologic property causing the appearance of withdrawal symptoms when the medication is stopped abruptly or following the administration of an antagonist, and tolerance is the requirement for increased doses of a drug to achieve the same effect. Finally, *pseudo addiction* is a term used to describe exaggerated behaviors seen in pain patients brought on by inadequate pain relief. Physical dependence and tolerance are involuntary mechanisms that occur in virtually all patients taking opioid analgesics for a prolonged period of time. They are easily managed in the patient with pain. Tolerance is managed with careful upward titration of the dose until adequate pain relief is attained. The effects of physical dependence are easily avoided by the gradual tapering of opioids on discontinuation of therapy, as opposed to abrupt withdrawal. Addiction, by contrast, is a voluntary mechanism that rarely occurs in patients taking opioid analgesics for pain.

Opioid analgesics are added to nonopioids to manage pain that is moderate to severe or that does not respond to nonopioids alone. Opioids are frequently combined with paracetamol or more recently with ibuprofen in treating acute dental pain. The combination of 600–650 mg of paracetamol with 60 mg of codeine produces very effective analgesia in postoperative pain patients. Opioid analgesics include both pure agonists, such as codeine and oxycodone, and agonist/antagonists, such as pentazocine. As a general rule, the agonist/antagonists should not be used as first-line therapy. There is no convincing evidence that these drugs offer any advantage over the pure opioid agonists. Agonist/antagonists become less effective at high doses and frequently cause dysphoria, confusion and hallucinations. In addition, they may cause withdrawal symptoms when given to patients physically dependent on opioid agonists.

The oral administration of opioid analgesics is preferred. It is convenient and inexpensive. Even severe postsurgical pain can be effectively treated with orally administered opioids in the proper doses. For the patient not able to swallow a pill or capsule, numerous liquid formulations of opioids are available (codeine, hydrocodone, oxycodone, and others). The drug reaches its peak levels (including side effects) in 1.5–2 hours after the oral administration of most opioids. Therefore, patients may take a second opioid dose safely 2 hours after the first dose if the pain persists and side effects are mild at that time. For patients unable to take medications by mouth, the intravenous, intramuscular, or rectal routes of administration may be considered. Use of the intravenous or intramuscular route to deliver analgesics should be limited to inpatient hospital settings.

Morphine and other opioid analgesics are the most efficacious analgesic drugs known for pain relief (Table 10.6). As emphasized earlier, these drugs provide only symptomatic relief of pain without influencing its underlying cause. The opioids, when administered at therapeutic doses to produce analgesia, also produce a drowsiness from which the patient is

Table 10.6 Drugs for pain control

Medication	*Recommended dose*	*Side effects*
Non-narcotics Nonopioids		
• Aspirin	650–1000 mg/4–6 hours, not to exceed 4 gm/day	Abdominal pain, nausea, and increased bleeding time
• *NSAIDs:* Ibuprofen (Advil)	400 mg/4–6 hours, not to exceed 2400 mg/day	Abdominal pain, nausea and increased bleeding time. Sometimes, it may also cause xerostomia (dry mouth)
• Acetaminophen (Paracetamol)	650–1000 mg/4–6 hours, not to exceed 4 gm/day. For severe pain, a narcotic may be combined with this	Best tolerated analgesic with few side effects. Overdose can cause liver damage
Opioids these are most effective when given in combination with non-opioids		Dizziness, drowsiness, vomiting and constipation. Alcohol consumption should be avoided
• Combination of acetaminophen and codeine	300 mg acetaminophen plus 30 mg codeine/ 4–6 hours (two tablets)	
• Aspirin with codeine	325 mg aspirin plus 30 mg codeine/4–6 hours (two tablets)	
• Acetaminophen with hydrocodone	500 md acetaminophen plus 5 md hydrocodone/4–6 hours (one or two tablets)	
• Ibuprofen with hydrocodone	200 mg ibuprofen plus 7.5 mg hydrocodone/ 4–6 hours (one tablet)	

generally easily aroused, as well as "tranquillization." There is without doubt a significant antianxiety or sedating component in the analgesic effect of opioids. Thus, although nausea and vomiting, respiratory depression, constipation, and tolerance and physical dependence can be drawbacks to their use, the opioids undeniably produce an important combination of desirable effects (e.g. analgesia and sedation) in the suffering patient.

Adverse Effects

Opioids are highly effective analgesics but they also have a high incidence of side effects. In treating acute dental pain, opioids are used in low dosages providing minor adverse effects at the cost of reduced analgesia. The opioids should not be considered as the analgesic of first choice in this setting. Instead, opioids should be used as adjuncts to nonnarcotics that are given at maximally effective dosages (i.e. 1000 mg paracetamol).

Like the pharmacologic effects, *the adverse reactions* of the opioid analgesics are proportional to their analgesic strength.

- *Respiratory depression:* The opioid analgesic agonists depress the respiratory center in a dose-related manner. This is usually the cause of death with an overdose.
- *Nausea and emesis:* Analgesic doses of opioid analgesics often produce nausea and vomiting. This is due to their direct stimulation of the chemoreceptor trigger zone (CTZ) located in the medulla. This side effect is reduced by discouraging ambulation.
- *Constipation:* The opioids produce constipation by producing a tonic contraction of the gastrointestinal tract. Small doses of even weak opioids frequently have this effect and its duration outlasts their analgesic effect. Even with continued administrations tolerance does not develop to this effect.
- *Urinary retention:* The opioids increase the smooth muscle tone in the urinary tract, thereby causing urinary retention. They also produce an antidiuretic effect by stimulating the release of antidiuretic hormone (ADH) from the pituitary gland.
- Central nervous system (*CNS) effects:* Occasionally, opioids may produce CNS stimulation exhibited by anxiety, restlessness, or nervousness.

Codeine

It is not advisable to use codeine alone and is added to other analgesics like paracetamol (as mentioned before) because neither codeine nor any of the other opioids have anti-inflammatory properties. It is not used often due to its side effect of constipation.

Dosage: 30–60 mg every 4 hours IM/PO combined with NSAIDs or analgesics.

Morphine

Morphine is widely used for pain control and can be given by virtually via any route of administration. The effects of morphine include analgesia, drowsiness, euphoria-dysphoria, respiratory depression, suppression of the cough reflex and pupillary constriction. The analgesia produced by morphine occurs without loss of consciousness. An additional significant feature of opioid analgesics is that they are generally more effective against continuous, dull aching pain than against sharp, intermittent pain. Neuropathic pain, such as trigeminal neuralgia, is less responsive to opioids. Sensitivity to pain decrease with age, whereas the elimination half-life of morphine does the opposite; thus, the pain relief provided by morphine typically increases with age.

Dosage: Dependent on previous analgesia but can start at 10 mg every 4 hours. A laxative and an antiemetic should also be prescribed along with this.

Corticosteroids

Steroids can be used in various forms like topical, oral, systemic, intra-lesional and parental. Systemic corticosteroids are rarely indicated in dentistry but they can at times be useful for the management of inflammation. They should also only be used when there are no signs of infection and no possibility of an infection developing. Such situations include emergencies (adrenal crisis, anaphylaxis and allergic reactions), severe postoperative swelling, and acute apical periodontitis following removal of an acutely inflamed pulp and for some oral ulcerations and mucosal lesions that cannot be managed with topical medications.

Corticosteroids can be either glucocorticosteroids or mineralocorticosteroids. Only glucocorticosteroids inhibit immune and inflammatory responses. Glucocorticoids are very effective in reducing the periapical inflammatory response following endodontic treatment. They also reduce bradykinin levels, postoperative pain and edema in the third molar extraction.

Topical steroids like triamcinolone and hydrocortisone are used to treat recurrent aphthous ulcers and lichen planus cases. Corticosteroids such as orabase-HCA, oracort, and oralone used to relieve discomfort and redness of the mouth.

Adverse Effects

Corticosteroids not only reduce inflammation but they also suppress the immune response. This may have adverse effects on the patient's health and well-being. The topical use of corticosteroids is preferred since the immunosuppressive effects are much less severe. The glucocorticosteroids should be avoided in patients with systemic fungal infection and known hypersensitivity to the drug. They should be used with caution in patients with ulcerative colitis, pyogenic infections, peptic ulcers, diabetes mellitus, and tuberculosis. They can cause mild psychological disturbances such as euphoria, insomnia and nervousness but can also cause severe problems such as manic depression and schizophrenic psychosis. These side effects are usually related to the size of the dose and the duration.

Dosage: A simple and relatively safe corticosteroid that can be used for oral and dental inflammatory conditions is dexamethasone. It should only be used as an adjunct to dental treatment and not as the sole means of managing the pain. Dexamethasone is available as 4 mg tablets. The usual oral dosing regime is an 8 mg loading dose, followed by 4 mg every eight hours for two to three days up to a maximum of five days.

Topical Steroids

Topical corticosteroids are frequently used in management of the oral mucodermatoses and other conditions (Table 10.7). Secondary oral candidiasis is of particular importance in patients being treated for oral mucosal disease. Candidiasis will aggravate the existing oral condition and may prevent successful treatment unless it is recognized and managed.

DRUGS USED TO TREAT DENTAL INFECTIONS

Antibiotics

An antibiotic is a substance which causes the death of or prevents successful replication of microorganisms. Antibiotics are indicated for the treatment of odontogenic infections, oral nonodontogenic infections, as prophylaxis against focal infection, and as prophylaxis against local infection and spread to neighboring tissues and organs. Antibiotic prescription is almost invariably associated with the prescription of NSAIDs (Table 10.8).

Antibiotics are typically prescribed in dental practice for some of the following purposes: (a) as treatment for acute odontogenic infections;

Table 10.7 Topical steroids

Forms available are:
• Hydrocortisone hemisuccinate (pellets)
• Triamcinolone acetonide (in adhesive paste)
• Fluocinonide (in adhesive paste)
• Betamethasone sodium phosphate (mouthwash)
• Triamcinolone mouthwash
• Beclomethasone dipropionate (spray)

Table 10.8 Prescription of antibiotics

Guidelines to be followed before prescribing antibiotics in dentistry:
• Make an accurate diagnosis. Always prefer to use a narrow-spectrum antibiotic rather than a broad-spectrum. Narrow-spectrum has a limited range of effect, usually against Gram positive bacteria. Broad-spectrum is active against Gram positive bacteria and sometimes mycoplasma. The narrower the spectrum, the better as this reduces the GI side effects by limiting the destruction of the normal flora. Use of a narrow-spectrum antibiotic also minimizes the overgrowth of opportunistic pathogens like *Candida albicans*
• Based on the diagnosis, use the appropriate type of antibiotic along with dose and duration of the course. An increasing problem is that some organisms are acquiring multiresistance. Example is the methicillin-resistant *Staphylococcus aureus* (MRSA). Therefore, the prescription should be carefully assessed and given only when absolutely necessary
• The interactions of antibiotics with the other drugs that the patient might be using should always be considered

(b) as treatment for nonodontogenic infections; (c) as prophylaxis against focal infection in patients at risk (endocarditis and joint prostheses); and (d) as prophylaxis against local infection and systemic spread in oral surgery.

Adverse Effects

Antibiotic prescribing may be associated with unfavorable side effects ranging from gastrointestinal disturbances to fatal anaphylactic shock and development of resistance. Blood dyscrasias are rare but include leukopenia and agranulocytosis. Nausea, vomiting and diarrhea are very common side effects of antibiotic regime. Antibiotic associated colitis (AAC) may occur during or after the use of antibiotics. This usually occurs following the use of broad-spectrum antibiotics. The cause is a toxin of *Clostridium difficile*, a gut organism. Abdominal pain, blood-stained diarrhea and fever are the common symptoms of AAC. Fluids and the electrolytes should be replaced in such a condition and hospitalization is required. Another side effect of broad-spectrum antibiotics is candidiasis. Itchy skin reactions to edematous swelling and full blown anaphylactic shock may occur in cases of hypersensitivity reactions.

THERAPEUTIC ANTIBIOTICS

Most oral diseases presented to the dentist are primarily inflammatory conditions that are associated with pain. Majority of the dental conditions do not require the use of antibiotics. A considerable percentage of dental pain originates from acute and chronic infections of pulpal origin, which necessitates operative intervention, rather than antibiotics. Nonindicated clinical cases for antibiotic use include acute periapical infection, dry socket, and pulpitis. Chronic inflammatory periodontal conditions are also not indicated for antibiotics; systemic antimicrobials should only be used in acute periodontal conditions where drainage or debridement is impossible, where there is local spread of the infection or where systemic upset has occurred. Another nonindicated condition is localized swelling. More common dental infections present in the form of pulpitis and periapical periodontitis, which require only operative measures like fillings, root canal therapy, or extraction if the tooth is not restorable.

Clinical situations that require antibiotic therapy are limited, and they include oral infection accompanied by elevated body temperature and evidence of systemic spread like lymphadenopathy and trismus. Facial cellulitis that may or may not be associated with dysphagia is a serious disease that should be treated by antibiotics promptly because of the possibility of infection spread via lymph and blood circulation, with development of septicemia.

There are also a limited number of localized oral lesions that are indicated for antibiotic use and these include periodontal abscess, acute necrotizing ulcerative gingivitis, and pericoronitis.

The antibiotic course prescribed is of two types: short duration course (2–3 days) or long duration course (7–10 days). This is decided on the basis of the severity of the infection, the type of organism, and the extent of the disease progression. Short duration courses are preferred where appropriate, as this reduces the chances of the resistant forms emerging. They are also preferred when treating children. The long duration antibiotic course may result in the reduction on the ability of the microflora to resist the colonization of the harmful bacteria which are not normal resident of the oral flora, thereby leading to superimposed infections by multiresistant bacteria and yeasts.

Penicillin

The most commonly used antibiotic in dental practice is penicillin (amoxicillin, followed by penicillin V, metronidazole, and potassium clavulanate). Penicillin is still considered the gold standard in treating dental infections. They act by interfering with the transpeptidase enzyme responsible for the bacterial cell wall rigidity. Gram positive bacteria are sensitive towards the penicillin group but the Gram positive bacteria are protected by an outer layer of lipopolysaccharide. Broad-spectrum antibiotics like amoxicillin are able to penetrate this outer cell wall layer. Phenoxymethylpenicillin (Pen V) is commonly used for all sorts of dental infections. Amoxicillin is more effective than Pen V but is more liable to cause GI side effects than Pen V. Amoxicillin may interfere with the action of oral contraceptives. Ampicillin is better absorbed in the gut and has a more rapid action.

Flucloxacillin is a beta-lactamase resistant form of penicillin and is used for skin organisms. Erythromycin is usually prescribed when patients have allergies to penicillin or amoxicillin. It is bacteriostatic in nature and active against penicillinase-producing organisms. Augmentin is a mixture of amoxicillin and potassium clavulanate—inhibits penicillinase and is active against most *Staphylococcus aureus*. It also inhibits lactamases and is therefore active against some Gram positive and penicillin-resistant bacteria but is contraindicated in penicillin hypersensitivity.

Dosage: Pen V-250–500 mg qds PO, Amoxicillin is 250–500 md tds PO. Tetracycline is given as 250–500 mg qds PO and should be taken before food as the absorption is inhibited by chelation with milk. Erythromycin is given as 250–500 mg qds PO/IV.

Metronidazole

This is an antimicrobial chemotherapeutic agent. It is effective against only anaerobes and acts by disrupting the DNA synthesis and causing the breakdown of the existing DNA. Metronidazole can be used to treat odontogenic conditions like dental abscess, pericoronal infections, acute necrotizing ulcerative gingivitis (ANUG) and wound infections. The classical dose for treating ANUG is 200 mg three times/day PO for 3 days. It is otherwise used as 400 mg twice daily/thrice daily. The most common side effects are nausea and vomiting specially if consumed with alcohol.

Clindamycin

Often is used in the treatment of serious infections caused by susceptible anaerobic bacteria and hence are effective for dental abscesses in bone and soft tissue that does not respond adequately to penicillin or erythromycin. Other uses include endocarditis prophylaxis and salivary gland infections. Clindamycin should be used with caution due to the risk of antibiotic induced colitis. It is useful in the treatment of Staphylococcal osteomyelitis in conjunction with metronidazole. Dose is 150–300 mg orally three times a day.

Chlorhexidine

This is an antibiotic used to control plaque and gingivitis in the mouth, or in periodontal pockets. Chlorhexidine comes as a chip, which is used as an adjunct to scaling and root planing procedures for reducing the depth of pockets around the teeth in patients with adult periodontitis or as a rinse, which provides antimicrobial activity between dental visits. Chlorhexidine may cause staining of the tooth, tooth filling, and dentures or other mouth appliances.

Tetracycline

This is a broad-spectrum antibiotic used mainly for antral infections and osteomyelitis. The major side effect is that it can become incorporated into the developing teeth causing staining. Therefore, it should not be prescribed during the period of tooth development. Tetracyclines like doxycycline and minocycline can be used to help treat periodontal disease.

PROPHYLACTIC ANTIBIOTICS

Prophylactic antibiotics, taken prior to a number of dental procedures, have been advocated to reduce the likelihood of postoperative local complications, like infection, dry socket, or serious systemic complications like infective endocarditis. For most dentoalveolar surgical procedures in fit, nonmedically compromised patients, antibiotic prophylaxis is not required or recommended.

In the case of bacterial endocarditis (IE), the absolute risk rate after dental treatment, even in at-risk patients, is considered very low. This is consistent with recent guidelines from the British Society for Antimicrobial Chemotherapy, and the American Heart Association, which recommend that only patients in the high-risk category require cover.

Prophylaxis of local infection is taken to comprise the administration of antibiotics on a pre-, intra- or postoperative basis, to prevent bacterial proliferation and dissemination within and from the surgical wound. Prophylaxis in oral surgery in a healthy patient was only recommended in the case of the removal of impacted teeth, periapical surgery, bone surgery, implant surgery, bone grafting and surgery for benign tumors. In subjects with risk factors for local or systemic infection including oncological patients, immune suppressed individuals, and patients with metabolic disorders such as diabetes, and splenectomized patients, prophylactic antibiotic coverage should be provided before attempting any invasive procedure. The use of antibiotics in endodontics should be reserved for patients with signs of local infection, malaise or fever. Prophylactic or preventive use should be reserved for endocarditis and the systemic disorders commented above avoiding indiscriminate antibiotic use.

Recommendations

Drainage is the recommended treatment for periapical periodontitis and for localized dentoalveolar abscess, with incisional drainage rather than via the root canal preferred. Empirical antibiotic therapy and drainage are recommended for more severe infections such as facial cellulitis, Pericoronitis, lateral periodontal abscess, and necrotizing ulcerative gingivitis. The type of antibiotic chosen and its dosing regimen are dependent upon the severity of infection and the predominant type of causative bacteria.

Dosage: Amoxicillin is recommended for dental infections in doses ranging from 250 to 500 mg, every 8 hours. Another antibiotic is coamoxiclav, which can be used in doses ranging from 375 to 625 mg every 8 hours. In patients allergic to penicillin, clindamycin can be used in doses ranging from 150 to 450 mg every 6 hours. For severe odontogenic infections, higher doses of a broad-spectrum antibiotic may be required. Patients who are allergic to penicillin should benefit from clindamycin as it is active against some oral anaerobes penetration. However, increasing the dose may increase the possibility of serious side effects such as pseudomembranous colitis, Sweet's syndrome, and neutropenia. Infections in which anaerobic bacteria are implicated (such as pericoronitis, periodontal abscess and necrotizing ulcerative gingivitis) are better treated with metronidazole.

In addition to the proper dosing regimens and professionally responsible prescribing practices, the general public needs to be educated about the importance of restricting the use of antibiotics to only cases of severe infection. Patients have become accustomed to being given an antibiotic for a range of medical complaints. Unfortunately, patients presenting at dental surgeries also routinely expect an antibiotic for the treatment of 'toothache'. Dental patients not only pressure their dentist to get an antibiotic prescription, they also self-medicate.

TOPICAL ANTIBIOTICS

Some topical antibiotics are available without a prescription and are sold in many forms, including creams, ointments, powders, and sprays. Some widely used topical antibiotics are bacitracin, neomycin, and polymyxin B. The value of topical antibiotics overweighs risks in some cases. Tetracycline is a useful topical antibiotic as at 2% solution it is often effective in reducing secondary infection (and thus the discomfort) in cases of aphthous stomatitis, primary herpetic stomatitis, and all oral ulcerative conditions. Use of topical antibiotics is also seen to be helpful in acute chronic gingivitis treatment. On the other hand, there are inherent disadvantages associated with the use of topical antibiotics (Table 10.9).

They can be used to prevent secondary infection (ulcers). The use of topical antibiotics cannot normally be practiced as long-term treatment, and it is better to be reserved for acute episodes. Long-term use increases the risk of overgrowth of resistant organisms, and chances of a *Candida* infection. However, in some rare cases a prolonged topical antibiotic treatment is justified (patients with severe and persistent oral lesions). In such cases, a tetracycline with triamcinolone combination is preferred.

Precautions with Antibiotic Use

- Kidney failure.
- Many antibiotics are actively eliminated through the kidneys. The presence of impaired renal function requires reduction of the drug dose

Table 10.9 Antibiotics used in dentistry

Drug	*Route of administration*	*Recommended dosage*	*Side effects*
Penicillin V, K	IM/IV	250–500 mg/day/ 6 hours for 7–10 days	Nausea, vomiting, hypersensitivity reactions, and diarrhea. Penicillin V, Penicillin K can turn the tongue black occasionally (black hairy tongue)
Amoxicillin	PO IV	500 mg/8 hours or 1 gm/12 hours	Diarrhea, nausea, vomiting, hypersensitivity reactions and yeast infections in women
Amoxicillin-clavulanic acid	PO IV	375–625 mg/ 8 hours or 2000 mg/12 hours 1000–2000 mg/ 8 hours	Diarrhea, nausea, candidiasis and hypersensitivity reactions
Erythromycin (usually prescribed to patients with penicillin allergy)	PO	250–500 mg/ 6 hours for 7–10 days	Same as penicillin but more common
Clindamycin	PO IV	300 mg/8 hours 600 mg/8 hours	Diarrhea, abdominal pain and pseudomembranous colitis
Metronidazole	PO	500–750 mg/ 8 hours	Anesthesia/ parasthesia of the limbs, incompatible with alcohol consumption
Ciprofloxacin	PO	500 mg/12 hours	Gastrointestinal disorders

Abbreviations: PO, Oral route; IM, Intramuscular route; IV, Intravenous route

in order to avoid excessively elevated plasma drug concentrations that could lead to toxicity.

- Liver failure.
- Some antibiotics are metabolized in the liver, followed by elimination in bile. In patients with liver failure, the use of such antibiotics should be restricted in order to avoid toxicity secondary to overdose. Erythromycin,

clindamycin, metronidazole and antituberculosis drugs are antibiotics requiring dose adjustments when administered to patients with liver failure. Regardless of the above considerations, some antibiotics are potentially hepatotoxic. As a result, and whenever possible, they should be avoided in patients with some active liver disorder.

- In patients with a previous history of infective endocarditis.
- In patients who have undergone cardiac valve replacements surgery.

ANTIFUNGAL AGENTS

Antifungals are used for the treatment of candidiasis in the oral cavity. Certain antifungal agents such as nystatin are used to treat *Candida albicans* infection in the mouth, including thrush, and denture stomatitis. They are available in various forms, such as lozenges, pastilles, creams, and suspensions (Table 10.10). Unfortunately, patient compliance is often poor with these preparations, which may take a while to dissolve in the mouth (for example, pastilles and lozenges) and have a distinctive taste.

Nystatin and Amphotericin

Nystatin (Mycostatin) comes in lozenges and oral suspension. When taking the oral suspension, patients are instructed to take one half of the dose in each side of mouth, retaining the suspension as long as possible by swishing it around, before swallowing. These agents act by inhibiting the ergosterol synthesis and the DNA synthesis and also by causing the disruption of the fungal plasma. In cases when the *Candida* infection is related to dentures, denture hygiene instructions should be stressed upon. A number of effective antifungal agents are available.

Table 10.10 Topical antifungal therapy

Pseudomembranous, erythematous hyperplastic candidiasis
• Amphotericin lozenges (10 mg) • Nystatin pastilles (100,000 units): These are dissolved slowly in the mouth, after meals: use 4 times/daily
Candida-associated denture stomatitis
• Amphotericin or nystatin (as above) and remove dentures • Miconazole gel applied to palatal surface of denture 4 times daily for 1 to 4 weeks • Chlorhexidine 0.2% rinse, 4 times daily (do not use with nystatin)
Candida-associated angular cheilitis
• Nystatin cream; apply to corners of mouth 3 to 4 times daily, until resolution • Miconazole cream (or gel); apply 3 to 4 times daily to angles of the mouth

The polyenes antifungal agents like nystatin and amphotericin B, are relatively free from side-effects when used locally. They attach to the fungal cell membrane and disrupt the permeability.

Amphotericin is available as 10 mg lozenges. Nystatin ointment (100,000 U/g) is used on fitting surfaces of dentures and corners of the mouth. It is available as a cream, rinse, or lozenge (sugar added to liquids). Amphotericin is used alone if the patient does not wear dentures, or in conjunction with nystatin ointment or miconazole if dentures are worn—for a period of three weeks. The ointment should be liberally applied to the fitting surface of the denture four times daily. At night, dentures should be removed and cleaned thoroughly and soaked twice weekly in a diluted solution (approximately 1:20) of either sodium hypochlorite (common bleach) or white vinegar. This latter step is most important as the denture will act as a reservoir of infection if not treated in this way.

Miconazole

This belongs to the imidazole group of antifungal agents. It is effective against Gram positive bacteria and has a mixed fungal/bacterial action. This makes it more effective in treating angular cheilitis than polyenes. The available forms are oral, cream and cream with 1% hydrocortisone. Oral gel (20 mg/mL) is to be used four times daily in a dose of half a measuring spoon dropped onto the tongue and swished around the mouth for as long as possible before swallowing. Alternatively, place on the fitting surface of the denture four times daily. Care should be taken with the use of miconazole as it can potentiate the effect of warfarin.

Triazoles

Itraconazole, fluconazole and ketoconazole are reserved for debilitated or immune-compromised patients. These agents act systemically and inhibit fungal enzymes associated with ergosterol synthesis. The available formulation is capsules given as 50 mg daily for 7–14 days.

ANTIVIRAL AGENTS

HSV-1 is the most common viral infection affecting dental profession's area of responsibility. Few drugs have been developed in past 5 years although there is no specific treatment for most viral infections affecting oral cavity (Table 10.11). Most of the antiviral agents are capable of interfering with the reproductive processes of viruses and are likely to be toxic to host cells.

Acyclovir

Although the antiviral agent acyclovir has been found to be of benefit in limiting the extent of primary genital HSV2 infections, it has had less effect

Table 10.11 Antiviral therapy

Dosage
• Herpes labialis (cold sore)—cream is applied to the site of the early lesion every 4 hourly for 5 days • Herpes stomatitis—200 mg PO 5 times daily for 5 days • Herpes zoster—800 mg PO 5 times daily for 7 days

on orofacial HSV1 primary infections in healthy individuals. However, it does have an important role in the management of primary and secondary HSV1 infections in immune compromised patients and acute attacks of herpes zoster. This acts by disrupting the viral DNA synthesis. This is available as tablets (200 and 800 mg), suspension (200 mg/5 mL), and cream (5%). Topical acyclovir is useful for recurrent herpetic infections, but must be started early in the prodromal phase to be effective. Acyclovir should be avoided in pregnancy, lactation and in renal disease. The recent drugs for the management of herpes zoster are valacyclovir and famcyclovir.

AGENTS USED TO CONTROL ANXIETY

Fear and anxiety of dentistry are common. The severity ranges widely, with mild apprehension to severe anxiety, leading to avoidance of dental treatment. Although mild fear may have only a minor impact on oral health, true phobia can cause patient to avoid treatment in spite of significant symptoms and to have detrimental consequences for their overall health. The usefulness and effectiveness of any given antianxiety agent will vary, depending on the patient, the clinical surroundings, the "chairside" manner of the dentist, the route of administration, and the properties of the chosen drug. The antianxiety agents summate with the anesthetics, antipsychotics, antidepressants, opioid analgesics, and sedative-hypnotics. The antianxiety agents are important in dentistry for the premedication of the apprehensive patient, the patient exhibiting mild neurosis associated with the mouth, and the uncooperative child. Antianxiety agents, particularly intravenous midazolam and diazepam, are used as adjuncts to local anesthesia.

Benzodiazepines

The benzodiazepines rank as one of the most widely used drug classes in the history of medicine. This popularity stems from the fact that they are more selective and have a greater margin of safety than drugs used earlier (e.g. barbiturates) for the treatment of anxiety. Currently, there are several dozen benzodiazepines being marketed throughout the world. The most important pharmacologic effects of the benzodiazepines are on the CNS.

They bind to the GABA receptors in the cerebral cortex and enhance their activity. The benzodiazepines have clinically useful antianxiety, sedative-hypnotic, anticonvulsant, and skeletal muscle relaxant properties. The clinical effects of these agents in humans are anxiety reduction at low doses and production of drowsiness, and even sleep at higher doses. They do not have any analgesic effect.

The benzodiazepines, particularly diazepam, have anticonvulsant activity (i.e. they increase the seizure threshold). Diazepam has been shown to be an effective anticonvulsant for the prevention of seizures associated with local anesthetic toxicity and for the treatment of status epilepticus. This is also used as a pre-medication to help anxious patients achieve sleep before their dental treatment and to relieve nervousness an hour or two before appointments. Diazepam is also used patients with myofascial pain dysfunction syndrome to relax the muscles of mastication. Drowsiness and sedation are common manifestations of this central depressant action and may be considered a side effect in some instances and therapeutically useful in others. As is true of any sedative drug, the benzodiazepines are respiratory depressants. In normal doses the benzodiazepines have little effect on respiration in the healthy person.

Adverse Effects

The most common side effect of the benzodiazepines is drowsiness. This may not necessarily be an unwanted side effect, but rather a desirable therapeutic response to anxiety states that cause insomnia. Other side effects that are a result of dose-dependent CNS depression include ataxia, incoordination, dysarthria, confusion, apathy, muscle weakness, dizziness, particularly in elderly people. Tolerance and psychological dependence occur rather frequently with the benzodiazepines, but true physical dependence is less common.

In cases of physical dependence, the severity of withdrawal depends on the dose of the drug being used and the drug half-life. The symptoms become more severe with high doses and prolonged treatment. Withdrawal can be minimized by reducing the dosage very gradually (10% or less per day over a course of 10–14 days) or by the use of longer-acting compounds. Despite these problems, one of the major advantages of the benzodiazepines, as compared to other sedatives, is their high margin of safety. Death is rare in cases of overdose and is usually the result of a combination of drugs (especially alcohol) with the benzodiazepines.

Precautions

Patients should be warned of the sedative effects and should be accompanied to and from the dental surgery. They should not drive a car or use domestic or industrial machinery/appliances. Alcohol should be avoided during the use of benzodiazepines as it enhances the effect of the drug.

OTHER DRUGS USED IN DENTISTRY

Topical Antiseptics

First Generation

The agents that do not exhibit any significant substantivity (only minutes) were categorized as first-generation antimicrobial agents and are composed of certain antibiotics, quaternary ammonium compounds (cetylpyridinium chloride), essential oil phenolic compounds fluorides including mono fluorophosphates and sodium fluoride, oxidizing agents, plant alkaloids and iodine including povidone iodine.

Second Generation

Second-generation antimicrobial agents are characterized by high substantivity, that is, retention of 25–30% after each 1-minute mouth rinse. Such compounds remain active *in situ* for hours and include bis-biguanides (such as Chlorhexidine), amine fluoride and stannous fluoride mouth rinse, triclosan when associated with a copolymer of polyvinyl methyl ether and maleic acid copolymer.

Chlorhexidine

The most effective antiplaque agent known today is chlorhexidine, which has been used for more than two decades. This is a biguanide antiseptic. The mode of action of chlorhexidine against bacteria is concentration dependent. Chlorhexidine has antibacterial activity. It can be used as a mouthwash, spray, or gel to control secondary infections in mucosal ulcerations. This is mainly effective against Gram positive bacteria. Chlorhexidine acts on the cell wall of the microorganisms by changing their surface structures. Because chlorhexidine has been shown to be able to break up existing dental plaque, it can be considered as a potent antibacterial agent, bactericidal at high concentration and bacteriostatic at lower concentration, such as when gradually diluted in saliva over time. This is mainly indicated in the treatment of periodontal pockets, and in cases of oral ulceration to prevent secondary infection and to promote healing. The side effects include staining on teeth and tongue which is largely dose dependent and reversible. Desquamation of the oral mucosa and perturbation of the taste can also occur with prolonged use of chlorhexidine and are usually concentration dependent.

Anesthetics

Topical anesthetics come in ointments, sprays or liquids. Topical anesthetics are used to prevent pain on the surface level of the lining of the mouth. They also can be used to reduce pain from superficial sores in the mouth or to numb an area before an injectable local anesthetic is given. Local anesthetics are injected into the deeper tissues of the mouth and work by inhibiting the impulses from pain-sensing nerves and hence are used to reduce pain especially in procedures involving drilling, and cutting of the tissue. Common local anesthetics are 2% lidocaine hydrochloride and 2% mepivicaine. General anesthetics are inhaled and include antianxiety agents, such as nitrous oxide, that help to ensure relaxation during dental visits and often may be used along with local anesthetics. Anesthetics are used for temporary pain relief, and should not be used for long durations of time.

Saliva Substitutes

Saliva substitutes are used for treating dry mouth, an occasional complication of autoimmune diseases or occasionally unassociated with other diseases. They usually come as sprays and are used as needed. The cause of dry mouth should always be established first and foremost without using/ prescribing these medicines.

PREGNANT PATIENT

Overestimation of the risk of teratogenicity in the fetus resulting from medical and dental drugs/procedures may cause a dentist to avoid necessary treatment of the pregnant patient. During pregnancy, dental treatment may be modified but need not be withheld, provided that the risk assessment is made before starting the procedure. Medications used during pregnancy still cause anxiety and misunderstanding amongst both members of the public and the dental health care professional. Primarily, dentists should be familiar with the risks and benefits of five types of medications namely: *analgesics, and anti-inflammatories, antibiotics, local anesthetics, sedatives and emergency medications.*

Teratogenic drugs are medications that may be associated with the development of structural abnormalities in a developing fetus (cleft lip and palate). The greatest risk to the fetus is from 3 to 8 weeks after conception. For example, use of NSAIDs may be associated with fetal renal dysfunction in the second and third trimester and premature closure of the ductus arteriosus in the third trimester. The aim when prescribing medicines to a pregnant patient is to balance the risks of the drug's adverse effects (on the fetus) with the benefit (on the mother) of treating the disease.

To determine the risks associated with the use of drugs in pregnancy, The United States Food and Drug Administration (FDA) has classified drugs based on the level of risk they may pose for the fetus (Table 10.12). Accordingly, drugs in categories A and B are considered safe for use, whereas drugs in category C may be used only if the benefits outweigh the risks (Table 10.13). Additionally, drugs in category D should be avoided except in exceptional circumstances. Use of category X drugs in pregnancy is strictly prohibited.

Table 10.12 Food and Drug Administration pregnancy risk factor definitions

Category	*Definition*
A	Controlled studies fail to demonstrate a risk to the fetus in the first trimester (and there is no evidence of risk in later trimesters), and the possibility of fetal harm appears remote
B	Either reproduction studies have not demonstrated a fetal risk but there are no controlled studies in pregnant women or animal reproduction studies which show an adverse effect (other than a decrease in fertility) that was not confirmed in controlled studies in women in the first trimester (and there is no evidence of risk in later trimesters)
C	Either animal studies have revealed adverse effects on the fetus (teratogenic, embryocidal, or other) and there are no controlled studies in women or studies in women and animals are not available. Drugs should be given only if the potential benefit justifies the potential risk to the patient
D	There is positive evidence of human fetal risk, but the benefits of use in pregnant women may be acceptable despite the risk (for example, if the drug is needed in a life-threatening situation or for a serious disease for which safer drugs cannot be used or are ineffective)
X	Studies in animals or human beings have demonstrated fetal abnormalities or there is evidence of fetal risk based on human experience, or both, and the risk of the use of the drug in pregnant women clearly outweighs any possible benefit. The drug is contraindicated in women who are or may become pregnant

Source: US Food and Drug Administration, Physicians' desk reference, 56 edn. Montvale, NJ: Medical Economics, 2002:342

Table 10.13 Pregnant woman

Clinical considerations for pregnant women:
• Use medication only if the expected benefit outweighs the risk • Try to avoid during the first trimester • Prescribe the minimum dose required for the desired effect

No antibiotic corresponds to category A. Category B (caution should be used with treatment during pregnancy) contains: Azithromycin, cephalosporins, erythromycin metronidazole and penicillin with or without beta-lactamase. Category C includes clarithromycin, and the sulpha drugs. Gate gory D contains aminoglycosides and tetracyclines (Table 10.14).

Local Anesthetics

There are no general contraindications to the use of lidocaine with epinephrine or prilocaine in pregnant patients provided that aspiration is performed to minimize the risk of intravascular injections. Both these drugs are category B listed. The use of long acting local anesthetic bupivacaine should be avoided during pregnancy to minimize the risk of fetal exposure and toxicity. Other commonly used local anesthetics like—articaine, bupivacaine and mepivicaine all are listed as category C drugs. Topical anesthetics fall like—benzocaine, lidocaine and tetracaine fall under the category C listing except for lidocaine which is B category. These local and topical anesthetics have been associated with a condition called methemoglobinemia. This is caused by the conversion of the iron molecule in hemoglobin from the ferrous to the ferric state, thus resulting in the inability of the hemoglobin molecule to transfer oxygen. Therefore, the use of benzocaine, tetracaine and prilocaine should be avoided in patients with a history of methemoglobinemia.

Analgesics and NSAIDs

Acetaminophen (also known as Paracetamol) is widely accepted for use during pregnancy as the choice of analgesic. The absorption and disposition of the drug is not altered during pregnancy. It does not prolong the bleeding time, unlike aspirin, and is nontoxic to the fetus. The use of NSAIDs is not favorable during pregnancy as these drugs may inhibit labor and prolong the length of pregnancy. Ibuprofen may cause embryonic implantation disturbances, inhibition of parturition and gastroschisis (a congenital malformation in which the fetal organs develop outside the abdominal wall). Glucocorticoids such as prednisone and dexamethasone have been associated with oral clefts if administered during the first trimester. Narcotics like codeine are also not recommended as they lack any anti-inflammatory property. Therefore, the risk outweighs the benefit of this drug. Despite being nonteratogenic, aspirin and the group of salicylates should be avoided during pregnancy. These drugs may cause maternal and fetal hemorrhage, as well as prolonged labor. Use of aspirin during pregnancy, (especially chronic use or intermittent high doses) is not recommended during the second and third trimester.

Table 10.14 Drugs used in pregnancy

Drug	*FDA Category*	*Safe use in pregnancy*
Analgesics		
Acetaminophen	B	Yes
Aspirin	C/D	Avoid if possible, do not use in the third trimester
Codeine	C	Use with caution, low dose of short duration is acceptable
NSAIDs (Ibuprofen)	B/D	Avoid in the third trimester
Local Anesthetics		
Lidocaine (with or without epinephrine)	B	Yes
Articaine	C	Yes but use with caution
Bupivacaine	B	Yes
Mepivacaine	C	Yes but use with caution
Prilocaine	B	Yes
Lidocaine (topical)	B	Yes
Benzocaine (topical)	C	Yes but use with caution
Antibiotics		
Penicillin	B	Yes
Amoxicillin	B	Yes
Amoxicillin + Clavulanic acid	B	Yes
Azithromycin	B	Yes
Clindamycin	B	Yes
Cephalosporins	B	Yes
Erythromycin	B	Yes
Tetracycline	D	Avoid (No)
Doxycycline	D	No
Metronidazole	B	Yes but use with caution
Nystatin	B/C	Yes
Fluconazole	C	Yes but use with caution, single-dose regimen
Chlorhexidine (topical and rinse)	B	Yes
Sedatives		
Benzodiazepines	D/X	No

Source: Data compiled from Briggs et al.

Antibiotics

Penicillin V and amoxicillin are the safest and most commonly prescribed antibiotic drugs during pregnancy. Some antibiotics can cross the placental membrane and get deposited in the growing embryo's teeth and bones at sites of active calcification. All the tetracyclines have this effect and can produce yellow staining of both the primary and the secondary dentition. These group of drugs fall under the risk category D including doxycycline. Metronidazole and erythromycin should be used with caution in breast-feeding patients as these drugs are concentrated in the human milk. The breast-feeding mother should be advised to discontinue breast-feeding for 12–24 hours to allow the excretion of the drug. Anti-fungals are not prescribed commonly by the dentist. If a need arises for such a prescription, then oral nystatin (category C) is the safest drug to use both in pregnant and breast-feeding patients.

Sedatives

Benzodiazepines are the most commonly used drugs in this category. Their effects during pregnancy may be related to fetal abortion, malformations, intrauterine growth retardation, functional deficits, carcinogenesis and mutagenesis, with the greatest risk between two and eight weeks after conception. If these drugs are used near term, fetal dependence and withdrawal may occur. Due to all the above mentioned reasons, this group of drugs has been listed as category D/X by the FDA.

Prenatal Fluoride

Fluoride use cannot be recommended to a pregnant patient since it seems ineffective and the scientific basis for its use is still lacking.

NEWER DRUGS OF USE IN DENTISTRY (APPROVED BY FDA IN 1996)

Amlexanox (Aphthasol)

This is a locally applied anti-inflammatory indicated for the treatment of signs and symptoms of canker sores (minor aphthous ulcers) (Table 10.15). It is supplied as a 5% paste. The recommended dosage is the application of a small amount directly to ulcers 4 times daily following oral hygiene, after meals, and before going to bed. The adverse effects are a stinging or burning sensation at the site of application.

Table 10.15 Newer drugs

Name	Use
Amlexanox	Aphthous ulcers
Penciclovir	Recurrent herpes labialis
Lidocaine patch	Local anesthetic
Tetracaine 2%	Cold sore (as an analgesic)

Penciclovir (Denavir)

This is a topical antiviral agent indicated for the treatment of recurrent herpes labialis (cold sores) in adults. It is supplied as a 1% cream in 2 g tubes. The recommended dosage is the application of a small amount at the first sign or symptom of a cold sore (e.g. tingling, swelling), and then every 2 hours, during waking hours, for 4 days.

Lidocaine Transoral Mucosal Dental Delivery System (Dent Patch)

This is a preparation of lidocaine available in a transoral patch to provide local anesthesia of the oral mucosa prior to oral injections and soft-tissue dental procedures. The recommended dose is one patch applied to a selected area of the oral mucosa. The onset of anesthesia is 2 minutes after patch application, with duration of 45 minutes.

Tetracaine 2% (Viractin)

This is used for cold sore and fever blister. It is available in 0.25 oz. cream and gel forms. The 2% tetracaine penetrates the skin to attack the source of pain.

CONCLUSION

This chapter highlights the common dental drugs to avoid and drugs that are relatively safe to use in dentistry. While prescribing, the dentist must weigh the balance between the risk associated and the benefit provided, and the appropriate conclusion should be made. Proper assessment, intervention, and patient education about various dental problems can help to enhance the desired outcome. Dentists should help the patients understand all of the risks and benefits before they use any prescribed medication.

BIBLIOGRAPHY

1. Ahmad N, Grad HA, Haas DA, Aronson KJ, Jokovic A, Locker D. The efficacy of nonopioid analgesics for postoperative dental pain: a meta-analysis. Anesth Prog. 1997;44:119-26.
2. Barsan WG, Jastremski MS, Syverud SA, Eds: Emergency drug therapy, Philadelphia 1991, WB. Saunders.
3. Briggs GG, Freeman RK, Yaffe SJ. Drugs in Pregnancy and lactation, 4th edn. Baltimore: Williams and Wilkins, 1994.
4. Dionne RA, Phero JC. Management of pain and anxiety in dental practice. New York, 1991, Elsevier Science.
5. Dray A, Urban L, Dickenson A. Pharmacology of chronic pain. Trends Pharmacol Sci. 1994;15:190-7.
6. Garcia-Martin E, Martinez C, Tabares B, Frias J, Agundez JA. Interindividual variability in ibuprofen pharmacokinetics is related to interaction of cytochrome P450 2C8 and 2C9 amino acid polymorphisms. Clin Pharmacol Ther. 2004;76: 119-27.
7. Hardman JG, Limbird LE, (Eds). Goodman and Gilman's the pharmacological basis of therapeu tics, 9 edn. New York, 1996, McGraw-Hill.
8. Hargreaves KM, Dubner R. Mechanisms of pain and analgesia. In Dionne RA, Phero JC, Eds. Management of pain and anxiety in dental practice, New York, 1991, Elsevier Science.
9. Hyllested M, Jones S, Pedersen JL, Kehlet H. Comparative effect of paracetamol, NSAIDs or their combination in postoperative pain management: a qualitative review. Br J Anaesth. 2002;88:199-214.
10. Ibuprofen. *http://www.rxlist.com/cgi/generic/ibup_cp.htm.* Accessed March 2013.
11. Joshi A, Parara E, Macfarlane TV. A double-blind randomized controlled clinical trial of the effect of preoperative ibuprofen, diclofenac, paracetamol with codeine and placebo tablets for relief of postoperative pain after removal of impacted third molars. Br J Oral Maxillofac Surg. 2004;42:299-306.
12. Nikkels AF, Pierard GE. Treatment of mucocutaneous presentations of herpes simplex virus infections. Am J Clin Dermatol. 2002;3:475-87.
13. Omoigui S. The pain drugs handbook, St Louis, 1995, Mosby-Year Book.
14. Oxford League Table of Analgesic Efficacy. *http://www.jr2.ox.ac. uk/bandolier/booth/painpag/Acutrev/Analgesics/lftab.html.* Accessed March 2013.
15. O'Brien TP, Roszkowski MT, Wolff LF, Hinrichs JE, Hargreaves KM. Effect of a non-steroidal anti-inflammatory drug on tissue levels of immunoreactive prostaglandin E2, immunoreactive leukotriene, and pain after periodontal surgery. J Periodontal. 1996;67:1307-16.
16. Pasternak GW. Pharmacological mechanisms of opioid analgesics, Clin Neuropharmacol. 1993;16:1-18.
17. Pearlman B, Boyatzis S, Daly C, et al. The analgesic efficacy of ibuprofen in periodontal surgery: A multicentre study. Aust Dent J. 1997;42:328-34.
18. Siegel MA. Diagnosis and management of recurrent herpes simplex infections. J Am Dent Assoc. 2002;133:1245-9.
19. Stoopler ET, Greenberg MS. Update on herpesvirus infections. Dent Clin North Am. 2003;47:517 32.
20. Therapeutic Guidelines. Analgesics Version 4. Melbourne: Therapeutic Guidelines Ltd. 2002.pp.117-8.
21. Therapeutic Guidelines: Analgesics Version 4. Melbourne: Therapeutic Guidelines Ltd. 2002.pp.30-2.
22. Titsas A, Ferguson MM. Impact of opioid use on dentistry. Aust Dent J. 2002; 47:94-8.

CHAPTER **11**

DRUG INTERACTIONS

Balaram Naik, Priyanka Jain

INTRODUCTION

A drug interaction is defined as the action of an administered drug on the effectiveness or toxicity of another drug administered earlier, simultaneously, or later. The problem of drug interactions can become serious because some drug combinations result in more than a mere decrease in effectiveness; they could be potentially lethal. A dentist is likely to see many patients, especially elderly, who are taking either self-prescribed medications or medications prescribed by their physicians for other ailments. As the number of medications taken by a patient increases, so does the possibility of serious drug interactions. A complete medical history with a list of all other medications taken by the patient along with dosages is necessary to minimize the problems of drug interactions.

Drug-Drug Interactions

Some drugs interact with or interfere with the actions of other drugs. An example of one drug interfering with the action of another is the use of certain types of antacids when taken at the same time as tetracycline (orally) (an antibiotic used in the treatment of infections). The antacid may chemically interact with tetracycline and impair its absorption into the bloodstream, thus reducing the effectiveness of tetracycline.

Drug interactions can also be antagonistic or synergistic. Antagonistic drugs may interact with food, chemicals, or other drugs and produce opposing effects. An example of a beneficial antagonistic drug effect is the reaction of histamine with antihistamine. Antihistamines may be used to counteract (antagonize) the effects of histamine, which is a substance produced by the body as a natural allergic reaction response. Other antagonistic drug effects may not be beneficial. The administration of one drug that dilates blood vessels along with a drug that constricts blood vessels greatly reduces the effects of both drugs because the drugs are antagonistic to one another.

A synergistic drug effect may occur when a drug interacts with another drug (or drugs) and produces an effect that is greater than the sum of the separate actions of the two or more drugs. In other words, they end up working as an overdose of the individual drugs. A synergistic drug effect is seen in the person who takes a hypnotic, (a central nervous system depressant) that induces sleep, along with alcohol (also a central nervous system depressant) at the same time or shortly before or after the hypnotic. As a result the action of the hypnotic is potentiated, or increased. On occasion a synergistic drug effect can be serious and even fatal.

Drug-Food Interactions

Some drugs must be taken on an empty stomach, and some must be taken with food to achieve the best effect. Depending on the oral drug that is given, food may impair or enhance its absorption. When a drug is taken on an empty stomach, it will be absorbed into the bloodstream at a faster rate than it will be when taken with food in the stomach. Some drugs, especially those capable of irritating the stomach, can cause nausea, vomiting, or epigastric distress and are best taken with food or meals. However, the following oral drugs should be given at least 30 minutes before food, as their absorption is otherwise delayed: aspirin, erythromycin, and paracetamol/acetaminophen, penicillin, rifampicin, and tetracyclines (except doxycycline).

Herbal Supplements

Herbal supplements can cause side effects on their own or when combined with prescribed medications (Table 11.1). Other side effects of herbal supplements include episodes of oral ulcers, lip irritation, swelling and gingival bleeding. There are also chances of increased gingival bleeding with ginkgo; and oral and lingual dyskinesia with the use of kava.

Some Examples: *Grapefruit juice* disturbs absorption of cyclosporin, calcium channel blockers (e.g. nifedipine). Grapefruit juice and drinks that contain grapefruit juice or fresh, canned, or frozen grapefruit, may also alter the metabolism of several drugs, increasing the toxicity of benzodiazepines, carbamazepine and corticosteroids. *Sour orange juice, real lime juice, cranberry, and tangelos* (a hybrid of grapefruit), may possibly also have this effect. The effect appears to last for at least three days following ingestion, and could perhaps be longer in some patients. *Citrus juice* improves iron absorption, but may cause some medications to dissolve prematurely in the stomach rather than in the intestine as intended.

Table 11.1 Herbal supplements

Supplement	*Stop using prior to dental surgery*
Garlic and ginseng	At least seven days
Ginkgo	At least 36 hours
Kava and ephedra	At least 24 hours

Calcium, in dairy foods and in calcium supplements, chelates tetracycline, which is passed out of the body without being absorbed. Therefore, avoid high-calcium foods (milk products or supplements) within two hours of taking the medication, to minimize this problem. *Iron magnesium* and *aluminum* in drugs can impair absorption of tetracycline. Iron reduces absorption of quinolones (e.g. ciprofloxacin). Aluminum can impair absorption of azole antifungals. Phytates present in chapattis (Indian bread) bind calcium and impair its absorption. *Warfarin* can be antagonized by vitamin K in foods such as liver, cabbage, spinach, cauliflower, green tea and broccoli. At the same time warfarin activity can be enhanced by garlic supplements, and cranberry juice.

Garlic in the food alters pharmacokinetic variables of acetaminophen, decreases blood concentrations of warfarin, and produces hypoglycemia when taken with chlorpropamide (oral antidiabetic) (Izzo AA, Ernst E. Drugs. 2001;61:2163-2175).

Ginkgo reacts with aspirin, (causes hyphema (blood in eye), acetaminophen (causes bilateral subdural hematomas), warfarin (causes intracerebral hemorrhage), and valproate (can cause seizures).

Analgesics, anesthesia, anesthetics, antibiotics, and vasoconstrictors are the drugs most likely to cause a reaction when used in conjunction with herbal supplements. Other frequently used medications in dentistry include antiseptics, anti-inflammatory medications, antifungals, fluoride, muscle relaxants, pain relievers, and saliva stimulants. To lessen interaction potential in surgical situations, many anesthesiologists recommend discontinuing the use of herbal supplements two to three weeks before surgery. It is recommended that dentists tell their patients to stop using the following herbal supplements prior to dental surgery of any type:

The most common side effect resulting from drug interactions between drugs used in dentistry and herbal supplements is bleeding. Increased bleeding during dental surgeries can cause a variety of complications, and sometimes hospitalization. Dental surgeries include procedures such as tooth extractions, periodontal surgeries, root planning, and biopsies. Bleeding can also complicate routine procedures such as prophylaxis, exams, and restorations.

Increased bleeding is not the only side effect of interactions between herbal supplements and dental medicines. Herbal supplements can have an impact on cardiac function, immunity to fight infections, metabolism of drug compounds, pain thresholds, recovery time, bruising, and sedation effects. These supplements can increase or decrease the potency of prescription medications, reducing their effectiveness or leading to the accumulation of otherwise beneficial drugs to toxic levels in the body.

Adverse Drug Reactions

An adverse drug reaction is a symptom that is usually not desired when a drug is introduced to the body. For example, nausea, vomiting, difficulty breathing, diarrhea, dryness of mouth, constipation, and headache. Almost all drugs can potentially cause one or more adverse reactions, some of which may be severe and, on rare occasions, fatal. Usually, adverse reactions occur in few individuals, making many drugs relatively safe. Adverse reactions, or side effects, may occur after the first dose or after several doses. Many adverse drug reactions occur without warning, but some adverse drug reactions are predictable. For example, drugs used in the treatment of cancer are toxic and are known to produce adverse reactions in most of the patients who receive them. These are predictable adverse reactions that cannot be avoided. In such instances the adverse reaction may need to be tolerated because the drug is necessary for the treatment of a specific disease or disorder. Sometimes adverse reactions can be controlled or nearly eliminated. For example, dryness of the mouth, although uncomfortable, may need to be tolerated by the patient who has an ulcer and is being treated with a drug that is known to cause this adverse reaction. Often, drinking sips of cold water or allowing hard candy to dissolve in the mouth decreases this adverse reaction to a tolerable level.

TYPES OF DRUG INTERACTIONS

When two or more drugs interact the result may be either the enhancement or the depression of the pharmacological effects of the agents. There are two types of drug interactions: pharmacokinetic and pharmacodynamic.

Pharmacokinetic

This is the study of the action of drugs within the body, which can, in many respects, be envisioned more accurately as the actions of the body on an administered drug. It includes studies of the mechanisms of drug absorption, distribution, metabolism, and excretion; onset of action; duration of effect; biotransformation; and effects and routes of excretion of the metabolites of the drug.

Absorption

This may be altered in three ways: (1) adsorbed on a large surface area, (2) bound or chelated, and (3) altered gastrointestinal tract (GIT) motility. The rate of absorption and the extent of absorption (the amount absorbed of total dose taken) are the two factors which need to be taken into consideration. The absorption of a drug will be decreased if an inactive or insoluble derivative is formed in the intestinal tract. For example, the effect of tetracycline is decreased if the patient is taking antacids, iron, or zinc sulfate. Milk and dairy products also decrease tetracycline effect. Change in pH also alters the disintegration and dissolution of some drugs which in turn affect their absorption. Any slight change in pH alters the proportion of drug in the ionized form which in turn would result in the change of absorption of the drug.

Distribution

After absorption, the drug reversibly bound to the plasma proteins. The bound portion of a drug is biologically inactive, whereas the free portion exerts the desired pharmacologic effect. Since many weak acids are bound to the same site on the plasma proteins, an acidic drug can displace a bound acidic drug from its plasma protein-binding site, increasing the plasma concentration of the displaced drug and indirectly increasing its pharmacologic effect and toxicity. For example, aspirin and warfarin are both acidic drugs that bind to the same site on the plasma proteins. Aspirin would displace warfarin from the protein binding site, thereby increasing the amount of free warfarin which would increase its pharmacologic effect and toxicity which can lead to hemorrhage.

Metabolism

Before a drug can be excreted by the kidney, it must be metabolized into more water-soluble derivatives in the liver for it to be effective. Microsomal enzymes present in the liver are responsible for metabolizing the drugs. If there is an increase in these enzymes, as a result of certain drugs, then drugs metabolized by these enzymes would have less effect. Phenobarbital, carbamazepine, phenytoin, and rifampin are common enzyme inducers. On the other hand, cimetidine inhibits hepatic microsomal drug metabolism and enhances the action of many drugs metabolized by that system. Erythromycin, allopurinol, metronidazole, and sulfonamides also inhibit the metabolism of other drugs.

Excretion

Glomerular filtration removes a portion of the free drug from the plasma. If another bound drug is administered, it could displace a drug already bound so that the amount of free drug is increased. Hence, two or more drugs may compete for the same site of excretion. Administering one drug, for example, probenecid would interfere with the excretion of another drug, for example, penicillin, excreted by the same mechanism. Tubular reabsorption is one method whereby the body retains some drugs.

Pharmacodynamic

This is the study of how a drug acts on a living organism, including the pharmacologic response and the duration and magnitude of response observed relative to the concentration of the drug at an active site in the organism. Both the adrenergic (sympathetic) nervous system and the cholinergic (parasympathetic) nervous system possess sites for drug interactions to occur.

ADVERSE ORAL AND DENTAL EFFECTS OF DRUGS

Xerostomia (Dry Mouth)

Dryness of the mouth, or xerostomia, results from diminished secretions of saliva. Drugs that produce xerostomia as a side effect include anticholinergic, antidepressants, antiparkinson's drugs, antihistamines/decongestants, antipsychotics, diuretics, hypnotics, systemic bronchodilators, muscle relaxants, methyldopa, laxatives, beta-blockers, and narcotics. Medications that produce xerostomia also may increase the incidence of root surface caries.

In the absence of medication use in a patient with xerostomia, the dentist should screen for medical disorders associated with dry mouth, such as diabetes mellitus. An in-depth review of the patient's medication history should be conducted. Furthermore, a complete history and physical examination, and lab testing may be necessary to properly diagnosis and treat xerostomia. Patients with xerostomia may complain of generalized mouth soreness, dry mouth, painful or burning tongue, reduced denture retention, taste changes, difficulty in chewing, and problems with talking and swallowing. Clinical presentation of xerostomia includes oral fissuring, ulceration, and epithelial atrophy. The condition can be managed symptomatically by increasing the patient's water intake, using saliva substitutes, and oral lubricants. Saliva stimulation is most important in the management of xerostomia. The patient can be instructed to suck on grape or lemon sugarless gum or candies in order to increase saliva. Agents such as citric acid and pilocarpine can also be used for the stimulation of saliva.

Intraoral Hemorrhage

Intraoral hemorrhage is another condition which can be drug-induced. A majority of bleeding episodes occur as a result of a decrease in the number of platelets or thrombocytopenia. Numerous agents have been implicated to cause thrombocytopenia including sulfonamides, quinine, thiazide diuretics, methyldopa, antineoplastic agents, digitalis, heparin and phenytoin. Antibiotics such as cephalosporin, penicillin, and tetracycline can also lead to intraoral hemorrhage. Patients who have cardiovascular disease and are on long-term aspirin, and who are on long-term antibiotic in therapy are at an increased risk of intraoral hemorrhage.

Alcohol also has the propensity to reduce platelet lifespan, which can lead to bleeding problems. Many patients may be stabilized on warfarin prophylaxis. Since warfarin interferes with hepatic synthesis of vitamin K dependent clotting factors, the international normalized ratio (INR) and prothrombin time (PT) must be closely monitored, especially in patients with intraoral hemorrhage. Thrombocytopenia clinically may present as petechiae, which are small round flat dark-red spots caused by bleeding beneath the mucous membranes. The petechiae in the mouth are most commonly found as very tiny bleeding points in the palatal mucosa.

Dysgeusia (Taste Changes)

Individuals taking any variety of medications may present with subjective complaints of taste changes. Patients may have complaints of a bitter, metallic, unpleasant or altered taste, "medication" taste, complete loss of taste, and decreased taste sensation. Drugs which can cause taste changes include clarithromycin, captopril, enalapril, penicillamine, metronidazole, chlorhexidine, lithium, vitamin D, and sulfasalazine. The most common complaint by patients taking medications is a sense of altered taste. There are three mechanisms by which drugs affect the taste sensations vary. First, there is the influence of saliva on taste, i.e. the drug itself may be secreted into the saliva, producing dysgeusia. Another mechanism is the effect of drug metabolite which could possibly interact with taste buds or saliva. Finally, drugs may directly damage the taste buds. There may be age-related effects on taste that can enhance medication taste disorders. The dentist should do a complete medication history in patients that present with complaints of taste changes.

Oral Candidiasis (Thrush)

Candidiasis is the most common oral opportunistic infection seen in dental practices. Patients usually present with creamy, white plaques on the tongue and buccal mucosa. When scraped the lesions leave a red, painful ulcerated surface exposed. Immunocompromised patients such as AIDS may be more susceptible to oral infections. Drugs either act locally or systemically to predispose patients to super infection with *Candida albicans*. Broad-spectrum antibiotics, antineoplastic agents (cancer chemotherapy), corticosteroids (including metered-dose inhalers), and immunosuppressive agents used to prevent rejection of transplant organs are all the various group of drugs which have the potential to produce oral candidiasis. Patients who present with an early *Candida* infection usually have mild symptoms (Table 11.2).

The diagnosis of candidiasis is based upon history and clinical examination findings, but is confirmed by the presence of yeast forms or pseudohyphae. Oral candidiasis related to drug therapy can present in various forms. The forms include acute atrophic candidiasis (antibiotic sore mouth), chronic atrophic candidiasis (denture sore mouth), or acute pseudomembranous candidiasis (thrush). Nystatin suspensions are extremely effective in treating oral candidiasis. High doses of inhaled the corticosteroids increases the risk of developing oral thrush via local deposition of glucocorticoid. This complication can lead to poor compliance with asthma medications. The use of a metered-dose inhaler (MDI) plus a spacer device, such as an aero chamber will decrease the incidence of oral and pharyngeal *Candida* super infections.

Table 11.2 Drug interactions of anti-infectives and antifungals of significance in dentistry

Dental drug	*Interacting medical drug*	*Outcome/result*
Anti-infectives		
Tetracyclines (doxycycline, minocycline)	• Food and dairy products	• Decreased absorption of tetracycline. Avoid administration within 2–3 hours
	• Antacids containing Al, calcium and magnesium	• Reduced serum concentrations of tetracycline. Space administration by 1–2 hours
	• Oral contraceptives	• Slightly increased risk of ovulation
	• Oral anticoagulants	• Increased effect of anti-infectives
Metronidazole	• Anticoagulants • Barbiturates • Disulfiram (antabuse) • Ethyl alcohol	• Risk of bleeding disorders may be increased in anticoagulated patients • Decreases the metronidazole levels. Therefore, dose of metronidazole may be increased • Central nervous system (CNS) toxicity, psychosis and confusion • Risk of disulfiram like reaction. Avoid
Antifungals		
Systemic azole drugs (fluconazole, itraconazole, ketoconazole)	• Anticoagulants • Rifampicin	• Increased risk of bleeding • Decreased levels of antifungals
Fluconazole	• Cimetidine • Oral contraceptives • Phenytoin	• Decreased effect of fluconazole • Decreased estrogen levels. Avoid • Increased effect of the medical drug. Monitor
Itraconazole	• Increased gastric pH • Isoniazid (INH)	• Decreased itraconazole levels • Decreased itraconazole levels
Ketoconazole	• Corticosteroids • Increased gastric pH • Isoniazid (INH)	• Possible increase in steroid levels • Decreased ketoconazole levels • Decreased ketoconazole levels

Gingival Hyperplasia (Enlarged Gums)

Patients may present to the dentist with gingival enlargement if they have been taking agents such as phenytoin, nifedipine, or cyclosporin A. Gingival hyperplasia occurs when there is an increased production and growth of normal gingival cells. The affected area becomes larger but maintains its normal form. The severity of gingival hyperplasia is related to the degree of local irritation and inadequacy of oral hygiene and not generally related to the duration of therapy or dosage. Patients who are started on a strict program of oral hygiene within ten days of initiation of therapy may be able to minimize the occurrence of gingival enlargement.

Phenytoin-induced gingival hyperplasia can also be treated surgically. Nifedipine produces alterations of the intracellular calcium levels in gingival cells and can produce local inflammatory factors to elicit gingival enlargement. Cyclosporin A is given to transplant recipients in order to prevent transplant rejection. Enlargement in this situation is correlated to gingival irritants, such as dental calculus, imperfections in dental restorations, dental plaques, and the effects of mouth breathing. Meticulous plaque control before initiation of therapy and during therapy is a preventive measure against gingival enlargement.

Tooth Discoloration

One of the main drugs to cause tooth discoloration in young adults is tetracycline. However, other agents such as minocycline, iron salts, ciprofloxacin, and chlorhexidine all have the potential to cause tooth discoloration. Some of these medications will cause only cosmetic problems with discoloration and others will cause permanent tooth staining. Tetracyclines have the ability to penetrate bony tissues, especially the developing dentition of young children. They are able to widely distribute throughout the body; therefore, are able to deposit in the growing dentition and other bony tissues. The teeth will become bright yellow upon development and the stains will eventually turn to gray or brown over time. These effects can also occur in the permanent teeth of children between the ages of two and eight years old who have received tetracycline. Depending on the specific tetracycline used, the type and severity of discoloration may vary.

Minocycline is often given to adult patients and adolescents to control acne. Oral iron solutions can cause superficial discoloration of teeth which is reversible and can be removed with proper oral hygiene.

Stomatitis

Stomatitis is an inflammation of the mucus lining of the mouth and is characterized as painful, generalized erythema. Severe cases of stomatitis can develop into ulcerations. The most common drugs associated with stomatitis are the chemotherapeutic agents. Oral/dental care is often overlooked in cancer patients until a problem such as stomatitis occurs. Mild forms of stomatitis can be managed by cleansing the oral cavity with a soft tooth brush and rinsing with a saline solution.

Oral Ulceration and Necrosis

Ulceration and necrosis of the oral mucosa occurs when patients use medications that are not intended for topical therapeutic use or they are taking medications incorrectly. The classic "aspirin burn" is a good example of what can happen when patients tries to self-medicate. Aspirin is one of the best-known locally toxic substances to oral mucous membranes. When a patient has a toothache they may try to relieve the pain by placing an aspirin in the mucobuccal fold opposite the toothache. However, the tissue exposed to the aspirin will become white and depending on the severity of tissue destruction, the lesions may be scraped off. Once the lesion is scraped off, the result is a painful bleeding area. Drugs capable of producing stomatitis can potentially produce reactions that are severe and lead to ulcerations. Drugs capable of causing ulceration or mucosal necrosis include aspirin, phenylbutazone, indomethacin, hydrogen peroxide, phenols, acids or alkalis, and potassium chloride.

DENTAL DRUG REACTIONS

Combinations of two or more drugs taken simultaneously can result in adverse effects that may not occur when the drugs are taken singularly. Some of these interactions occur in dental patients when a medical drug and dental drug are combined. Among these, some dental drug interactions have the greatest potential for serious adverse effects. These are described below.

Aspirin and Oral Anticoagulants (Coumarins)

Aspirin and products that contain aspirin increase the risk of bleeding in patients who are using anticoagulants (Table 11.3). Small doses of aspirin inhibit platelet function. Large doses (more than 3 g per day) can cause a hypoprothrombinemic effect. Aspirin may displace oral anticoagulants from plasma protein-binding sites.

Management: Aspirin and products that contain aspirin must not be administered to patients who are on oral anticoagulant medication. Acetaminophen and narcotic analgesics can be administered safely in patients using oral anticoagulants.

Table 11.3 Drug interactions of aspirin of significance in dentistry

Interacting medical drug	*Outcome/result*
• Anticoagulants	• Increased effect of the medical drug, thus chances of bleeding/hemorrhage
• Steroids	• Decreased salicylate levels
• Antacids	• Decreased salicylate levels
• Insulin	• Enhances hypoglycemic response. Increases bleeding time
• Antihypertensives (ACE inhibitors, β-blockers and diuretics)	• Reduces the effect of the antihypertensives

Epinephrine

With Propranolol

Epinephrine can lead to serious cardiovascular problems in patients who were using propranolol. There is a marked hypertensive episode followed by a reflex bradycardia. Propranolol blocks the beta-2 effect of epinephrine in blood vessels of skeletal muscle. Thus the alpha-receptor response to epinephrine predominates, resulting in hypertension due to increases in systolic and diastolic blood pressure.

Management: When and if possible, epinephrine should not be administered to patients who are using propranolol and other nonselective β-blockers. No risk appears to be associated with selective β-blockers. Local anesthesia without adrenaline can be administered.

With Tricyclic Antidepressants

Use of epinephrine as a vasoconstrictor in local anesthetic injections may cause a hypertensive reaction in patients who are using tricyclic antidepressants (TCAs). TCAs increase norepinephrine in synapses in the central nervous system and periphery. Epinephrine may add to the effects of norepinephrine to cause vasoconstriction and transient hypertension.

Management: When possible, epinephrine should not be used in patients taking TCAs. If adrenaline is necessary, consider using one-third of the normal amount with extra care to avoid any intravascular injection. Felypressin is a good alternative.

Erythromycin

With Carbamazepine (Tegretol)

Erythromycin may interact with carbamazepine, an anticonvulsant agent, to increase blood levels, resulting in carbamazepine toxicity (Table 11.4). Symptoms include drowsiness, dizziness, nausea, headache, and blurred vision. Erythromycin inhibits the hepatic metabolizing enzymes that normally convert carbamazepine to inactive products.

Management: Erythromycin should be administered with caution to patients who are using carbamazepine and only if there is no alternative. Such patients *should be monitored closely.*

With Ketoconazole-Terfenadine (Seldane)

Erythromycin and ketoconazole may cause cardio toxic effects in patients who are using terfenadine, a drug used to treat hay fever. Both erythromycin and ketoconazole may block the metabolism of terfenadine. The resulting nonmetabolized terfenadine stimulates the heart and can cause ventricular arrhythmias.

Management: Erythromycin and ketoconazole are absolutely contra-indicated in patients who are using terfenadine.

Table 11.4 Drug interactions of antibiotics of significance in dentistry

Dental drug	*Interacting medical drug*	*Outcome/result*
All penicillin	Bacteriostatic antibiotics (clindamycin, erythromycin, tetracyclines)	The static drug may impair the action of penicillin
Cephalosporins (all agents)	• Anticoagulants	Increased risk of bleeding. Use with caution
	• Bacteriostatic antibiotics	The static drug may interfere with the action of cephalosporins
Clindamycin	• Erythromycin	Chances of antagonism (avoid)
Macrolides (clarithromycin, erythromycin)	• Anticoagulants	Risk of bleeding disorders may be increased in anticoagulated patients. Monitor
	• Benzodiazepines	Increased benzodiazepine levels resulting in CNS depression
	• Clindamycin	Chances of antagonism (avoid the combination)
	• Carbamazepine	Increased carbamazepine levels. Azithromycin is okay

Theophylline

Erythromycin can interact with theophylline, a bronchodilator, to result in symptoms of theophylline overdose, including nausea, vomiting, and seizures. Erythromycin forms a complex with the hepatic enzyme that metabolizes theophylline. This impairs the metabolic deactivation of theophylline; higher blood and tissue levels of the drug result.

Management: Erythromycin should be administered to patients who are using theophylline only if there is no alternative. Such patients should be monitored closely.

Ibuprofen

Lithium

Administration/prescribing of ibuprofen in a patient on lithium may produce symptoms of lithium toxicity, including nausea, vomiting, slurred speech, and mental confusion (Table 11.5).

Management: Ibuprofen and naproxen should not be administered to patients who are using lithium. Administration of other nonsteroidal anti-inflammatory drugs (NSAIDs) also should be avoided. Acetaminophen and narcotic analgesics do not interact with lithium and can be used.

Table 11.5 Drug interactions of analgesics (non-narcotic analgesics-NSAIDs and opioids/narcotic) of significance in dentistry

Dental drug	*Interacting medical drug*	*Outcome/result*
Nonsteroidal anti-inflammatory drugs (NSAIDs)	• Oral anticoagulants	• Increased effect of the medical drug. Risk of bleeding
	• Antihypertensives (ACE inhibitors, β-blockers and diuretics)	• Decreased antihypertensive effect. Monitor the blood pressure
	• Salicylates	• Decreased NSAID levels with increased glycemic index (GI) effects
	• Cyclosporin	• Nephrotoxicity
All opioids	• Alcohol, CNS depressants, local anesthetics, antidepressants, antipsychotics, antihistamines, cimetidine	• Additive and increased CNS depression may occur. Use with caution

Oral Anticoagulants (Coumarins)

Bleeding may occur when ibuprofen is administered to patients who are using coumarins-type anticoagulants. Inhibition of prostaglandins by ibuprofen results in decreased platelet aggregation and interferes with blood clotting thus enhancing the anticoagulant effect of coumarins.

Management: Ibuprofen, naproxen, diflunisal and perhaps other NSAIDs should not be administered to patients who are using coumarins-type anticoagulants.

LOCAL ANESTHESIA INTERACTIONS

Drug interactions with local anesthetics may be a concern with lidocaine and procainamide when they are used to treat arrhythmias. When administered at high doses by intravenous infusion to treat cardiac arrhythmias, the combination of these two local anesthetic agents theoretically could produce an additive interaction and, subsequently, toxicity. Maximum safe dosage recommendations for local anesthesia permit volumes of solutions usually adequate for adult patients undergoing dental procedures (1.8 mL cartridges of 2% lidocaine with epinephrine is 13.9 mL; for 3% mepivacaine the maximum number of cartridges is 7.4 mL). Most dental procedures, even complex procedures involving multiple quadrants, can be completed comfortably using this volume of local anesthetic. Drug interactions and local anesthetic toxicity become a concern when young children are being treated, when additional anesthetic is required for completing prolonged dental procedures, when excessive topical anesthesia using ointments is necessary to supplement regional anesthesia, or when a long acting local anesthetic is administered for postoperative pain management. Although rarely encountered, the local anesthetic drug interaction is well documented and severe. Fortunately, most dental practitioners are aware of this interaction and prevent its occurrence by limiting the total dose of local anesthetics administered.

Amides

Amides with Epinephrine

- 2% lidocaine
- 4% prilocaine
- 0.5% bupivacaine
- 4% septocaine.

Amides without Epinephrine

- 3% mepivacaine
- 4% prilocaine.

Esters

Propoxycaine: This is ideal for patients with cirrhosis.

Ester Local Anesthetics with Sulfonamides

Sulfonamides act by competing with para-amino benzoic acid, or para-aminobenzoic acid (PABA), a substrate required for bacterial synthesis of folic acid. Procaine and tetracaine, two local anesthetics containing ester linkages, are broken down by plasma esterase to PABA. Metabolism of these ester local anesthetics may increase the concentration of PABA available to bacteria, thereby antagonizing the sulfonamide inhibition of bacterial growth. This adverse drug interaction may cause a reduction in sulfonamide antibacterial activity after the use of procaine for dental anesthesia. Additionally, this drug interaction is dose-dependent and transient and would have, at most, a minor effect on the overall course of the sulfonamide. This type of a reaction is mild in severity. Nevertheless, because alternative local anesthetics are available, the use of procaine for local anesthesia with patients receiving sulfonamide therapy should be avoided when feasible.

Amide Local Anesthetics

After absorption, amide local anesthetics such as lidocaine and mepivacaine are broken down primarily in the liver. Impaired hepatic function, stemming from chronic liver disease or concomitant drug therapy, may decrease the rate of local anesthetic elimination, resulting in an elevation of peak plasma concentrations. This is most significant with multidose therapies, such as when intravenous lidocaine is used to manage cardiac arrhythmias. These adverse drug interactions results from changes in liver amidase activity, and decreased hepatic blood flow or both.

- *Interaction with cimetidine*: Cimetidine is a histamine H_2-receptor antagonist known to inhibit the hepatic oxidative enzymes needed for the metabolism of many drugs, including lidocaine. Following administration for dental anesthesia, blood concentrations of lidocaine during its terminal elimination phase may remain elevated for an extended period. This inhibition is not seen with other histamine H_2-receptor antagonists such as ranitidine or famotidine. Classic local anesthetic overdose reactions theoretically are possible, only when high doses of lidocaine are used or when reinjection is necessary. Increased risk of lidocaine toxicity after administration of a single dose for dental anesthesia resulting from interaction with cimetidine is.
- *Interaction with propranolol*: The β-adrenergic blocker propranolol can decrease hepatic blood flow and reduce the clearance of lidocaine. As with the previously discussed drug interaction with cimetidine,

lidocaine blood concentrations may remain elevated for an extended period. The β-blockers atenolol and pindolol do not appear to inhibit lidocaine metabolism significantly.

Local Anesthetics with Opioid Sedation

During conscious sedation, the use of local anesthetic is essential. Local anesthetics are absorbed, and because they are membrane depressants, they alter central nervous system (CNS) and cardiovascular function.

The opioids may induce a mild respiratory acidosis that decreases protein binding of local anesthetics, thereby permitting free drug to distribute to the CNS. Additionally, the elevation of arterial carbon dioxide tensions that occurs with opioid premedication is known to increase CNS sensitivity to local anesthetic. Classic local anesthetic overdose reactions are CNS excitation, convulsions, respiratory depression and cardiac arrest. This can lead to serious major outcomes. This interaction may be particularly significant in general practice settings, because convulsions and respiratory depression are life-threatening and difficult to manage outside a hospital setting. Practitioners using drug therapies for pediatric sedation should have anesthesia training and be prepared to manage the serious reactions that are possible.

This complication can be managed by prevention and be adjusting the doses of local anesthetic.

Local Anesthetic-Induced Methemoglobinemia

When administered in excessive doses, the dental anesthetics prilocaine and benzocaine (and, rarely, lidocaine and articaine) have been associated with the development of drug induced methemoglobinemia. Agents like nitroglycerin, the antimicrobials dapsone and sulfonamide, and the analgesic phenacetin can cause the oxidation of the iron atom within hemoglobin, producing methemoglobin. The risk factors for this reaction include extremes of age, anemia, respiratory disease, hereditary deficiencies in glucose 6-phosphate dehydrogenase and methemoglobin reductase deficiencies, as well as ingestion of combinations of these oxidant drugs. The topical administration of a eutectic mixture of prilocaine and lidocaine, EMLA may also be responsible for this condition. It is recommended that the dose of local anesthetics be calculated carefully and should not be exceeded.

Avoid the use of local anesthetics with epinephrine in conjunction with:

- Tricyclic
- Antipsychotics
- Digitalis
- Patients with severe cardiopulmonary disease.

SEDATIVE AND ANXIOLYTIC DRUGS

The combination of two or more central nervous system (CNS) depressant drugs is known to produce increased levels of CNS depression. The use of combinations of CNS drugs also increases the risk of unexpected over-sedation and respiratory depression, particularly if opioids are used. Because of the severe consequences that may occur with the combination of CNS depressants, dentists routinely inform patients to restrict alcohol consumption after receiving general anesthesia or sedation. Alcohol consumption after sedation therapy should be restricted too, because it can result in severe drowsiness and significant impairment of psychomotor performance, including driving skills.

Chloral Hydrate

Chloral hydrate is an oral sedative commonly used for sedation of pre-school children in pediatric dentistry. Chloral hydrate, when administered with other sedatives, may increase levels of CNS depression.

- *With alcohol:* The combination of chloral hydrate with alcohol potentiates the effect of alcohol by altering its metabolism. Chloral hydrate and its primary metabolite, trichloroethanol, competitively inhibit alcohol-metabolizing dehydrogenases, thereby elevating alcohol blood concentrations. This combination, commonly known as "a Mickey Finn" or "knockout drops," can induce severe alcohol intoxication with stupor, coma or death. In dentistry, chloral hydrate is used almost exclusively in pediatric sedation, and alcohol usually is not a concomitantly administered agent in such patients. This drug combination, although rarely encountered in dentistry, is significant and may result in severe, potentially life-threatening CNS depression.
- *Anticoagulants (warfarin):* Chloral hydrate may modify the response to the oral anticoagulant warfarin sodium increase free warfarin plasma concentrations by interfering with warfarin's protein binding capacity. This may result in hypoprothrombinemia which is transient and may be clinically insignificant, particularly with single dose therapy of chloral hydrate. If sedation is necessary, use of a benzodiazepine such as diazepam is recommended.
- *Diuretics (furosemide):* The interaction may result in diaphoresis, hot flashes, variable blood pressure, tachycardia and hypertension. The mechanism may relate to enhanced sensitivity to a chloral hydrate metabolite. Although the use of furosemide is rarely encountered in pediatric patients, who are premeditated with chloral hydrate, this is a moderately severe reaction and can occur when furosemide is administered within 24 hours of chloral hydrate. Alternative sedation regimens are recommended.

Barbiturates

Barbiturates are less specific in providing relief from the fear and anxiety associated with dental procedures. Drowsiness and ataxia are frequent side effects of barbiturate sedation. The disadvantages of barbiturate use include the induction of hepatic microsomal oxidative enzymes that can alter other drug actions and the chance for abuse. Although barbiturate use in dentistry is infrequent, the most important barbiturate drug interactions are discussed.

- *Valproic acid:* Valproic acid is an antiepileptic drug for the management of various partial and generalized seizures. When administered in combination, valproic acid may reduce the metabolism of phenobarbital. This would result in enhancement and prolongation of sedative effects. Oral benzodiazepines provide effective sedation and anxiolysis and are an appropriate alternative to barbiturates.
- *Warfarin:* Barbiturates, when administered for a period of one to two weeks, induce hepatic oxidative drug-metabolizing enzymes. When barbiturates are administered in combination with warfarin, doses of warfarin may need to be increased to maintain therapeutic prothrombin times. When prolonged barbiturate therapy is discontinued and warfarin's enhanced rate of metabolism returns to normal, the anticoagulant concentrations increases and so does the risk of a serious bleeding.

Benzodiazepines

Oral benzodiazepines commonly used in dentistry include diazepam, triazolam, lorazepam, alprazolam, and oxazepam. Midazolam is frequently administered intravenously for conscious sedation. Benzodiazepines are metabolized by hepatic oxidative enzymes. The resulting oxidative metabolites are conjugated and eliminated primarily through renal excretion. Benzodiazepines rates of absorption, distribution and metabolism vary greatly among patients (Table 11.6).

Table 11.6 Drug interactions of benzodiazepines of significance in dentistry

Interacting medical drug	*Outcome/result*
• Alcohol	• Additive CNS depression
• Antacids (ranitidine)	• Decreased absorption of benzodiazepines, effect is unpredictable
• Oral contraceptives	• Decreased effect of benzodiazepines
• Smoking	• Decreased effect of benzodiazepines enhances hepatic metabolism
• Levodopa	• Decreased levodopa effect, increases parkinsonism

Drugs that Increase the Metabolism of Benzodiazepines

- *Rifampicin:* Rifampicin induces the metabolic enzymes of the gut wall and liver responsible for the metabolism of diazepam, midazolam and triazolam. Due to this interaction, the bioavailability of oral midazolam is reduced. Use of an alternative sedative such as oral oxazepam or inhaled N_2O is recommended as this interaction, results in the loss of the benzodiazepine's anxiolytic activity and, therefore, in poor sedation. It is not life-threatening and can be considered a minor adverse drug interaction.
- *Carbamazepine:* The anticonvulsant carbamazepine can induce hepatic enzymes for the oxidative metabolism of benzodiazepines. After oral administration of these agents, benzodiazepine plasma concentrations may be decreased and sedative effects may be greatly reduced. This interaction may be important in medicine because of loss of seizure control, but it is of minor importance in dentistry.

Drugs that Inhibit the Metabolism of Benzodiazepines

- *Calcium channel blockers:* Calcium-channel blockers like verapamil and diltiazem are popular cardiovascular drugs used for the management of angina, arrhythmias and hypertension. Both agents inhibit the liver enzymes required for the metabolism of triazolam and orally administered midazolam. Avoidance of this combination is recommended, particularly in elderly patients known to be sensitive to benzodiazepines.
- *Cimetidine:* Cimetidine inhibits the oxidative metabolism of diazepam, triazolam and alprazolam. Increased and prolonged sedation after oral administration may occur because of a significant decrease in first-pass metabolism.
- *Erythromycin, clarithromycin and azole antifungal agents:* These antimicrobial agents have the potential to inhibit the specific liver enzymes required for the metabolism of triazolam and oral midazolam and thus may increase their blood concentrations.
- *Protease inhibitors such as indinavir and nelfinovir:* Protease inhibitors are antiviral agents used for the management of human immunodeficiency virus (HIV) infections. They bind to the active site of the HIV protease enzyme and interrupt the maturation process of newly formed viral particles. They are capable of inhibiting the hepatic oxidative enzymes required for the metabolism and elimination of triazolam, alprazolam and oral midazolam. This may result in severe sedation and respiratory depression. Patients being managed for human immune deficiency virus infections often have complex medical and drug histories, and consultation with their physicians may be required and is recommended.

Red-flag drugs in dentistry

Drug	*Comments*
• Alcohol	• Avoid especially with benzodiazepines
• Erythromycin, cimetidine	• Inhibits metabolism and increases the other drug's effects
• Oral hypoglycemic agents	• Highly protein bound
• Oral contraceptives	• Avoid with antibiotics even though the event for risk is very small
• Anticoagulants	• Narrow therapeutic index and is influenced by many drugs

CONCLUSION

Adverse drug interactions associated are reported rarely in dentistry. In general, the potential for encountering the most serious adverse drug interactions can be minimized by administering local anesthetics, anxiolytics, sedatives and other medicines at doses that are within accepted guidelines. By avoiding the most significant reactions discussed in this chapter, dentists can maintain their patients' safety.

BIBLIOGRAPHY

1. Burney RG, DiFazio CA, Foster JA. Effects of pH on protein binding of lidocaine. Anesth Analg. 1978;57:478-80.
2. Ciancio SG (Ed). ADA guide to dental therapeutics. Chicago: ADA Publishing Co.; 1998.
3. Eckenhoff JE, Helrich M. Study of narcotics and sedatives for use in pre-anesthetic medica ion. JAMA. 1957;167:415-22.
4. Heylen R, Miller R. Medications commonly used in the treatment of adult HIV positive patients: part 2. Genitourinary Med. 1997;73:5-11.
5. Ilyas M. Delirium induced by a combination of antiarrhythmic drugs. Lancet. 1969;2:1368.
6. Lambertsen CJ, Wendel H, Longenhagen JB. The separate and combined respiratory effects of chlorpromazine and meperidine in normal men controlled at 46 mm Hg alveolar pCO_2. J Pharmacol Exp Ther. 1961;131:381-93.
7. Lloyd CJ. Clinically induced methemoglobinemia in a neonate. Br J Oral Maxillofac Surg. 1992;30(1):63-5.
8. McKee KC, Nazif MM, Jackson DL, Barnhart DC, Close J, Moore PA. Dose response characteristics of meperidine sedation in preschool children. Pediatr Dent. 1990;12:222-7.
9. Moore P. Adverse Drug Interactions In Dental Practice: Interactions Associated With Local Anesthetics, Sedatives and Anxiolytics, Clinical Pharmacology part four. JADA. 1999.pp.13-9.
10. Page M. psychotropic drugs and dentistry. Australian prescriber. 2007;30:98-101.

11. Porter SR, Scully C. Adverse drug reactions in the mouth. Clin Dermatol. 2000;18 (5):525-32.
12. Requa-Clark BS, Holroyd SV. Applied Pharmacology for the Dental Hygienist. 3rd (edn). Mosby, St Louis (1995).
13. Sanders LD, Whitehead C, Gildersleve CD, et al. Interaction of H_2-receptor antagonists and benzodiazepine sedation. Anaesthesia. 1993; 48:286-92.
14. Wynn RL. Dental non-steroidal anti-inflammatory drugs and prostaglandin based drug interactions, part two. Gen Dent. 1992;40:104-10.
15. Wynn RL. Epinephrine interactions with β-blockers. Gen Dent. 1994;42:16-8.
16. Yagiela JA. Adverse drug interactions in dental practice: interactions associated with vasoconstrictors. J Am Dent Assoc. 1999;130:701-9.

CHAPTER 12

DENTAL CONSIDERATIONS IN MEDICALLY COMPROMISED PATIENTS

Priyanka Jain

INTRODUCTION

This is the management of patients in whom the dental treatment may need modification according to their medical condition. Within the mass of humanity, is a substantial number of people that are elderly and individuals with systemic medical conditions that can affect oral health and dental treatment. The dental management of these medically compromised patients can be problematic in terms of oral complications, dental therapy, and emergency care.

This chapter focuses on a number of medical problems that dentists might encounter in daily practice that necessitate extra knowledge and care to prevent potential complications causing otherwise unnecessary morbidity and mortality.

The medically compromised patient represents a greater treatment risk than average, and thus merits particular attention for safe management, as well as effective sedation. A method of safe management developed at the USC (University of South Carolina, USA), School of Dentistry is very effective. This treatment system is explained by the acronym *RAM-E, R* representing recognition of common risk disease through a comprehensive yet manageable medical history, *A* representing assessment of treatment risk by using a basic, popular physical status classification system, and *M* representing safe management by using simple treatment modifications for safety. *E* represents medical emergency care that would be most uncommonly required when following the RAM-E principles. In order to provide safe comprehensive care for the medically compromised patient who cannot tolerate, care designed for the healthy patient, dentists must supply knowledgeable treatment modification for safety and comfort.

Recognition

The first step in managing the patient with medical problems is acquiring a thorough health history followed by the clinician to fully understand the significance of the disease. Each identified condition can affect dental care in a unique manner. For example, medication prescribed for a medical condition might produce a problem during the administration of a local anesthetic, or it could interact with pain medication prescribed postoperatively. The dentist needs to understand the potential complications that can occur as a consequence of dental treatment of a medically compromised patient.

Recognition of common risk disease is provided primarily through the routine pretreatment medical history. Good detailed medical history of the patient should be taken and updated during each visit. Any medical condition should be mentioned in the consent form. This should include documentation via questionnaire as well as a verbal history. Any problem in previous dental treatment should be reported along with any previous hospitalization of the patient and the reason for it. The dental history should also include questions related to current oral conditions such as periodontal disease or oral ulceration and past dental treatment and potential complications from prior intervention including treatment failure and the delivery of anesthesia or post-treatment medication.

Certain medically compromised patients should only be treated in a hospital setting where in case of an emergency, can be immediately treated. For example, patient with a significant bleeding problem or thrombocytopenia arising as a primary condition or secondary to medication, radiation, or leukemia is best managed in a hospital setting as replacement of platelets can be provided before the procedure or afterwards, if spontaneous bleeding occurs.

Assessment

Assessment of the patient's condition follows the physical status classification system of the American Society of Anesthesiologists (ASA) (Table 12.1). The ASA system is used for all patients before surgery or outpatient procedures requiring anesthesia. The ASA physical status class is also required when a patient is scheduled for hospital inpatient or outpatient treatment under anesthesia. Examination of the patient with a history of medical problems should be more extensive than that associated with the healthy patient. In patients that present with problems identified at examination that have not previously been reported to a health care practitioner, the dentist can be instrumental in defining potential pathology and making the appropriate referral for additional medical evaluation. Such patients should be referred for medical assessment prior to dental treatment. In the patient with pre-existing disease, preparation for dental treatment should include determination of disease status.

Table 12.1 American Society of Anesthesiologists (ASA) classification

ASA physical status classification	*Considerations in dentistry*
A normal healthy patient	Stress reduction measured if needed
A patient with mild-to-moderate systemic disease	Stress reduction as indicated
A patient with severe systemic disease that limits activity but is not incapacitating	Modify the treatment as required, reduce stress/anxiety levels, discuss with the physician before starting the treatment
A patient with severe systemic disease which limits activity and is a constant threat to life	Only urgent care delivered in consultation with the physician, and consider a hospital setting
A dying patient not expected to survive 24 hours with or without operation	Treatment, if absolute necessary should be provided in the hospital only

Management

Planning the dental treatment in the medically compromised patient primarily involves having an understanding of the nature of the patient's disease and how it can impact their physiology and his/her response to dental management and postdental treatment healing. Knowing how to manage potential complications is also important and is presented in the later part of the chapter.

Management of treatment for safety can be categorized as stress reduction, ischemia-based modifications, and/or adjuvants. Pain, anxiety, and stress are a common feature in the medically compromised patient. Stress reduction elements (SREs) can be used in such cases, if the need arises. They are mere common sense. The dentist must remind the patient to obtain proper preoperative rest or to take a sedative. Intraoperative sedation should be used, if necessary, and special effort should be made to ensure effective pain control. Always try to schedule the patient's appointments during morning hours. Prescriptions should be offered as indicated. Sound judgment will determine logical applications in the interest of safety of the patient.

Since most disease states of significant risk in dentistry, share the ischemia factor on a general or local basis, specific treatment modifications aimed at improving tissue oxygenation should be designed and incorporated in the treatment plan. Sedation by an appropriate route is of great benefit to the medical-risk patient, if anxiety or fear is significant.

Nitrous oxide/oxygen, which is often used when mild-to-moderate sedation is indicated, supplies supplemental oxygen as well. A maximum of 50% nitrous oxide is suggested for these patients, as disorientation and excitement can be harmful; effective sedation is often accomplished with 30% nitrous oxide. A semireclining chair position, with the backrest at 45° is comfortable for most of the patients. This chair position ensures the patient's comfort and safety edema. The supine position, if used will decrease the vital capacity and further can compromise a patient. Patients in the supine position will also have difficulty clearing bronchial secretions during treatment. A rubber dam may be contraindicated in a patient with severe ischemia-based disease. If a dam cannot be tolerated, the patient should be warned about the danger of swallowing or aspirating a foreign body. Caution and care is also indicated in treating the patient with a recent significant change in life/lifestyle such as serious illness, loss of a job, bankruptcy, serious marital concerns, or death or divorce of a spouse/family member.

Adjuvants

This involves the other considerations such as drug allergy or the need for antibiotic prophylaxis. Nitroglycerin premedication applies only to a history of angina pectoris within the past 6 months. Effective prophylaxis helps in the stress management. If a patient has a pacemaker, the dentist should be cautious regarding the use of electrocoagulation during a procedure or performing surgery. An anticoagulant may merit special attention, or at least a warning about the possibility of increased postoperative bleeding. A preoperative warning is required of all complications that are not remote and generally considered to be remote.

MEDICAL HISTORY AND ASSESSMENT

It is essential to try and obtain as much relevant information as possible especially when invasive procedures or the use of potent drugs are being considered. The main objective of a thorough medical history is to try and acertain whether the patient is fit to undergo the dental procedure being considered and if any drugs are contraindicated (Table 12.2). It also helps to exclude any oral disease.

Table 12.2 Significant medical conditions

The medical history should elicit any systemic diseases relevant to dentistry like:
A Anemia
B Bleeding disorders
C Cardiac disorders
D Drug allergies
E Endocrine disorders
F Fits
G Gastrointestinal disorders
H Hospitalizations
I Infections
J Jaundice
K Kidney disease
L Liver disease

The history must be updated before any surgical procedure or the start of a new treatment procedure. A careful examination and assessment of the patient's appearance, behavior, speech can also give a hint of a significant condition. The history should include the date of the last physical examination along with a list of all the medical conditions being treated and the list of the medications with it. Confidentiality must be respected with regard to the patient's history.

Determine the status of the disease. For example, in case of a diabetic patient, is it well-controlled or uncontrolled? In case of a hypertensive patient, assess the BP and categorize as Stage 1, Stage 2, or Stage 3 hypertension (Table 12.3).

SIGNIFICANT INVESTIGATIONS IN DENTISTRY

Hematological Tests

- *CBC* (Complete blood count) with platelets and WBC differential (Tables 12.4 and 12.5)
- *ESR* (Erythrocyte sedimentation rate)
- *Coagulation tests:* PT/INR (Prothrombin time/international normalized ratio), PTT (partial thromboplastin time) (Tables 12.6 and 12.7).

Renal Assessment Tests

- Serum creatinine
- Blood urea nitrogen.

Diabetes Assessment Tests

- *FBS* (Fasting blood sugar)
- *PPBS* (Postprandial/post meal blood sugar)
- *HbA,C* (Hemoglobin A,C).

Table 12.3 Classification of blood pressure (according to the Joint National Commission (JNC 2203) BP classification)

Category	*Systolic BP (mm Hg)*	*Diastolic BP (mm Hg)*
Normal	<120	<80
Prehypertension	120–139	80–89
Stage 1	40–159	90–99
Stage 2	≥160	≥100
Stage 3	≥180	≥110

Table 12.4 Complete blood count (CBC)

Cells	*Normal values*
WBC	4000–10,000/mm^3
RBC	4.2–5.9 million/mm^3
Hemoglobin (Hb):	
• Males	14–18 d/dL
• Females	12–16 g/dL
Hematocrit (packed cell volume or PCV measures the percentage of the formed elements in the blood namely RBC, WBC and platelets)	
• Males	40–54%
• Females	37–47%
Mean corpuscular volume (MCV)	78–99 fL
Mean cell hemoglobin (MCH)	27–31 pg
Platelet count	150,000–400,000/mm^3
WBC differential	
• Neutrophils (engulf bacteria and cellular debris)	3 x 10^9/L
• Lymphocytes (produce antibodies and regulate the immune response)	2.5 x 10^9/L
• Monocytes (associated with engulfing cellular debris)	1–10%
• Eosinophils (associated with parasitic infection and allergic response)	0.15 x 10^9/L
• Basophils (associated with hypersensitivity and histamine release)	0–2%
ESR	0–15 mm/hour

Liver Assessment Tests

- Hepatic serology
- Liver function tests (LFTs).

Bone Assessment Tests

- Serum calcium
- Serum phosphorous
- Alkaline phosphates.

Table 12.5 Interpretation of the blood picture

Cells	*Levels increase in*	*Levels decrease in*
Hemoglobin	Polycythemia	Anemia
PCV	Dehydration	Anemia
MCV	Vitamin B_{12} deficiency, liver diseases, alcoholism	Iron deficiency, thalassemia
RBC	Polycythemia	Anemia
MCH	Pernicious anemia	Iron deficiency
WBC total	Pregnancy, exercise, infection, trauma	Anemia
WBC differential		
• Neutrophils	Acute bacterial infection Treatment:antibiotics	Viral infections
• Lymphocytes	Viral infections, Treatment: Antiviral agents	Immune defects
• Monocytes	Chronic bacterial infections (bacterial endo-carditis, tuberculosis), acute exacerbation of inflammation, treatment: defer routine dental treatment for 4–6 weeks	
• Eosinophil	Allergies, parasitic infections, skin disease	Immune defects
• Basophils	Chronic myeloid leukemia, polycythemia	
Platelets	Chronic inflammation, acute infections, postsurgery, myeloproliferative disease	Thrombocytopenia, aplasia, marrow invasion and cirrhosis
ESR	Pregnancy, infections, anemia, inflammation, trauma	

Table 12.6 International normalized ratio

INR normal value	*Comments*
2.0–3.0	Therapeutic range
Under 2.0	Associated with minimal bleeding
3–4.5	Associated with excessive bleeding

HIV/AIDS Status Assessment Tests

- CD4 count and viral load
- CBC
- LFTs and hepatic serology
- PT/INR.

Table 12.7 Differences between PT and PTT

Prothrombin time (PT/INR)	*Partial thromboplastin time (PTT)*
Measures the extrinsic pathway	Measures the intrinsic pathway
Normal range: 10–12 seconds	Normal range: 25–38 seconds
Affected by coumarin intake	Affected by heparin and excessive coumarin intake
Prothrombin time (PT) is maintained at 1.3–1.5 times the normal during anticoagulation	Partial thromboplastin time (PTT) is maintained at 1.5–2.0 times normal with intravenous heparin

Table 12.8 Normal values

FBS: <125 mg/dL
Post prandial (PP)/Post meal: <140 mg/dL
HbA,C: <7% in controlled patients
HbA,C: >8% in uncontrolled diabetes in the past 2–3 months

International Normalized Ratio

International normalized ratio (INR) is checked every 4–6 weeks. INR of 3.0–4.5 is required for patients with a history of:

- Valves
- Deep vein thrombosis
- Recent myocardial infarction
- Atrial fibrillation associated with stroke or MI
- Pulmonary embolism.

BLOOD TESTS FOR RENAL FUNCTION

Normal serum creatinine level is 0.4–1.2 mg/dL. Renal failure is associated with increased serum creatinine. Blood urea nitrogen (BUN) levels increase with changes in the plasma volume, protein metabolism, hemorrhage, shock and renal failure. But serum creatinine is a more specific indicator of renal disease than blood urea nitrogen. Serum creatinine and BUN are not useful in detecting early renal dysfunction and their levels do not give abnormal values till 50% of the renal function is lost.

BLOOD TEST FOR DIABETES

The well controlled patient (Table 12.8):

- *FBS:* <125 mg/dL
- *PP:* <140 md/dL
- *HbA,C:* <7%
- For pain control and analgesia, we can safely use *(Maximum)* 2 carpules of epinephrine with 1:100,000.

The Moderately Controlled Patient

- *FBS:* 125–140 mg/dL
- *PP:* 140–200 mg/dL
- *HbA,C:* Between 7% and 8%
- For analgesia, use (maximum) 2 carpules of prilocaine or bupivacaine only
- It is recommended to use full dose of antibiotics, following any major procedure/management of infection.

The Uncontrolled Patient

- *FBS:* >140 mg/dL
- *PP:* >200 mg/dL
- *HbA,C:* >8%
- Treat only acute infections
- For analgesia, it is recommended to use mepivacaine without epinephrine only
- A low dose antibiotics course is recommended to promote healing.

LIVER FUNCTION TESTS AND HEPATIC SEROLOGY

Enzymes

Serum Glutamic-Pyruvic Transaminase (SGPT/ALT): This enzyme is specifically associated with the liver cells only (Table 12.9). Increase in their levels is an indication of liver cell inflammation.

Serum Glutamic-Oxaloacetic Transaminase (SGOT/AST): This enzyme is associated with the liver, heart and the brain tissues. An increase/decrease suggest cell necrosis.

Serum Gamma-Glutamyl Transferase (SGGT): This particular enzyme is associated with alcoholism.

HIV/AIDS ASSESSMENT TESTS

These tests must be assessed before proceeding with the dental procedure.

CD4 Count and Viral Load

These are significant for efficient monitoring of the HIV patient. The CD4 count provides an estimate of the patient's immune system status and is also used to determine the patient's response to therapy. HIV RNA level is a strong predictor of the disease progression. If HIV RNA levels are below 50/75 copies/mL they are undetectable. These are done at an interval of 3 months.

Table 12.9 Liver function tests

Enzyme/ component	*Normal range*	*In hepatitis*	*In cirrhosis*	*Comments*
Total protein	62–80 g/L	Normal	↓	Levels ↑ in connected tissue diseases and liver diseases and ↓ in pregnancy and malnutrition
Albumin	35–55 g/L	Normal	↓	Levels ↑ in dehydration and ↓ in malabsorption
Globulin	22–36 g/L	Normal	↑	Levels ↑ in chronic infections and ↓ in malnutrition and chronic lymphatic leukemia
ALT	3–60 IU/L	↑ into 1000s	Increased up to a maximum of 300 IU	Levels ↑ in liver disease and infectious mononucleosis
AST	3–40 IU/L	↑ into 1000s but ALT is always >AST	Increased up to a maximum of 300 IU. AST > ALT	Levels ↑ in trauma and myocardial infarction
Alkaline phosphatases	30–110 IU/L	↑ 1–2 times normal	↑ 1–2 times normal	Levels ↑ in puberty and pregnancy and ↓ in hypo-thyroidism and malnutrition
SGGT	5–42 IU/L	↑ with alcoholic/ biliary hepatitis, but normal, if hepatitis is due to other causes	↑ with alcoholic/ biliary cirrhosis, but normal, if cirrhosis is due to other causes	↑ in diabetes and myocardial infarction
Total bilirubin	1–17 μmol/L	Normal or ↑	Normal or ↑	Levels ↑ in puberty and pregnancy and ↓ in hypo-thyroidism and malnutrition

Abbreviation: IU, International unit

INFECTIVE ENDOCARDITIS, SURGICALLY CORRECTED HEART DISEASE AND ANTIBIOTIC COVERAGE

The pathogenesis of infective endocarditis (IE) is complex and involves a number of different factors. Vessel turbulence leading to platelet deposition and damage to the endothelium of the cardiac valve or surgically constructed pulmonary shunt or conduit exists, combined with a bacteremia arising from oral trauma with microorganisms that are capable of adhering to the site (i.e., typically streptococci, staphylococci, and enterococci), and bacterial proliferation at the site of adherence.

The American Dental Association and its council on Scientific Affairs (2007) have reduced the classes of patients for whom antibiotic prophylaxis is recommended because the risk of morbidity resulting from antibiotic use outweighs its probable benefits. Most cases of endocarditis are not attributable to an invasive procedure; therefore, cardiac conditions are classified into high, moderate, and negligible risk categories based on potential outcome, if endocarditis develops. For oral/dental procedures, a follow-up antibiotic dose is no longer recommended, and erythromycin is no longer recommended for penicillin-allergic individuals but clindamycin and other alternatives are offered.

ENDOCARDITIS PROPHYLAXIS RECOMMENDED

Cardiac conditions associated with the highest risk of adverse outcome from endocarditis for which prophylaxis with dental procedures is recommended are:

High-risk Category

- Prosthetic cardiac valves
- Previous bacterial endocarditis
- Complex congenital heart disease (CHD)
- Surgically constructed systemic-pulmonary shunts or conduits.

Moderate Risk Category

- Most other congenital cardiac malformations (other than above)
- Rheumatic heart disease
- Hypertrophic cardiomyopathy
- Mitral valve prolapse with vulvar regurgitation.

ENDOCARDITIS PROPHYLAXIS NOT RECOMMENDED

Negligible risk category (No greater risk than the general population)

- Atrial septal defect
- Surgical repair of atrial septal defect and ventricular septal defect

- Previous coronary artery bypass graft surgery
- Mitral valve prolapse
- Physiologic, functional, or innocent heart murmurs
- Previous Kawasaki disease without vulvar dysfunction
- Previous rheumatic fever (RF) without vulvar dysfunction
- Cardiac pacemakers.

DENTAL PROCEDURES FOR WHICH PROPHYLAXIS IS RECOMMENDED

Endocarditis Prophylaxis Recommended (High or Moderate risk category): All dental procedures that involve the manipulation of the periapical region of the teeth or perforation of the oral mucosa require antibiotic prophylaxis (Table 12.10).

- Dental extractions
- Periodontal procedures including surgery, scaling and root planning
- Dental implant R
- Reimplantation of avulsed teeth
- Endodontics
- Subgingival placement of antibiotics/strips
- Initial placement of orthodontic bands but not brackets
- Intraligamentary local anesthetic injections
- Prophylactic cleaning of teeth where bleeding is anticipated.

Table 12.10 Suggested antibiotic prophylaxis regimen for a dental procedure

Situation	*Agent*	*Regimen: 30 minutes–1 hour before the procedure*
Oral	Amoxicillin	• Adults: 2 gm • Children: 50 mg/kg
Unable to take oral medications	Ampicillin	• Adults: 2 mg IM/IV • Children: 50 mg/kg IM/IV
Allergic to penicillin or ampicillin (Oral)*	Clindamycin	• Adults: 600 mg • Children: 20 mg/kg
	Azithromycin/ Clarithromycin	• Adults: 500 mg • Children: 15 mg/kg
	Cephalexin	• Adults: 2 gm • Children: 50 mg/kg
Allergic to penicillin or ampicillin and unable to take oral medication	Clindamycin	• Adults: 600 mg IM/IV • Children: 20 mg/kg IM/IV
	Cefazolin	• Adults: 1 gm IM/IV • Children: 25 mg/kg IM/IV

Abbreviation: IM/IV, Intramuscular/Intravenous

* Cephalosporin should not be given to individuals with a history of hypersensitivity reactions to penicillin.

Endocarditis prophylaxis is not recommended in:

- Restorative dentistry with/without retraction cord
- Local anesthetic injections (nonintraligamentary)
- Intracanal endodontic treatment; post placement and buildup
- Placement of removable prosthodontic/orthodontic appliances
- Electrosurgery
- Taking impressions
- Fluoride treatments
- Taking radiographs
- Shedding of primary teeth
- Bleeding from trauma to the lips or oral mucosa.

ANTIBIOTIC PROPHYLAXIS FOR DENTAL PATIENTS WITH TOTAL JOINT REPLACEMENTS (ADA)

Antibiotic prophylaxis is not indicated for patients with pins, plates and screws undergoing dental procedures, nor is it routinely indicted for most dental patients with total joint replacements. However, it is advisable to consider premedication in a small number of patients (patients with rheumatoid arthritis, systemic lupus erythematous) who may be at potential increased risk of hematogenous total joint infection (Table 12.11). Patients who are about to have a total joint arthroplasty should be in good dental health prior to surgery. Patients who already have had a total joint, arthroplasty should perform effective daily oral hygiene procedure to establish and maintain good oral health. The risk of bacteremia is far more substantial in a mouth with ongoing inflammation than in one that is healthy and employing these homeoral hygiene devices.

Bacteremia can cause hematogenous seeding of total joint implants, both in the early postoperative period and for many years following

Table 12.11 Antibiotics

Antibiotic premedication indications
• Prosthetic heart valves
• Heart murmurs, with a history of rheumatic fever (RF), rheumatic heart disease (RHD)
• Patients with congenital heart disease
• Dialysis patients
• Organ transplant patients
• Chemotherapy patients, including bone marrow transplant
• Artificial joint patients
• Poorly controlled diabetic patients
• Radiation therapy patients, depending on procedure
• Down syndrome patients (many have cardiac defects)
• Immunosuppressed patients (depending on treatment)

implantation. The most critical period is up to 2 years after joint placement. In addition, bacteremia may occur in the course of normal daily life and concurrently with dental and medical procedures. It is likely that many more oral bacteremia are spontaneously induced by daily events than the dental treatment induced.

Suggested antibiotic prophylaxis regimens (no second dose is required)

- *Patients not allergic to penicillin:* Cephalexin, cephradine or amoxicillin 2 grams orally 1 hour prior to dental procedure
- *Patients not allergic to penicillin and unable to take oral medications:* Cefazolin or ampicillin, cefazolin 1 gram or ampicillin 2 grams intramuscularly or intravenously 1 hour prior to the dental procedure
- *Patients allergic to penicillin:* Clindamycin 600 mg orally 1 hour prior to the dental procedure
- *Patients allergic to penicillin and unable to take oral medications:* Clindamycin 600 mg IV 1 hour prior to the dental procedure.

DENTAL MANAGEMENT IN SPECIFIC ILLNESSES

Anemia

Disease Nature

Anemia is a fall in the level of the circulating hemoglobin level below the normal reference level l for age and sex. It is classified on the basis of red cell (erythrocytes) size as normocytic, microcytic, and macrocytic (Table 12.12). The most common type of anemia is microcytic in nature, which is due to iron deficiency. Macrocytic anemia is usually caused by vitamin B_{12} or folate deficiency. It may additionally be seen in patients with liver diseases. Normocytic anemia results from leukemia, chronic disease pattern, liver diseases, renal failure, malignancy, or infections. In the early stages, anemia is frequently asymptomatic.

Deficiency anemia can be caused by lack of iron, vitamin B_{12} or folate. Different deficiencies produce different effects on the erythrocyte, hence, microcytic/macrocytic anemia. These deficiency states can be corrected by replacement therapy. Iron deficiency may be due to either dietary factors or loss of blood. Vitamin B_{12} deficiency (pernicious anemia) is caused by poor absorption of the vitamin due to the defective intrinsic factor function caused by antibody attack. Pernicious anemia is of interest to the dentists, as it is one of the complications of nitrous oxide abuse.

Hemolytic anemia can be a result of extrinsic factors like malaria or problems with the circulating hemoglobin. These could be sickle cell disease, thalassemia, or glucose 6-phosphate dehydrogenase deficiency (G6PD).

Table 12.12 Anemias by RBC patterns

Type	*RBC pattern*	*Cause*
Microcytic hypochromic	Decreased Hb, PCV (hematocrit), MCV and MCH. MCV is below 78 fl	Iron deficiency anemia, thalassemia
Macrocytic/megaloblastic	Decreased Hb, PCV Increased MCV and MCH. MCV is more than 99 fl	Vitamin B_{12} or folic acid deficiency
Normochromic, normocytic pattern	Normal MCV and MCH MCV is between 79–98 fl	Acute hemolysis Aplastic anemia Chronic disease

Dental Management

Hypoxia, infection or acidosis can lead to crisis in patients with anemia. Always provide stress management using oxygen and nitrous oxide. Use antibiotics to prevent/treat infections and promote healing.

Anemia and Anesthetics

Local anesthesia is the safest method of pain control.

- *Mild anemia (Hb decreased by 25% from normal):* Use lidocaine with epinephrine (Maximum of 2 carpules)
- *Moderate anemia (Hb decreased by 25–50% from normal):* Use bupivacaine with 1:200,000 epinephrine for major procedures (as it is long acting) and mepivacaine without epinephrine for minor procedures
- *Severe cases (Hb drops by more than 50%):* Defer dental treatment until the patient is stabilized.

It is preferred to avoid prilocaine with respect to all anemias, as it may precipitate methemoglobinemia.

Anemia and Analgesics

Drugs that can potentially cause hemolysis such as aspirin and NSAIDs should be stopped. If used, there is an increased risk of platelet dysfunction, gastritis and acidosis. Acetaminophen, with or without codeine can be prescribed as analgesics. But avoid acetaminophen with codeine sulphate in patients with G6PD. In such cases, use codeine phosphate.

Anemia and Antibiotics

Prophylactic antibiotics like penicillin V or clindamycin should be given for surgical procedures. Penicillin should be used with caution in patients with iron deficiency anemia. Infections must be treated as fast as possible and vigorously, as the patient may be immune compromised, if the spleen is nonfunctional. No sulfa containing drugs should be prescribed to patients with G6PD deficiency.

BLEEDING DISORDERS

Disorders of hemostasis cause management problems in dentistry due to prolonged postoperative bleeding (Table 12.13). This is majorly due to local causes like excessive trauma to the soft tissues, inflamed mucosa, and/or poor compliance with the postoperative instructions. Thrombocytopenia exists when the platelet count falls below 150,000/mm^3. This causes petechiae, ecchymosis and postoperative hemorrhage. Idiopathic thrombocytopenic purpura (ITP), an autoimmune disorder is one of the most common bleeding disorders.

Dental Management

When faced with a bleeding patient, it is very essential to establish whether the situation is urgent and if there could be an underlying bleeding tendency. The situation is considered urgent, if the patient is losing large quantities of blood, or is hypotensive. To stop bleeding, press firmly with a gauze pad over the socket for 10–15 minutes and suture the socket under local anesthesia.

Table 12.13 Bleeding in relation to surgery

Immediate type of bleeding	*Delayed type of bleeding*
Oozing occurs beyond 24 hours postoperatively	Deep tissue bleeding occurs 4–10 days postoperatively
Defect in the primary hemostasis	Defect in the secondary hemostasis
Often associated with superficial bleeding	Associated with deep tissue bleeding
Small bruises and petechiae can be seen on the skin	Large bruises may occur
Mucous membrane bleeding can occur	Bleeding into the joints can occur (hemarthrosis)
Tests of significance: • Bleeding time • Platelet count	Tests of significance: • PT/INR • PTT

The main complication in such cases is hemorrhage. Therefore, it is essential to take a complete family history to determine whether the bleeding disorder is inherited or due to an acquired problem. A recent and updated medical report and consultation with the hematologist is required. Bleeding parameters can change frequently; therefore, investigations are needed closer to the time of the dental treatment. Dental procedures should be limited according to the medical condition. Patients with congenital bleeding disorders should be treated in specialist centers. Regional anesthetic block injections are contraindicated, if the platelet levels are below 300,000/mm^3.

Prothrombin times are reported as INR. It is the ratio of the patient's one-stage prothrombin time to that of the controls. A normal healthy patient has an INR of 1. A traumatic removal of one or two teeth in patients on anticoagulants can be carried out using local measures (unless the INR is greater than 3.5) to control bleeding or the use of tranexamic acid/ desmopressin. Absorbable hemostatic agents such as oxidized regenerated cellulose (Surgicel), synthetic collagen or microcrystalline collagen may be put in the socket to assist clotting. Hemostasis after a minor surgery is usually adequate, if the platelet levels are above 500,000/mm^3. For major procedures, platelet levels over 750,000/mm^3 are desired.

Drugs that affect platelet function, particularly aspirin and NSAIDs, should be avoided (Table 12.14). It is also recommended to avoid erythromycin and ketoconazole in patients taking warfarin (as these drugs inhibit warfarin metabolism).

CARDIAC PROBLEMS

Dental procedures or drugs used in dentistry, can aggravate heart disease, precipitate angina, or even provoke a heart attack. Changes in the heart rate and the blood pressure are related more to the anxiety/ pain experienced during the procedure rather than to the administration of the local anesthetic. Moreover, a dental procedure can occasionally be the main factor in precipitating a potentially lethal form of heart disease, namely infective endocarditis. Cardiovascular problems that warrant special attention and dental treatment plan modification include infective endocarditis, cardiovascular lesions, ischemic heart disease, myocardial

Table 12.14 Platelet count levels required in various dental procedures

- *For periodontal or oral surgery:* Platelet counts should be above 75,000/mm^3
- *For major surgical procedures:* Platelet counts should be above 100,000/mm^3
- *Spontaneous bleeding occurs:* When the platelet count is less than 20,000/mm^3

infarction, cardiac arrhythmias, and congestive heart failure. In patients with cardiovascular disease, the most important considerations during treatment include the maintenance of blood pressure, pulse, cardiac output, and myocardial oxygen and the prevention of bacteremia via prophylactic antibiotic.

Generally, best practice suggests that a comprehensive dental evaluation should involve a thorough medical history and premedical evaluation, if required, and an examination that includes assessment of vital signs (e.g. pulse, blood pressure, the rate and depth of respiration, and temperature). Dental treatment should include short morning appointments, good procedural pain control, stress and anxiety reduction that could include preoperative or intraoperative conscious sedation good postoperative follow-up with pain control using appropriate medication, and pretreatment and post-treatment antibiotic coverage for specific conditions.

Dental Considerations

Patients should be instructed always to maintain good oral hygiene. Effective painless local analgesia (LA) is essential, and an aspirating syringe should be used. Epinephrine containing LA should not be given in excessive doses to patient taking beta blockers, as it may induce hypertension and cardiovascular complications. Citanest is not recommended to be used for cardiac or hypertensive patients. Assure the patient. Stress free short, morning appointments are recommended. Antibiotic prophylaxis is recommended for cardiac patients to prevent infective endocarditis. Flu-like symptoms within 2–4 weeks following procedure may be a signs of bacterial endocarditis, even if prophylaxis was taken.

Hypertension

Hypertension is the persistently raised blood pressure resulting from increased peripheral arteriolar resistance. Dental management can be complicated, since any procedure causing stress can further raise the blood pressure and may precipitate acute complications like cardiac arrest.

In cases of abnormal situations where the:

- Diastolic pressure is
  - <85—do periodic biannual checks
    - 85–89—recheck annually
    - 90–104—confirm within 2 months
    - 05–115—evaluate or refer immediately to physician, within 2 weeks, no dental treatment
    - >115—evaluate or refer immediately to physician, no dental treatment.

- Systolic
  - <140—do periodic biannual checks
  - 140-200—confirm promptly, within 2 months limited dental treatment
  - >200—evaluate or refer immediately to physician, no dental treatment.

Since the blood pressure rises with anxiety, steps should be taken to make the patient relaxed and fully at rest. Common medication side effects when prescribed to a hypertensive patient can cause xerostomia and frequent urination (with diuretics), and postural hypotension (with beta-blockers). Vital organ status must be evaluated prior to deciding on the type of local anesthetic in a hypertensive patient. Prilocaine/Bupivacaine may be used for mild hypertension. Mepivacaine without epinephrine may be used for moderate hypertension. Lidocaine with epinephrine may be used in well-controlled ASA-1 or ASA-11 patients.

Preoperative assurance is important and sedation may be helpful. Patients are best treated in the morning with continuous BP monitoring and given short appointments. Adequate analgesia must be provided but NSAIDs are best avoided. Gingival retraction cords containing epinephrine should be avoided. Common medication side effects of antihypertensive drugs are xerostomia, frequent urination, postural hypotension (with beta blockers), salivary gland swelling or pain, lichenoid reactions, gingival hyperplasia , and/or sore mouth.

Stroke (Cardiovascular Attack)

In such a scenario, side of body affected is contralateral to location of injury and may affect speech, understanding, and visual perception. Gag reflex may be compromised and oral hygiene may be poor on affected side. Patient may be on anticoagulants and hypertensive.

Ischemic Heart Disease with Angina

Angina attacks may be precipitated by dental treatment. This can lead to infarction and cardiac arrest. This patient will benefit from empathy, short morning appointments, premedication with anxiolytics or prophylactic nitroglycerin, nitrous oxide-oxygen sedation, and slow delivery of an anesthetic with epinephrine (1:100,000). The patient should be reminded to have with them their nitroglycerin tablets in case of an attack during treatment. Patients will also benefit from being placed in a semireclined position in the dental chair. This group of patients may also be taking Beta-adrenergic blocking agents and calcium channel blockers. The prevention of complications relies on the above considerations.

Local analgesia should be given with an aspirating syringe. Adrenaline containing LA solutions may be used but no more than 4 mL of solution in 1:80,000 adrenaline. Gingival retraction cords containing adrenaline should be avoided. Mepivacaine 3% is preferable for use in patients on beta-blockers.

Myocardial Infarction

Although relatively uncommon in the dental setting, cardiac arrest as a result of myocardial infarction (MI) can occur. In patients with a history of MI, dental treatment should not be pursued for at least 6 months after the cardiac event. The patient's physician should be contacted prior to treatment and verification sought regarding the patients current cardiac status. As with the ischemic patient, short morning appointments are best. The combination of an MI with congestive heart failure increases risk to the patient, so only emergency treatment should be provided on an outpatient basis. The onset of chest pain and shortness of breath during dental treatment should be immediately followed by discontinuing of the procedure and immediate medical consultation or hospitalization.

A patient post myocardial infarction may be on anticoagulant medication and the dose may need to be reduced, if dental extractions or periodontal surgery is necessary. Even prolonged aspirin use can affect bleeding time. Potential complications can be avoided by acquiring a prothrombin time on the day of surgery. Potential adverse reactions need to be taken into account after treatment (e.g., the interaction between NSAIDs, penicillin, tetracyclines, metronidazole, and anticoagulants) because prophylactic antibiotic may need to be considered to prevent infection. Cardiac patients may also be prescribed digitalis, which can increase nausea as well as exacerbate the gag reflex. Epinephrine is contraindicated, if the patient is on digitalis as it can cause digitalis toxicity. Recommended use of mepivacaine without epinephrine for the first 6 months of dental treatment and then evaluate, if LA with epinephrine can be given.

Cardiac Arrhythmias

Patients with cardiac arrhythmias are at greater risk for more serious cardiac complications including cardiac arrest. Most patients presenting for dental treatment will know, they have an arrhythmia and will be taking controlling medication such as procainamide, quinidine, or propranolol. Medical consultation should be sought before dental treatment to verify the patient's cardiac status and confirm the medications. Complications during dental treatment can be prevented by reducing stress and anxiety and providing short morning appointments. If the patient's cardiac status is unclear, treating in a more controlled hospital environment may be best. It is best to avoid excessive anesthetic with epinephrine.

Congestive Heart Failure

The challenges in treating the patient with congestive heart failure are numerous. A determination must be made via physician consultation on the status of the disease prior to treatment (i.e., is it stable or unstable?). The condition is often complicated by hypertension, a history of MIs, renal failure, thyrotoxicosis, and chronic obstructive pulmonary disease (COPD). Antibiotics will need to be prescribed following treatment to prevent infection. The dentist should always be prepared for potential complications. Only urgent dental needs should be provided in patients with uncontrolled cardiac failure and medical attention comes before dental treatment. For the patient who is deemed stable and without significant complications, routine conservative dental care can be performed in and outpatient setting. Prior to treatment, a prothrombin time should be obtained, and, during treatment, the patient should be placed in an upright position to prevent additional pulmonary fluid collection. Bupivacaine should be avoided. Placing the patient supine will worsen dyspnea and should therefore, be avoided. NSAIDs should be avoided in patients taking ACE inhibitors, since they increase the risk of renal damage.

Heart Transplants

No treatment should be carried out within first 6 months (except emergency care). A thorough dental evaluation and treatment is done prior to transplant. There is an increased risk for infection due to immunosuppressive drug therapy and increased candidiasis and herpes incidence. Therefore, antibiotic prophylaxis is indicated for surgical procedures, as well as extended post-treatment to promote healing. Minimize and control stress, monitor vital signs, and manage pain/anxiety. Use local anesthetic without epinephrine.

Pacemakers

Consult with the physician as antibiotic prophylaxis may be indicated. Additionally, in patients with pacemakers, electrocautery and the use of a cavitron should be avoided. It is best to avoid using epinephrine in anesthesia.

Coronary Artery Bypass Grafts

Avoid routine dental treatment for the first 6 months after surgery, and only emergency dental care should be performed. Antibiotic prophylaxis is usually needed only during these first 6 months. It is best to consult with the physician. Routine treatment can be carried out after 6 months. Like with all cardiac problems, it is best to generally avoid epinephrine (Table 12.15).

Table 12.15 Basic rules for cardiac patients

Medically: • Consult physician • Obtain good health history • Obtain accurate and correct medication history • Monitor vital signs each visit • Antibiotic coverage when and if needed • Minimize stress and pain *Dental considerations:* • Control pain and infection • Maximize oral hygiene abilities • Evaluate for anticoagulant medications • Keep appointment short and in the mornings • Use la without epinephrine

Medications of Concern in Patients with Cardiac Problems

- *Warfarin (Coumadin):* Anticoagulant, check prothrombin time (desired maximum level 18–20 seconds) (INR should be under 2.5)
- *Aspirin:* Decreases platelet aggregation, check bleeding time
- *Heparin:* Anticoagulant, check PTT (desired maximum level 45–50 seconds).

ENDOCRINE CONDITIONS

Diabetes Mellitus

Disease Nature

Diabetes mellitus (DM) is a complex syndrome characterized by abnormalities in carbohydrate, lipid and protein metabolism that result either from profound or an absolute deficiency of insulin, related to autoimmune destruction of the insulin producing pancreatic beta cells (Type 1), or from target-tissue resistance to its cellular metabolic effects, related commonly to obesity (Type 2) or both conditions. Other types of diabetes include gestational diabetes and diabetes occurring secondary to other diseases. Complications in the diabetic patient that can occur during and after dental treatment include hypoglycemia, coma, infection and delayed healing.

Dental Management

A carefully constructed questionnaire and thorough medical history can give some indications that a patient could be at risk of being diabetic or be an undiagnosed diabetic, especially Type 2. The classical symptoms of DM include (3P's): polydipsia, polyuria and polyphagia. The following findings are also indicative of possible diabetes: recent weight loss, irritability, dry mouth, frequent infections and a history of poor wound healing. A patient suspected by the dentist to be diabetic, should be referred to a physician for proper evaluation and diagnosis. Properly controlled Type 1 and Type 2 diabetic patients usually can undergo all dental treatments without special precautions.

Consultation with the patient's physician is a must when:

- The patient has systemic complications of diabetes such as heart or renal disease
- The patient has difficult to control diabetes or is under high insulin dosage
- The patient has an acute oral infection such as periapical or periodontal abscess.

Blood sugar level should be checked and monitored regularly. Early morning appointments are preferred which will minimize the risk of stress-induced hypoglycemia. LA can usually be safely used. Drugs that can disturb diabetic control (aspirin and steroids) must be avoided. Routine dental treatment or short minor surgery under LA can be carried out with no special precautions apart from ensuring that it does not interfere with eating (Table 12.16).

In patients with controlled diabetes, no special treatment is required for routine dentistry including prophylaxis and dental restorative care. The patient should be told to continue with their normal eating and injection regimen. Morning appointments are recommended because cortisol levels are highest at this time and will provide the best blood glucose level. The appointments are best scheduled after breakfast. No more than two carpules of lidocaine 1:100,000, prilocaine HCL (1:200,000), or bupivacaine with 1:200,000 epinephrine should be used.

In the moderately-controlled diabetic patient, a maximum of two carpules of bupivacaine or prilocaine should be used and, if a major procedure is planned (e.g., multiple extractions, periodontal surgery), an antibiotic should be prescribed following therapy. Following surgery the patient's food intake should include the proper caloric content and protein/carbohydrate/fat ratio to maintain glucose balance.

Table 12.16 Diabetic patients

DM-dental management
• Always treat a diabetic on a full stomach • Never forget to ask if the patient has eaten • Always compensate for the snack time between 10 am and 3 pm • Use stress management when needed • Maintain hygiene recall visits at 3–4 or 4–6 months interval • Since diabetics heal slowly, so use nonabsorbable suture material • Always consult with the physician, if blood sugar levels are raised • Avoid the chronic use of NSAIDs

In the uncontrolled or brittle diabetic patient, only acute dental infection should be treated. Local anesthetic should not include epinephrine. Antibiotics should be prescribed following treatment to promote healing and treat infections. Delay the treatment, if there is no dental emergency, as the diabetes needs to be brought under control first.

The most common in-office complication that occurs during treatment of the diabetic patient is hypoglycemia resulting from a severely depressed glucose level (as normal pattern of food intake gets disrupted). Symptoms may include mood change, hunger, and weakness and signs include sweating, tachycardia, and mental disturbance. The patient usually senses that they are becoming hypoglycemic and request a source of sugar such as orange juice.

HYPER/HYPOTHYROIDISM

Hyperthyroidism

A hyperthyroid patient is on antithyroid drugs like Propylthiouracil (PTU). While starting any dental procedure on such a patient, stress management protocol should be followed. For local anesthesia, only mepivacaine is recommended. Once the hyperthyroid patient is off the antithyroid medication, then lidocaine or prilocaine, or bupivacaine may be used (maximum 2 carpules). Nitrous oxide may be used for sedation. Before starting with the treatment, check the CBC with platelet count and INR as the antithyroid drug causes agranulocytosis, and thrombocytopenia.

Hypothyroidism

In the controlled hypothyroid patient, lidocaine, prilocaine or bupivacaine may be used with a maximum of 2 carpules. As like before, stress management measures are important. Acetaminophen may be used to control pain. In the uncontrolled hypothyroid patient, use only mepivacaine as the choice of local anesthetic. It is best to avoid codeine, and morphine.

PATIENT ON CORTICOSTEROIDS

Corticosteroids are stress fighting hormones. Always determine the maximum dose of steroid the patient has taken in the last 2 years. Consult with the physician to determine the amount of steroid boost needed, if any major surgical procedure is being performed. These patients benefit being treated as the first appointment of the day. Schedule the surgery on the day of the steroid intake. Double the routine dose of the patient. Always confirm with the physician prior to the dental treatment to confirm the amount of steroids needed (Table 12.17). Aspirin and other NSAIDs should be avoided, as they may increase the risk of peptic ulceration in these patients.

Table 12.17 Suggested guidelines for a patient on steroids

- Conservative dentistry or minor surgery (single tooth extraction). No cover required
- 1–2 quadrant flap surgery or up to 4–16 extractions. Use 20–40 mg on the day of the surgery
- Major surgery or trauma. Use 60 mg on the day of the surgery

EPILEPSY

Epilepsy is a term that describes a group of disorders characterized by chronic, recurrent, and paroxysmal changes in neurologic function (seizures) that are caused by abnormal electrical activity in the brain. Seizures may either be accompanied by motor manifestations or manifested by sensory, cognitive or emotional changes in neurologic function. The first step in the management is identification, which is best accomplished by the medical history and seizure history: type, age at onset, cause and medications. Make sure patient has taken his medication. Try to schedule the appointment early morning. It is important to appreciate the fact that epileptics can have good and bad phases and that various factors can precipitate seizures in susceptible patients. Dental treatment should therefore, be carried out in a good phase, when attacks are infrequent. Poorly controlled patients may require additional anticonvulsant or sedative medications. For these patients, a consultation with the physician is advised before dental treatment.

A strong mouth prop is to be kept in position and the oral cavity as free as possible of any debris. Keep equipment and apparatus as much as possible away from the area of the patient. Be alert and on your guard for any feature that may indicate the start of seizure. Aspirin and NSAIDs should not be administered to patients taking valproic acid (medicine used in treatment of epilepsy). Erythromycin should not be administered to patients taking carbamazepine. Oral complications include gingival overgrowth associated with phenytoin. The anterior labial surfaces of the maxillary and mandibular gingivae are most commonly and severely affected.

RENAL DISEASE

Renal disease in children mainly comprises the so-called nephritic syndromes which may progress to chronic renal failure (CRF). Progression to CRF leads to the need for dialysis and possibly transplantation. CRF patients may be taking corticosteroid and other immunosuppression drugs. This can make medical management difficult for these patients. The main concern is the bleeding tendency. Careful hemostasis should be ensured, if surgery is necessary.

Local anesthesia is safe, unless there is severe bleeding tendency. Prophylactic antibiotics should be prescribed due to immunosuppression for all invasive procedures. Dental treatment is best carried out on the day after dialysis. Avoid prilocaine or septocaine, as the erythropoietin level is low. Tetracycline should be avoided in chronic renal failure, as they can cause increase in the nitrogen retention and acidosis. Aspirin and NSAIDs should be avoided, as they affect renal function and can cause bleeding. Codeine and dyhydrocodeine are favored as analgesics (Table 12.18).

PULMONARY DISEASES

Bronchial Asthma

Bronchial asthma is a generalized airway obstruction which in the early stages is paroxysmal and reversible. The obstruction, leading to wheezing, is due to bronchial muscle contraction, mucosa swelling and increased mucus production. Exposure to allergens and/or stress can induce an attack. Infrequent attacks of asthma can be managed by salbutamol inhaler or can be used prophylactically, if an attack is predicted, e.g. before exercise or prior to a stressful event such as dental treatment. If the attacks are more frequent, then salbutamol should be used regularly.

Dental Management

Avoid anxiety which may precipitate an asthmatic attack. Patients are advised to bring their regular medication with them. Elective dental care should be deferred in severe asthmatics, until they are in a better phase. Patient should not be treated during sickness, e.g. flu-like symptoms. Allergy to penicillin may be more frequent. Drugs which may precipitate an asthma attack should be best avoided like aspirin, NSAIDs and penicillin. Epinephrine, erythromycin, clindamycin and azithromycin are contraindicated for patients on theophylline. Avoid the use of LA containing vasoconstrictor because some asthmatic patients may react to sulphites which are present in the local anesthetic solution as preservatives.

Table 12.18 Drugs for use for patients with renal disease

Safe to prescribe	*Fairly safe (dose reduction only in severe cases)*	*Less safe (dose reduction required) and best to avoid*	*Contraindicated*
Antimicrobials			
• Doxycycline • Erythromycin • Flucloxacillin • Ketoconazole • Penicillin	• Ampicillin • Amoxicillin • Clindamycin • Metronidazole	• Acyclovir • Fluconazole	• Sulphanamides • Tetracycline
Local anesthetics			
• Lignocaine • Codeine	• Codeine	• Paracetamol	• Aspirin/NSAIDs

CHRONIC OBSTRUCTIVE PULMONARY DISEASE AND TUBERCULOSIS

Chronic obstructive pulmonary disease (COPD) is most frequently caused by chronic bronchitis and emphysema. Stress management measures should be carried out and inhalants can be used as prophylactic measures. Wherever possible, dental treatment should be carried out under local anesthesia but without epinephrine. Patients are best treated in the upright position as they may become breathless, if laid flat. It may also be difficult to use a rubber dam in these patients as they may not be able to tolerate the additional obstruction to breathing.

It is recommended to use universal precautions in all patients suffering from tuberculosis being treated in the dental environment. Patients with open pulmonary tuberculosis are clearly contagious and dental treatment is thus deferred, until the tuberculosis (TB) has been treated. An open case can safely be treated after two weeks of continuous antiTB treatment. Use lidocaine with epinephrine with a maximum of two carpules. Avoid aspirin and NSAIDs. Penicillin and clindamycin are safe to use antimicrobials, should the need arise.

LIVER DISORDERS

Liver disorders are important to the dentist due to a potential bleeding tendency, intolerance to drugs (e.g. general anesthetics, benzodiazepines) and the possibility of underlying infective causes for the liver dysfunction. Signs of liver disease includes jaundice, spider naevi, leukonychia, finger clubbing, palmar erythema, dupuytren's contracture, sialosis and gynecomastia. Patients with liver disease have impaired hemostasis and can present serious bleeding problems. Disorders associated with an early rise in serum levels of conjugated bilirubin can cause dental hypoplasia and greenish discoloration of the teeth.

Dental Management

Local analgesia (LA) is safe given in normal doses, prilocaine or articaine are preferred to lidocaine. In patients with cirrhosis, minimize the bleeding and use the suction judiciously. Patients should not be allowed to swallow blood, as encephalopathy may occur. Severe bleeding can occur after dental extractions in patients with chronic liver disease and hence, the clotting status must be tested, as they may have decreased platelets and/or decreased clotting factors. The most common liver function test (LFT) involves the measurement of aspartate transaminase (AST) and alanine transaminase (ALT). ALT may also be raised in cardiac or skeletal muscle damage and is therefore, not specific for liver disease.

Hepatic impairment will lead to failure of metabolism of many drugs that can result in toxicity. In some cases dose reduction is required; other drugs should be avoided completely. The antifungal drug miconazole is contraindicated, if there is hepatic impairment and fluconazole requires dose reduction. Erythromycin, metronidazole and tetracyclines should be avoided. Antimicrobials such as penicillin, cephalexin and cefazolin can be safely given in normal doses. Acetaminophen can be used for pain control. Aspirin and NSAIDs should be avoided because of the risk of gastric hemorrhage (Table 12.19).

INFECTIOUS DISEASES

Infectious conditions that are problematic in terms of dental management include hepatitis B (HBV), hepatitis C (HCV), HIV, and tuberculosis. Less likely to cause a problem but of additional concern are viral infections such as that seen in severe acute respiratory syndrome (SARS) or methicillin-resistant *Staphylococcus aureus* (MRSA). There are several potential complications that can occur during dental treatment with this group of infections such as the risk of transmission, medication interactions in patients being treated for active disease, management of the patient with organ disease or other complications related to viral infection or associated with medication management (e.g., susceptibility to bleeding, oral disease, or respiratory infection). In addition, the transmission of cold and flu virus

Table 12.19 Drugs in liver disorders

Drugs	Comments
Local anesthesia	
• Lidocaine	Contraindicated in patients suffering from cirrhosis of liver. Maximum two carpules may be used with hepatitis.
• Prilocaine	Choice of local anesthetic for cirrhosis
Analgesia	
• Aspirin/NSAIDs	Contraindicated in all liver disease, hepatitis or cirrhosis
• Acetaminophen	Can be used in lower than normal doses Cirrhosis—<1–1.5 gm/day Hepatitis—2–2.5 gm/day
Antimicrobial	
• Amoxicillin	Safe to use
• Tetracycline, metronidazole and macrolides	Contraindicated
• Doxycycline	Regular dose with hepatitis; 50% reduction with cirrhosis, doxycycline cannot be used in a patient having both kidney and liver disease
• Clindamycin	Regular dose with hepatitis; 50% reduction with cirrhosis

from staff to patients with immune suppression resulting from treatment of the viral infection is also a concern.

Viral Hepatitis

This is important and of relevance in dentistry, since it is due to blood-borne viruses which pose an infection risk and there is an associated liver dysfunction. Viral hepatitis relevant to dentistry may be caused by hepatitis B virus (HBV), C (HCV), D (HDV), or G (HGV). Hepatitis B may be associated with hepatitis D and cause a fulminant hepatitis (Table 12.20). The main problems are: highly infective disease, bleeding tendency and drug sensitivity. Pure saliva does not contain HBsAg, but serum via gingival exudates does.

Dental Management

Dentist should treat the patient within the current regulations for cross infection control. Patients with active acute hepatitis B should have dental treatment after complete recovery only, which may take about three months after symptomatic recovery. Needle stick injury can transmit the virus. An injection of hepatitis B immunoglobulin (HBIG) within 24 hours of contact may protect from developing hepatitis. Any patients with signs or symptoms of hepatitis should be referred to a physician. If emergency care becomes necessary, it should be provided as for a patient with acute disease.

The only oral complication associated with hepatitis is the potential for abnormal bleeding in cases of significant liver damage. If surgery is required, it is advisable to check the prothrombin time (discuss with the patient's physician), and monitor the bleeding time to check platelet function (if it is not less than 20 minutes, discuss with the patient's physician).

Patients identified as having such illness at check-in may be rescheduled. Only "urgent" dental care be provided in a room with a closed door, and staff should wear personal protective garments. When performing procedures on the patient, a good fitting surgical face mask should be worn, so that the spray or spatter potentially occurring during the dental procedure be minimized. It also goes without saying that sick personnel should not come to work, until fever free.

Table 12.20 Various forms of hepatitis

Water/food borne	*Blood borne*
Hepatitis A: 2–6 weeks Hepatitis E: 2–9 weeks Hepatitis A and E are acute types of hepatitis	Hepatitis B: 2–6 months Hepatitis C: 15–150 days Hepatitis B, C and D are chronic types of hepatitis

A potential problem associated with the treatment of patients with infectious disease is that while millions of people worldwide are, per published data, infected and thousands may be infected every year, a large number of these people are unaware of their disease. For this reason, best practices include "Universal" (now termed "Standard" by the CDC) versus selective precautions.

Note that although dental procedures may contaminate the saliva with blood, the relative risk of disease transmission to dental personnel is considered extremely small. Occupational exposure, however, no matter how small the risk, remains an important concern for dental staff including assistants, hygienists, lab technicians, and dentists. Hence, education of all staff, whether administrative or clinical, is extremely important, if patients with infectious disease are to be managed in an outpatient setting.

Precautions

Wounds and needle sticks following dental procedures that result in oral bleeding and subsequent instrument or materials contamination represent the biggest problem with respect to potential viral transmission to clinical staff. Two other areas of concern with respect to viral contamination include potential backflow associated with dental restorative equipment (e.g., high speed hand-pieces that use water and compressed air and their cross-connections) and aerosols and salivary/water droplets produced during restorative dental procedures. The latter is of concern with respect to potential airborne transmission of some diseases (e.g., tuberculosis, N1H1).

Dental health care personnel are encouraged to read literature about this as a first step in providing appropriate precautions in the clinical setting. Staff training updates are recommended. To avoid complications from medication interactions in the patient with infectious disease, prior to treatment, the patient's physician should be contacted and queried regarding current medications, precautions related to immune suppression or thrombocytopenia, which would necessitate a platelet count and bleeding time prior to invasive (e.g., extraction or periodontal surgery) intervention, and the extent of potential organ damage (e.g., liver).

Hepatitis B immunization is recommended for all dental clinical staff. This vaccine is a recombinant vaccine of HBsAg, which gives protective antibody levels after three doses in healthy adults for at least 3 years.

HIV/AIDS

Treat the patient as a "normal" patient, if the WBC count is normal. Check if the patient has neutropenia by assessing the absolute neutrophil count. Neutrophil counts below 1500 cells/mm^3 predict the risk for mild/moderate infection. Fever is usually the only symptom present. Minimal or no pus formation occurs with oral infections. Pain and erythema may be the only signs of infection.

Mild/Moderate Neutropenia

Neutrophil count is 1000–1500 cells/mm^3 in mild neutropenia, whereas in moderate cases the neutrophil count is 500–1000 cells/mm^3. The patient has a mild risk of infection and may undergo major or minor dental procedures. Premedication is required only for major surgical procedures. Patients are advised to use a nonalcoholic mouth rinse prior to all dental procedures. Antibiotics may be prescribed for 3-5 days post major surgeries. It is recommended to use cidal/static agents.

Severe Neutropenia

Neutrophil count is less than 500 cells/mm^3. There is a risk of life threatening infection. Patients should be isolated and hospitalized. The signs and symptoms of the oral infections may be masked. Only palliative dental treatment should be provided.

CONCLUSION

In order to provide safe comprehensive care for the medically compromised patient who cannot tolerate care designed for the healthy patient, dentists must apply knowledgeable treatment modification for safety and comfort.

BIBLIOGRAPHY

1. American Dental Association Bureau of Economic and Behavioral Research Survey: 1988 Survey of Dental Practice, ADA News. 1989;20:15-6.
2. American Dental Association Bureau of Economic and Behavioral Research Survey: GPs keeping up with inflation. ADA News. 1989;20:14.
3. DiBaggio JA. Hospital training for dental students: problems and potentials. J Dent Educ. 1973;37:13-8.
4. Gregg JM. The nature and control of pain, anxiety, and stress, in emergencies in Dental Practice, In: McCarthy FM (Ed), ed 3, Philadelphia, WB Saunders, 1979.
5. Guntheroth WG. How important are dental procedures as a cause of infective endocarditis? Amer J. Cardiol. 1984;54:797-801.
6. Jacobsen JJ, Schweitzer SO, DePorter DJ, Lee JJ. Antibiotic prophylaxis for dental patients with joint prostheses? A decision analysis. Int J Tech Assess in Health Care. 1990;6:569-87.
7. McCarthy FM. Essentials of safe dentistry for the medically compromised patient, ed 1, Philadelphia, WB Saunders, 1989.
8. McGowan DA. Dentistry and endocarditis. Br Dent J. 1990;169:69.
9. Norden CW. Prevention of bone and joint infections. Amer J Med. 1985;78 (Suppl 6B):229-32.
10. Pallasch TJ, Slots J. Antibiotic prophylaxis and the medically compromised patient. Periodontology 2000. 1996;10:107-38.
11. Tsevat J, Durand-Zaleski I, Pauker SG. Cost-effectiveness of antibiotic prophylaxis for dental procedures in patients with artificial joints. Amer J Pub Health. 1989;79:739-43.

CHAPTER **13**

MEDICAL EMERGENCIES

Priyanka Jain

INTRODUCTION

Medical emergencies can occur at any time in the dental office. They can happen to anyone, like the anxious patient in the reception room to the receptionist with a seizure disorder or to the dentist experiencing prolonged chest discomfort. The best way to handle an emergency is to be prepared in advance. Whether the medical emergency never occurs or occurs this afternoon, preparation is the key. All health care providers including dentists should be prepared to recognize and handle medical emergencies in the office. Staff should be trained and frequently updated in first aid and cardiopulmonary resuscitation (CPR) procedures. An emergency plan should be available, and all staff members should be thoroughly familiar with it including their responsibilities in an emergency like training of office personnel in handling emergencies, and maintenance of an emergency kit fully equipped and ready for immediate use.

PREPARATION FOR EMERGENCIES/MEDICAL RISK ASSESSMENT

Medical emergencies in the dental office are rare. Most emergencies can be prevented by adequate preparation of the patient and staff. The following are suggested guidelines:

- Obtain a medical and the drug history for every patient and update it at each visit. Obtain physician consultation where and when necessary. This reduces the chances of a problem arising during treatment.
- When confirming appointments, remind patients to take their normal medications on the day of their appointment. Procedures should be scheduled around meal times for diabetics. Patients using inhalers or nitroglycerin should have these with them should an asthma or angina attack is precipitated by the stress of dental treatment.
- Dentists should also assess all the patients using the ASA (American Society of Anesthesiologists) classification. This will help the dentist to identify patients with a higher risk for medical emergencies occurring during treatment.

- It is important to monitor and interpret vital signs . These should be taken at the initial visit as a "baseline reading" and at each subsequent visit for those patients whose medical history indicates they may be "at risk" (Table 13.1).
- All staff members should be trained in basic first aid procedures and basic life support (CPR) (Flow charts 13.1 and 13.2).
- The office should have a written emergency plan (Table 13.2). Each staff member should know and practice their particular function in an emergency, and emergency telephone numbers should be posted at each phone.
- Office personnel should be aware of the signs and symptoms indicating an emergency. Each office should have an emergency kit readily available and each staff member should know where it is located. All staff should be aware of their legal responsibilities when responding to an office emergency.

The "best handled" medical emergency
is always be the one that never happened.

Table 13.1 Vitals

Baseline vitals	
Body temperature	
Location	*Normal*
Oral	98.6°F
Rectal	99.6°F
Axillary	97.6°F
Pulse rates	
Age	*Beats/Minute*
0–1 years	100–150
1–10 years	60–140
10 + and adults	60–100
Blood pressure	
Normal	120/80 or lower
Prehypertension	Between 120–140 systolic and/or 80–89 diastolic
Hypertension	Anything over 140 systolic and/or 90 diastolic
Respiratory rates	
Age	*Respiratory rate*
Adults	12–20
Teenagers	15–25
Toddlers	20–30
Infants	25–40

Flow chart 13.1 Adult basic life support algorithm

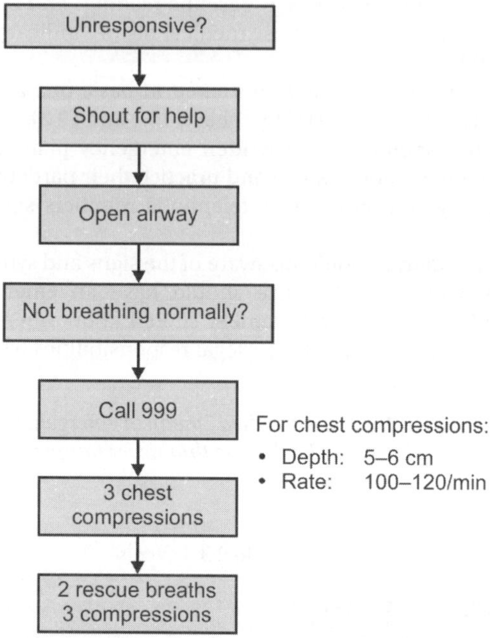

- The following minor modifications to the above sequence may be made
- Give five initial rescue breaths before starting chest compressions.
- If you are on your own perform cardiopulmonary resuscitation (CPR) for 1 minute before going for help.
- Compress the chest by one-third of its depth. Use one or two hands

Source: Reproduced with the kind permission of the Resuscitation Council (UK)

EMERGENCY TRAINING

Every member of the dental team should have completed a basic first aid course and have annual training in cardiopulmonary resuscitation (CPR). The CPR course for health care providers is recommended because it includes two-person CPR, child and infant CPR, and the use of a mask. Ideally, the entire staff should take the CPR refresher course together, so they will feel comfortable working with each other if the need arises. Masks with one-way valves should be used in training. Pocket masks are much easier to use, provide effective ventilations, and have ports for the addition of supplemental oxygen.

Flow chart 13.2 Adult and child choking algorithm

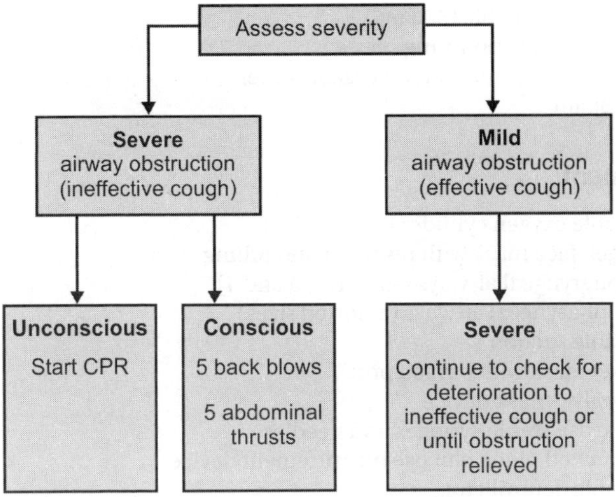

This algorithm is suitable for use in children over the age of 1 year

Source: Reproduced with the kind permission of the Resuscitation Council (UK)

Table 13.2 Emergency situations

Procedures for all emergency situations
• Supine position • If conscious, make them comfortable • Reassure the patient • Provide oxygen when not in hyperventilation phase • Monitor vitals/maintain open airway • Be prepared

Emergency drugs are standardized and should be immediately available in all dental surgery premises. They are:

Pharmacological Agents

- Oxygen
- Nitrous oxide
- Hydrocortisone injection
- Oral glucose
- Glyceryl trinitrate (GTN) spray (400 micrograms/dose)

- Salbutamol aerosol inhaler with spacer (100 micrograms/actuation)
- Adrenaline (Epinephrine) injection (1:1000, 1 mg/mL)
- Aspirin dispersible (300 mg)
- Glucagon injection 1 mg
- Oral glucose solution/tablets/gel/powder
- Diazepam.

Equipment

- Portable oxygen cylinder (E or D size)
- Oxygen face mask with reservoir and tubing
- Oropharyngeal airways (sizes 1, 2, 3 and 4)
- Nasopharyngeal airways (assorted sizes)
- Portable suction
- Pocket mask with oxygen port
- Bag-valve-mask device
- Single use sterile syringes and needles
- Automated blood glucose measurement device
- Portable defibrillator.

Other Equipment

- Gauze
- Tape
- Alcohol swabs
- Blood pressure monitoring device
- Stethoscope.

Drugs in solution should always be in a pre-filled syringe. All drugs should be stored together and the box marked as emergency drugs. Where possible all emergency medical equipment should be single use and latex free. An automatic external defibrillator (AED) is an adjunct piece of equipment every dental office would benefit from as part of the office emergency kit. The AED is a computerized defibrillator that recognizes the presence of ventricular fibrillation or rapid ventricular tachycardia and then allows the operator to administer "shocks" to convert the patient's heart rhythm back to normal. For every minute that lapses before defibrillation, the survival rate decreases by 10%. The AED is equipped with a voice prompt to lead the operator through its usage and requires no special training. Adult AEDs can safely be used on children over 8 years old. Some AED's have pediatric pads that permits them to be 'attenuated' to make them more suitable for use in children between 1 and 8 years of age. These modifications may be considered for practices that regularly treat children.

DRUGS

Epinephrine 1:1000 Concentration

This is used for severe allergic reaction and acute asthmatic attacks. Adult dose is 0.3 mg. The pediatric dose for adrenaline is based on the child's approximate age or weight. The method of delivery is via an auto-injector like epipen. Epipen is a preloaded dose of epinephrine injection delivering a dose of 300 micrograms (0.3 mL adrenaline injection 1:1000). Epinephrine is the treatment of choice for allergic reactions, as it reverses all the histamine induced symptoms and blocks the further release of histamine. The effect usually lasts for about 15–20 minutes. Pediatric size auto-injectors are also available.

Use: Epinephrine may be used to reverse hypotension , bronchospasm, and laryngeal edema that result from an acute anaphylactoid type reaction. It may also be used to reduce bronchospasm resulting from an acute asthmatic episode that is refractory to inhaler therapy. Epinephrine is available in the form of vials, ampules, or preloaded syringes in concentration of 1:1000, 1 mg/mL.

Epinephrine causes vasoconstriction that in turn increases blood pressure, heart rate, and force of contraction and reduces histamine release.

Adverse Effects of Epinephrine

- *Cardiovascular:* Tachycardia, tachyarrhythmia's, and hypertension
- *Central nervous system:* Agitation, headache, and tremors
- *Endocrine system:* Increased blood glucose
- *Pregnant female:* Can decrease placental blood flow
- *Drug interactions:* Use with nasal decongestants, antihistamines, and asthma inhalers will increase incidence of adverse effects. Can be ineffective if the patient is taking beta-blockers.

Glucagon

Glucagon mobilizes glucose from the last stores of glycogen in the liver. This helps the patient in regaining consciousness in case of an emergency crisis. Glucagon effect lasts for about 15 minutes and once the patient is conscious, oral glucose can be administered.

Diphenhydramine (Benadryl) 50 mg Injection

This may be used to reduce the effects of histamine release that is associated with allergic reactions, anaphylaxis, and acute asthma attack precipitated by exogenous causes. Benadryl is an antihistamine that blocks the release of histamine in the body. *It does not prevent the action of the histamine once released and thus must be given quickly.* This also prevents histamine responses such as bronchospasm, hypotension, rash, and edema.

Adverse Effects

- *Cardiovascular:* Tachycardia
- *Central nervous system:* CNS depression (sedative effects including drowsiness, lethargy, and mental confusion)
- *Gastrointestinal:* Xerostomia (dry mouth)
- *Drug interactions:* Any drugs causing CNS depression will increase the sedative effects of benadryl.

Nitroglycerin (GTN)

This is a venous and arteriolar dilator that results in increased cardiac output and reduced left ventricular filling pressure. If exposed to oxygen/light it is only effective for 12 weeks. It has a shelf-life of only 6 months. When using it should produce a bitter taste or impart a sting if still effective.

PROPOSED OFFICE EMERGENCY PLAN

Because it is impossible to know when an emergency may occur or what form it may take, it is important that every dental office have an established, written, and practiced routine for handling emergencies. Emergency numbers such as 911 (USA), 999 (UK), 102 (India), or an ambulance number should be posted conspicuously at every phone in the office. Other numbers for emergencies might include the hospital emergency department, an oral surgeon, a physician, and so forth. During an emergency, alert other staff to the existence of an emergency and avoid possible upset to the other patients in the clinic. The office emergency plan should be updated and practiced regularly at periodic staff meetings. Mock scenarios of various emergency situations can be developed which will allow each staff member to act out their assigned roles. With careful planning and frequent practice of the office emergency plan, confusion and panic can be significantly reduced during an actual emergency.

Anxiety Reduction

Stress may be considered as the major factor causing medical emergencies in the dental office. Syncope, hyperventilation, seizures, asthma attacks, and angina are some of the more common emergencies and all can be precipitated by stress and anxiety. Anxiety related problems are fairly easy to prevent. The first step is to identify the patient likely to experience anxiety. Anxious patients tend to startle easily, exhibit pale and clammy skin, and appear apprehensive. In pretreatment conversations, they may relate their phobia about the treatment or indicate a fear of pain. Once a stressed patient is identified, steps can be taken to manage the anxiety proactively. A first step can be to minimize the amount of waiting prior to any procedure. The procedure should be explained to the patient in a thorough and detailed manner beforehand, so that he or she experiences no surprise in the operatory. In more extreme cases, patients may need to be premedicated with antianxiety agents. Adequate pain control should be used and longer procedures may be divided into shorter dental appointments.

Recognition of an Emergency and Initial Emergency Procedures

A systematic approach to recognizing the acutely ill patient based on the 'ABC' principles is recommended. Documentation of the patient's medical history should allow those 'at risk' of certain medical emergencies to be identified in advance of any proposed treatment (Table 13.3). Physical signs and symptoms that may indicate a medical emergency may include chest pain, pale skin, sweating, vomiting, irregular respiratory rate, altered or unusual sensations, hemorrhage, and changes in pulse and blood pressure. When an emergency situation is recognized, dental treatment should be stopped immediately and assistance summoned. If the patient was receiving nitrous oxide, it should be discontinued.

In an emergency, stay calm. Ensure that you and your staff are safe. Look at the patient generally to see if they 'look unwell'. In an awake patient ask, "How are you?" If the patient is unresponsive, shake him and ask, "Are you all right?" If they respond to your questions normally, then that means that they are breathing and have no obstruction in their airway. If they speak only in short sentences, they may have breathing problems.

Table 13.3 Medical emergencies

Emergencies in dental practice:

- Syncope
- Allergic reactions
- Seizures
- Hyperventilation
- Postural hypotension
- Angina pectoris
- Asthma attack
- Epinephrine reaction
- Hypoglycemia
- Cardiac arrest
- Anaphylactic reaction
- Myocardial infarction

The ABC approach should always be followed and used in cases of emergency. **A**irway, **B**reathing, **C**irculation, approach (ABC) is the best way of assessing the patient experiencing difficulty in your dental operatory. This is the best way to identify and treat life-threatening problems. Assess the effects of any treatment given. Call for help early. Use all members of your dental team. This will allow you to do several things at once. Organize your team and communicate effectively.

Airway (A)

Airway obstruction is an emergency.

- *Look for the signs of airway obstruction:* In most cases, only simple methods of airway clearance are needed like airway opening maneuvers—head tilt/chin lift or jaw thrust and remove visible foreign bodies, debris or blood from the airway
- A face mask with oxygen inlet may be used to give oxygen.

Breathing (B)

Diagnose and treat immediately life-threatening breathing problems, e.g. acute severe asthma. Look, listen and feel for the general signs of respiratory distress: sweating, central cyanosis (blue lips and tongue), use of the accessory muscles of respiration (muscles of the neck) and abdominal breathing.

Circulation (C)

Simple faints or vasovagal episodes are the most likely cause of medical emergency problems in dental practice. These usually respond to laying the patient flat raising the legs. Common causes of unconsciousness include hypoxia, hypercapnia (raised carbon dioxide levels), cerebral hypoperfusion (low blood pressure), or the recent administration of sedatives or analgesic drugs. The cause of unconsciousness should, therefore, be singled out accordingly. A complete medical history of the patient taken before the start of the procedure would help in doing so. Assessment of the patient's conscious level should be done using the AVPU method: **A**lert, responds to **V**ocal stimuli, responds to **P**ainful stimuli or **U**nresponsive to all stimuli.

The most important aspect of nearly all medical emergencies in the dental office is to prevent, or correct insufficient oxygenation of the brain and the heart. Therefore, oxygen is the most important drug for use. Oxygen "E" cylinder is almost three feet tall and contains enough oxygen to ventilate a nonbreathing adult for approximately 30 minutes.

In all emergency situations, proceed rapidly and when in doubt, "do". Always stay in the sequence while doing your assessment of the patient and know what to look for, recognize and treat. Always look for likely, treatable problems and make decisions based on your direct examination. Be careful to initiate only simple test and procedures.

HANDLING SPECIFIC MEDICAL EMERGENCIES

Specific medical emergencies are depicted in Table 13.3.

AIRWAY OBSTRUCTION

Foreign bodies falling into the hypopharynx can lead to partial or complete airway obstruction. Blockage does not allow adequate air exchange in the lungs. The patient may complain of a foreign body sensation in the throat, be coughing and dyspneic, exhibit stridor, or become apneic and cyanotic. They may grasp their throat with their hand (choking symbol) and, in the case of complete airway obstruction, will be unable to speak. If not corrected immediately, respiratory arrest may occur and can lead to cardiac arrest within minutes. Dental patients are susceptible to choking with the potential risk of aspiration. They may have blood and secretions in their mouths for prolonged periods.

Symptoms and Signs

- The patient may cough and splutter
- Choking, gagging, violent expiratory effort, not able to speak, panic, labored breathing, rapid then decreased pulse, respiratory and/or cardiac arrest
- Breathing may become noisy with wheeze (usually aspiration) or stridor (usually upper airway obstruction)
- They may become cyanosed and lose consciousness.

Management

If the patient is coughing forcefully, allow them to continue to cough, as this is their best chance for clearing their airway. If the patient is conscious, but continues to choke and is unable to breathe, abdominal thrusts may be used (Stand behind the patient, and place the thumb side of the fist into the abdomen above the umbilicus and below the rib cage. Administer slow, inward and upward thrusts until the object pops free or the patient loses consciousness).

With loss of consciousness, help the patient to the floor in a supine position, open the airway and sweep out any obstructions which can be reached with the finger. Attempt to ventilate. If the patient cannot be ventilated, the airway is still obstructed. Continue the steps for CPR—checking mouth and ventilating at the appropriate time. This will not only provide circulatory support but also the pressure generated within the chest by performing chest compressions may help to dislodge the foreign body.

- In cases of aspiration, allow the patient to cough vigorously. Symptomatic treatment of wheeze with a salbutamol inhaler may help (as for asthma).
- If any large pieces of foreign material have been aspirated, e.g. teeth or dental amalgam, the patient should be referred to hospital for a chest X-ray and possible removal. Where the patient is symptomatic following aspiration they should be referred to hospital as an emergency.

Prevention

- Utilize rubber dam
- Assure all equipment is fastened tightly
- Keep the patient in an upright position while taking impressions
- Use high volume suction where required
- Use of appropriate chair and head position
- Floss should attached when able to (like tying the floss around the clamp during the use of rubber dam).

Because total airway obstruction usually occurs during inspiration, there is usually adequate oxygen in the cerebral blood to permit up to two (2) minutes of consciousness. If foreign body is not recovered or passes, refer patient as soon as possible for radiographic examination for the object localization.

ASTHMA/BRONCHOSPASM/CHRONIC OBSTRUCTIVE PULMONARY DISEASE

Asthma is an allergic response of the small airways (bronchioles). It is a slow progressing bronchospasm. Asthma affects people of all ages, but is more common in younger people. Chronic obstructive pulmonary disease (COPD) is a mixture of emphysema and bronchitis seen in older adults. Common to both is the propensity of the small airways to spasm (bronchospasm). In patients with COPD, the retention of carbon dioxide (CO_2) is a complicating factor.

In both cases, patients may respond to anxiety with bronchospasm. Many cases can be prevented by pretreatment with the patient's metered dose inhaler (puff) of bronchodilator medication. The inhaler should also be readily available at chairside. The patient may abruptly develop bronchospasm which may be evident by wheezing, coughing, and difficulty breathing, and may also complain of chest tightness. The patient should be placed in an upright position with arms forward to facilitate breathing and oxygen should be administered by mask.

Causes

- *Extrinsic:* This is an allergic type of asthma and can be classified as a Type 1 hypersensitivity reaction. It is more common in the younger people.
- *Intrinsic:* This type of asthma is mainly caused by respiratory infections or nonallergic factors such as cold temperatures, exercise or emotional stress/anxiety. This is more common in older patients and usually occurs after the age of thirty-five.

Symptoms and Signs

Acute severe asthma in adults:

- Inability to complete sentences in one breath
- Respiratory rate >25 per minute
- Tachycardia (heart rate >110 per minute)
- Labored breathing, tightness in chest, coughing spasms, wheezing, anxiety, and gagging are all the symptoms of acute asthma.

Life-threatening asthma in adults:

- Cyanosis or respiratory rate <8 per minute
- Bradycardia (heart rate <50 per minute)
- Exhaustion, confusion, decreased conscious level.

Management

Patients with asthma (both adults and children) may have an attack while at the dental surgery. Most attacks will respond to a few 'activations' of the patient's own inhaler such as salbutamol (100 micrograms/actuation or puffs). Repeat doses may be necessary. If the patient does not respond rapidly, or any features of severe asthma are present, an ambulance should be summoned. If the patient is unable to use the inhaler effectively, additional doses should be given through a large-volume spacer device. If the response remains unsatisfactory or if the patient develops tachycardia, becomes distressed or cyanosed (blueness around the lips or extremities), arrangements must be made to transfer them urgently to hospital.

Put the patient in an upright comfortable position (erect). Reassure the patient but do not crowd near him and give him some breathing space. Allow the patient to use his/her own inhaler if they have. Whilst awaiting ambulance transfer, oxygen (15 liters per minute) should be given. Salbutamol inhaler (2–4 puffs initially, repeat in 15 minutes) should be given using a large-volume spacer device until an ambulance arrives. This causes the relaxation of the smooth muscles of the bronchioles. If any patient becomes unresponsive always check for 'signs of life' (breathing and circulation) and start CPR in the absence of signs of life or normal breathing.

Signs patient is deteriorating

If the breathing does not improve, if the patient is tiring or if the breathing slows down dramatically are all signs of patient deterioration.

Prevention

- Identify any family history or patient's own of asthma
- Know what a typical attack is like for them and discuss how to manage it in case of its emergency
- Have inhaler accessible at all times near the operating chair
- Avoid inhalation of irritating agents or any stress from the procedure. Also the dentist should avoid prescribing any medicine which may cause dry mouth.

ALLERGY

An allergic reaction is the result of an antigen-antibody reaction to a substance to which the patient has been previously sensitized. Histamine and other complex chemicals are released from body cells causing symptoms in the patient. These symptoms may be confined to a single organ system or become generalized (anaphylaxis). In the dental office, the most likely causative factors are exposures to latex, local anesthetics, or antibiotics, but foods the patient may have eaten prior to their visit such as nuts, shellfish, milk products, and strawberries can also trigger this reaction.

The allergic reaction is frequently seen only in the body system which first came into contact with the allergen. Wheezing may be the result of something the patient may have inhaled which affects the lungs. A reaction may also be due to an injection of local anesthetic or antibiotic, resulting in a skin rash with intense itching. In other cases, ingested foods may lead to swelling of the upper airway and stridor. In its most severe form, an allergic reaction can progress to anaphylaxis, a condition in which several body systems are affected simultaneously.

Pathophysiology

This is an antigen-antibody reaction. It may be systemic or generalized and may be characterized by:

- Angioneurotic edema (pharynx and upper airway)
- Asthma (respiratory tract)
- Urticaria-pruritus (integumentary system)
- Anaphylaxis (all of the above with circulatory collapse).

The treatment of all types of allergic reactions is the same i.e. provide supportive care and administers epinephrine. Maintain the patient's airway, administer oxygen, and monitor the vital signs. Administer epinephrine 1:1000, 0.3–0.5 mg subcutaneously, often into the upper arm or thigh. Call emergency services immediately as anaphylaxis may be a life-threatening emergency.

ANAPHYLAXIS

Anaphylaxis is a severe, life-threatening, generalized or systemic immediate type of hypersensitivity reaction. It is characterized by rapidly developing life-threatening airway and/or breathing and/or circulation problems usually associated with skin and mucosal changes. Symptoms can develop within minutes and early and effective treatment may be lifesaving.

Risk Factors

- Multiple intermittent exposures in a patient
- Children have less chances of developing reactions to medicines due to shorter exposure times
- Women may show higher incidences of reactions (cutaneous) secondary to their increased exposure to cosmetics and latex
- Patients with multiple illnesses, prominent drug history
- Patients with allergies to food-stuff.

Hypersensitivity Classification (Gell and Coombs)

- *Type 1:* IgE mediated hypersensitivity. This is life-threatening and symptoms are evident within few minutes of the reaction.
- *Type 2:* IgM or IgG antibodies mediated hypersensitivity (cytotoxic/ cytolytic antibody mediated).
- *Type 3:* This is immune-complex mediated hypersensitivity and the antibodies involved are soluble metabolites of IgG and IgM. The symptoms take about 1–4 weeks to become apparent.
- *Type 4:* This is a delayed hypersensitivity reaction mediated by sensitized T-cell lymphocytes.

Symptoms and Signs

The lack of any consistent clinical manifestation and a wide range of possible presentations can cause diagnostic difficulty. Clinical assessment helps to make the diagnosis.

Signs and symptoms may include:

- Apprehension and anxiety
- Sudden hypotension due to hypervolemia caused by vasodilatation
- Labored breathing
- Respiratory and circulatory failure
- Shock
- Swelling of the tongue and oropharynx
- Urticaria (wheal and flare). Trunk, face and extremities are affected
- Erythema can be localized or generalized. The main symptom is flushing
- Pruritus may be specific for lesions or may be generalized. There may be mild to severe itching

- Angioedema (localized) affects mainly the face, lips and the periorbital area. There is localized skin swelling, edema and puffiness. Lesions may be painful or some patients may even experience a burning sensation of the skin
- Abdominal pain, vomiting, diarrhea and a sense of impending doom
- Facial flushing is common, but pallor may also occur
- Marked upper airway (laryngeal) edema and bronchospasm may develop, causing stridor, wheezing and/or a hoarse voice
- Cool, pale and clammy skin.

Typical Progression

This may occur rapidly with considerable overlap. Clinically this includes the appearance of skin reactions, smooth muscle spasms (GI, GU, respiratory), respiratory distress and cardiovascular collapse.

Management

The drug used in allergic reactions is mainly epinephrine, diphenhydramine, and dexamethasone. It is advisable to use an ABC approach to recognize and treat any suspected anaphylactic reaction. First-line treatment includes the termination of the dental treatment and removing the irritant, managing the airway and breathing and restoration of blood pressure (laying the patient in a supine position, raising the feet) and the administration of oxygen (15 liters per minute). For severe reactions, adrenaline should be given intramuscularly (anterolateral aspect of the middle third of the thigh through the clothes) in a dose of 500 micrograms (0.5 mL adrenaline injection of 1:1000).

The dose is repeated if necessary at 5 minutes intervals according to blood pressure, pulse and respiratory function and until a response is noted. Monitor the vitals. Proceed with basic life support as needed. In less severe cases any wheeze or difficulty in breathing can be treated with a salbutamol inhaler as detailed above in the section on *asthma*. All patients treated for an anaphylactic reaction should be sent to hospital for further assessment, irrespective of any initial recovery and kept under observation as a relapse is common in such situations.

ACCIDENTAL ANESTHETIC OVERDOSE

Rapid administration, excessive dosage, or inadvertent intravascular administration may all result in increased drug effects. Prevention is the most important key in avoiding adverse drug reactions. Use the minimum amount required to achieve the desired effect and administer the drug slowly. While administering blocks, always try to use an aspirating syringe.

For children, a child's body size and weight should be considered during dosing and anesthetic administration.

Local anesthetic reactions could be in the form of *local anesthetic toxicity, drug interactions, and vasoconstrictor interactions.* Anesthetic overdose can occur due to a majority of reasons. Some of them are discussed in brief below.

Rapid Intravascular Injection

The likelihood of occurrence of this type of overdose is common. Onset of the signs and symptoms is most rapid and occur within seconds of administration of the drug (intra-arterial is faster than intravenous). The symptoms are quite intense and last for about 2–3 minutes. Both amides and ester group of local anesthetics can cause an overdose. This overdose reaction can be prevented by aspirating and injecting slowly.

Too Large a Dose

This is the most common type of anesthetic overdose reaction occurring. It takes about 3–5 minutes for the signs and symptoms to occur. There is a gradual onset of the symptoms with increased intensity and may prove to be quite severe. The symptoms last for about 5–30 minutes depending on the dome and the ability of the individual's body to metabolize or excrete. The amide group of local anesthetics is the main culprit with esters rarely. The preventive method is to administer minimal doses.

Rapid Absorption

This type of overdose reaction occurs most likely with "high normal" dosages if no vasoconstrictors are used. The signs and symptoms take about 3–5 minutes to occur and gradually increase in intensity. They last for about 5–30 minutes. Again, this type of a reaction occurs with the usage of amide group of drugs. Always use a vasoconstrictor and limit the topical anesthetic use to a minimum.

Slow Biotransformation and Elimination

These types of reaction are uncommon/least common. The occurrence of the signs and symptoms to occur may take anywhere from 10 to 30 minutes to 10 minutes to hours. There is a gradual onset of the symptoms with slow increase in its intensity. The symptoms may last for potentially longest duration due to the inability of the body to metabolize or excrete. This can occur with both amide and ester group. Adequate physical evaluation of the patient before starting the treatment is very important and necessary.

Clinical Signs and Symptoms

Low to Moderate Doses

- Confusion, apprehension and restlessness
- Ringing or buzzing in the ears
- Blurred vision and unable to focus
- Slurred speech and generalized stutter
- Muscle twitching and tremor of the face and extremities
- Numbness of the tongue and perioral tissues
- Disorientation and a flushed/chilled feeling
- Nystagamus
- Increased blood pressure, heart rate, and respiratory rate
- Loss of consciousness.

High Overdose Levels in the Blood

Generalized tonic-clonic seizures followed by:
- Generalized CNS depression
- Depressed blood pressure, heart rate, and respiratory rate.

Management

The patient should be treated supportively until the effects of the drug wear off. Stop the administration of the drug, maintain the airway, monitor vital signs, and contact emergency services if the patient fails to show prompt improvement.

Mild Reaction: Slow Onset

As there is no specific antidote for lidocaine toxicity, provide supportive care. Maintain the airway, administer oxygen, and treat other problems as they arise. Reassure the patient. Allow for the recovery and get help if required.

Severe Reaction: Rapid Onset

Stop all treatment and place the patient in a supine position with feet up. Establish the airway and give oxygen. If the patient experiences convulsions, protect them by removing any harmful and dangerous object from around them. Summon medical help.

ACUTE ADRENAL INSUFFICIENCY

This type of a medical emergency arises if the patient is on long-term administration of oral corticosteroids. A patient with adrenal insufficiency may become hypotensive when under physiological stress. This is a rare occurrence in a dental surgery, but however if a patient collapses during dental treatment other causes should be considered first and managed before diagnosing adrenal insufficiency. A complete and thorough medical and drug history of the patient would show the use of oral corticosteroids.

Acute adrenal insufficiency can often be prevented by administration of an increased dose of corticosteroid prior to treatment. Usually, simple dental extractions and restorative procedures, including endodontics, are not a cause for concern, but surgical extractions or implant placement should be considered as a risk as they might put the patient under undue stress. Doubling the patient's steroid dose before significant dental treatment under local anesthesia and continuing this for 24 hours is also recommended.

CARDIAC EMERGENCIES ANGINA PECTORIS (CHEST PAIN)

Angina is the *Latin* term for spasmodic, choking or suffocating pain. Pectoris means chest in *Latin*. The central chest discomfort usually results from stressful situations in patients with coronary artery disease. In angina episodes, the coronary artery (narrowed by atherosclerosis) is unable to supply the heart muscle with adequate amounts of oxygenated blood, thus causing chest pain. The onset of this type of chest pain is usually related to exercise, stress, and anxiety. The decreased oxygen supply to the heart muscle is usually of short duration (less than five minutes) and no permanent damage occurs.

Signs and Symptoms

- Crushing or squeezing pain in chest, "intense" of short duration
- Excessive sweating
- History of angina pain (lasting more then 3–5 minutes but shorter than 20 minutes)
- Radiating pain to left arm/jaw
- Feeling of indigestion
- Prompt relief with rest and/or nitroglycerin.

The relevant factors which aid in diagnosing are: *Onset* (the time and the associated event causing stress and anxiety to the patient), *location of the pain, site of radiating pain* (less frequent sites include right shoulder and arm, left jaw, and epigastrium), *type of pain* (deep, visceral, superficial, or pleuritic), and *exacerbating/alleviating factors.*

Management

Stop all treatment. Place the patient in a comfortable semi-upright position. Administer oxygen and nitroglycerin sublingually (may be repeated in

3–5 minutes intervals, maximum of 3 times). It is very important to monitor vitals to have baseline. If pain lasts longer then 8–10 minutes or is atypical for patient, call for the emergency services immediately. Nitroglycerin comes in the form of 0.4 mg tablets or 0.4 mg metered dose spray. Their use is to relieve or eliminate chest pain associated with angina pectoris, and to differentiate between angina and a myocardial infarction. Patient should be sitting or supine when nitroglycerine is administered. Antihypertensive drugs may exaggerate the hypotensive effect of nitroglycerine.

Dose

- *Tablet:* One tablet sublingually and repeat after two minutes if no relief up to three doses.
- *Metered dose spray:* One spray sublingually repeat after two minutes if no relief up to three doses.

Prevention

A complete medical history should be taken and updated at each visit. Always have nitroglycerin pills available. Try to make the patient feel comfortable and alleviate any anxiety or stress he/she may have related to the procedure.

MYOCARDIAL INFARCTION (HEART ATTACK)

In myocardial infarction (MI or heart attack), a blood clot develops in one of the coronary arteries completely cutting off blood supply to a portion of the heart muscle. Without a blood supply, the heart muscle dies within a few hours. The ischemic heart is susceptible to cardiac arrhythmias and thus the patient is susceptible to sudden death. Whenever and wherever a myocardial infarction is recognized, emergency services must be called immediately (Table 13.4). This is critical, as about 50 percent of patients experiencing a myocardial infarction will die in the first two hours.

In both cases (angina pectoris and myocardial infarction), the patient will complain of chest pain usually described as a pressure or weighty sensation. This pain or numbness may radiate into either of their shoulders, arm, the neck, jaw, straight through to the back or to the upper part of the abdomen. Complaints of shortness of breath, nausea or vomiting are common, and the patient's skin may be pale and sweaty. If the patient has experienced angina in the past, they will be able to determine if this pain is different in character.

Table 13.4 Treatment considerations

Dental treatment considerations in the patient with a history of myocardial infarction (MI)
Review changes in the patient's medical history including medication doses. Stress reduction is a very important part of the procedure. Use adequate pain control measures and minimize the duration of the appointment-late morning, early afternoon. Only emergency procedures should be carried out if there is a history MI within six months, then a medical consultation is recommended. All other procedures/ treatments should be deferred until later.

Probable Causes

- Stress and anxiety
- Exertion
- Heredity, age (50–70)
- Smoking, obesity, and uncontrolled hypertension.

Symptoms

- Severe central crushing or squeezing pain in chest, "Sharp"
- Sudden onset of pain and the patient breaks into a cold sweat
- Radiating pain to left arm/jaw, back
- Nausea, vomiting, light headed
- Dull, heavy, pressure sensation
- Dyspnea, syncope, and sudden death
- Pain not relieved by nitroglycerin or rest and is of long duration
- Women tend to be fatigued and complain of back pain/upper abdominal pain
- Shortness of breadth
- Skin becomes pale and clammy.

Management

Stop all treatment and position the patient comfortably (sitting position in a conscious patient with short of breath, patients who feel weak/faint may be laid flat). Constantly reassure the patient. Give sublingual GTN spray. Have the patient chew to crush an aspirin—if not allergic (325 mg adult dose). High flow oxygen may be administered (15 liters per minute) if the patient is cyanosed (blue lips) or conscious level deteriorates. Continue to monitor the vitals every 5 minutes. If the patient becomes unresponsive always check for 'signs of life' (breathing and circulation) and start CPR in the absence of signs of life or normal breathing (Table 13.5).

Table 13.5 Differences between angina pectoris and myocardial infarction

Acute myocardial infarction	*Angina pectoris*
Pain lasts for 30 minutes to hours	Pain lasts 3–5 minutes
Associated with arrhythmias	Not associated with arrhythmias
Pain during exertion or rest	Pain follows exertion or rest
Pain is not relieved by rest	Pain is relieved by rest
Pain returns after administering nitroglycerin	Pain is relieved by nitroglycerin
Patient may have reduced or normal BP	Pain is uncomfortable in nature but not acute

Prevention

As in all cases, a thorough medical history should be taken. Stress should be as little as possible. Appointments should be scheduled in late morning/afternoon. Obtain a medical clearance from the patient's general physician. Do not treat a patient with history of MI attack within 6 months.

HEART FAILURE/SUDDEN CARDIAC ARREST

Heart failure results when one of the ventricles is unable to completely pump all of the blood filling the chamber forward into the arteries. Heart failure may involve either the left ventricle (left ventricular failure-LVF) or the right ventricle (right ventricular failure-RVF). Of the two, left ventricular failure is the more serious and occurs first. In LVF, blood backs up into the lungs causing pulmonary congestion and shortness of breath, particularly when the patient is lying flat. In RVF, the blood backs up into peripheral circulation causing swollen legs and ankles resulting in pitting edema.

Left ventricular failure is frequently precipitated by an acute myocardial infarction. Place the patient in whatever position is most comfortable for them, usually sitting bolt upright. Administer oxygen by mask and monitor vital signs. If the patient complains of chest pain, nitroglycerin may be given.

DIABETES

Diabetic emergencies are the result of diabetes mellitus, a chronic disorder of carbohydrate metabolism in which insufficient insulin is produced or insulin is not used effectively. The emergency conditions associated with diabetes include hypoglycemia, the most acutely life-threatening, and the slower onset hyperglycemia. There are two types of diabetes. They are:

1. Type I, insulin—dependent diabetes mellitus. This represents about five percent of all cases of diabetes. It is more common in adolescents, but can occur in adults. In this form virtually no insulin is produced.
2. Type II, noninsulin dependent diabetes mellitus. This is mostly seen in adults but may occur in some children.

A medical emergency of diabetes mellitus is precipitated by factors that increase the body's need for insulin. Dental therapy is a potential threat since stress increases insulin needs, which in turn can precipitate hyperglycemia even in a person who is normally well controlled. Simply having a dental appointment may cause the person to alter normal eating habits that could create an insulin imbalance.

HYPOGLYCEMIA

Hypoglycemia occurs when there is insufficient glucose in the bloodstream to meet the metabolic demands of cells. True hypoglycemia is seen only in insulin dependent diabetics (Type I) or in Type II diabetics using oral hypoglycemic agents. Hypoglycemia occurs when blood sugar levels drop below 80 mg/dL and typically becomes more acute in the 20–30 mg/dL range.

Risk Factors

- Omission of meals
- Overdose of insulin
- Alcohol consumption
- Excessive exercise
- Reduced meals
- Medication error
- Other illnesses.

Clinical Features

The lack of glucose results in immediate dysfunction, causing the patient to appear confused and restless. Patients may also complain of a headache or exhibit bizarre behavior. Their skin becomes pale, cool and clammy, and their heart rate increases. On occasion, a patient may exhibit seizure activity or transient stroke-like symptoms. If a source of glucose is not administered immediately, permanent damage may result.

- Shaking and trembling
- Sweating

- Difficulty in concentration/vagueness
- Slurring of speech
- Unconsciousness.

  Children may not have such obvios features but may appear lethargic.

Management

Stop all treatment. Position the patient comfortably, possibly semireclining. Maintain open airway and administer oxygen. Give glucose, carbohydrate (icing, juice). This step may be repeated after 10–15 minutes. Brain can only survive 5 minutes without glucose. If the patient becomes unconscious, summon medical help without delay. In such cases, glucagon may be given via the IM route (1 mg in adults and children >8 years old or >25 kg, 0.5 mg if <8 years old or <25 kg). It may take 5–10 minutes for glucagon to work and it requires the patient to have adequate glucose stores. Keep monitoring the blood glucose levels and the vitals. Check for 'signs of life' (breathing and circulation) and start CPR in the absence of signs of life or normal breathing. Once patients are alert and able to swallow after injecting glucagon, they may be given a drink containing glucose. The patient should be accompanied home.

Prevention

Hypoglycemia can be prevented by making sure the insulin dependent diabetic has eaten before treatment, by scheduling appointments in the morning, and by having a glucose source readily available at chairside. If the patient exhibits signs and symptoms of hypoglycemia, administer an oral carbohydrate such as regular cola, sugar, or even a spoonful of honey or icing to raise blood glucose levels. Patients with diabetes should eat normally and take their usual dose of insulin or oral hypoglycemic agent before any planned dental treatment.

HYPERGLYCEMIA/DIABETIC KETOACIDOSIS

Diabetic ketoacidosis occurs when there is not enough insulin available to move glucose into cells and there is too much glucose in the blood. This causes the cells to use fats and proteins for energy, leaving behind waste products which build up in the blood. Over time, from hours to days to sometimes weeks, the blood sugar level continually increases. Frequently an underlying medical problem such as heart attack, infection, or stroke may precipitate diabetic ketoacidosis even in diabetics who are normally in good control. This may be due to obesity, or may be heredity.

The signs and symptoms of diabetic ketoacidosis are related to high blood sugar, and the body's attempt to compensate for the acidosis. Patients may hyperventilate and have a fruity odor to their breath; extreme thirst due to severe dehydration and polyuria are the common features. Because of the loss of fluids, the skin is warm, red, and dry to the touch. Patient may feel fatigued with a weak/rapid pulse. Blood sugar levels may increase and the patient finally may lose consciousness. Treatment includes maintaining the airway by placing the patient on their side to prevent aspiration. This is a serious emergency and medical help should be immediately summoned. The patient may require hospitalization.

SYNCOPE (FAINTING)

Fainting or syncope results from the psychological response to fear, anxiety, stress, pain, or unpleasant situations. Syncope accounts for over 50% of reported emergencies in the dental office. The psychological reaction causes an abrupt slowing of the heart rate and pooling of blood in the extremities. Within seconds the patient may complain of a flushed sensation, followed rapidly by loss of consciousness. Inadequate cerebral perfusion (and oxygenation) results in loss of consciousness (Table 13.6). This most commonly occurs with low blood pressure caused by vagal over activity.

Therefore, simple faint/syncope is the loss of consciousness caused by a reversible disturbance in cerebral function owing to decreased circulation of blood to the brain. This is the most common emergency in the dental office and the patient may recover in seconds and may take up to 2–3 minutes.

Table 13.6 Types of syncope

Cause	*Type*	*Comments*
Circulatory	• Vasodepressor	• Often precipitated by stress/ anxiety
	• Hypovolemia	• Occurs with vomiting, diarrhea or hemorrhage
Central nervous system	• Cerebrovascular	• Transient ischemic attacks, stroke
	• Seizures	• Warning aura, postictal confusion
	• Emotional	• Anxiety
Metabolic	• Hypoglycemia	• Confusion
	• Anemia	–
	• Hypoxia	–
Cardiac	• Arrhythmias	• Dizziness, bradycardia/ tachycardia

It is very important to rule out any other causes of unexpected loss of consciousness and be able to differentiate a simple faint from them. Other causes of loss of consciousness in a dental office may be:

- *Postural hypotension:* This is due to low BP and can be attributed to the patient in a supine position for more then 15–20 minutes. Some drugs may also be the cause of loss of consciousness due to postural hypotension like nitroglycerin (as it lowers the blood pressure, so should not be administered), and niacin supplements which are used to lower the body cholesterol. Late stage pregnancy, advanced age, venous defects in legs-varicose veins, exhaustion, starvation, and nitrous oxide are all other possible causes of postural hypotension.
- *Hypoglycemia:* This is more often seen in starving diabetic patients with insulin overdose caused by stress and lack of meal.
- Cerebral vascular accident
- *Steroid crisis:* This is mostly seen only in patients taking systemic steroids.
- Seizure
- Arrhythmias
- *Anxiety attack:* This could be a simple faint though usually the patient would have some premonitory symptoms of faintness before losing consciousness. Recovery is quite rapid in these situations.
- Anaphylaxis
- *Hyperventilation:* Many anxious patients may hyperventilate under stress and may feel faint and light headed but do not usually lose consciousness. Reassure the patient in such cases.
- Adrenal insufficiency
- *Myocardial infarction:* Patient would usually have a history of angina, hypotension or any other risk factor.

Clinical Features

Presyncopal Phase

- Nausea and a feeling of warmth
- Perspiration and loss of color
- Prodromal pallor, light headedness, dizziness or weakness
- Baseline blood pressure
- Slow pulse rate
- Pupillary dilation and peripheral coldness
- Visual disturbances.

Syncopal Phase

- Loss of postural tone
- Sudden collapse and loss of consciousness
- Any syncope lasting for more than a few minutes may induce seizures and cerebral ischemia.

Management

When faced with a fainting episode, place the patient in a *Trendelenburg position* (supine position with legs elevated and head down). For the pregnant patient, place them in left lateral position. Try to assess the consciousness of the patient by using the ABC protocol. Once supine, the patient should regain consciousness almost immediately. Administer oxygen and loosen any tight clothing. Monitor their vital signs and maintain an open airway. Cold compresses to the forehead, and neck also might be useful. If the patient is unresponsive to any of the above mentioned measures, check for signs of breathing and circulation and initiate CPR. It is recommended that treatment be stopped and rescheduled for another date. Call for medical help if loss of consciousness continues for more than 5 minutes or if recovery period is more than 20 minutes.

Prevention

Syncope can be prevented by identifying the patient prone to anxiety or who is using anti-anxiety agents. Fearful and anxious patients may be prescribed a premedication to help them relax. Keep the patient supine if possible; with older patients, allow them time to slowly adjust to an upright posture after procedures are completed as in the elderly, rapid changes in posture can result in postural (orthostatic) hypotension.

SEIZURES

Convulsions or seizures are caused by waves of abnormal electrical activity in the brain and are a manifestation of brain dysfunction. There is excessive neuronal cortical damage in such cases. Seizures could occur secondary to toxins, drugs, cerebral hypoxia, or metabolic disturbances. Seizures are most commonly seen in patients with known seizure disorders such as epilepsy. Such patients may have stopped taking or missed a dose of their anti-seizure medication or they may experience a seizure as a result of exposure to a triggered or stressful situation. It is important to note that otherwise "normal" patients may seize if the conditions are right, particularly with hypoglycemia or hypoxia. In cases of partial/petit mal seizure, the patient remains conscious whereas in cases of tonic clonic/grand mal seizure, there is loss of consciousness. It is very important to take a detailed and a thorough medical history in such patients and update it regularly.

The questions to ask during the history taking could be like:

- What kind of a seizure disorder do you have?
- What happens when you have an episode? Do you have an "Aura"?
- Are you taking any medications for the disorder?
- How long do they typically last?
- When was your last seizure? If within the last one week, it is very important to call their physician and get medical clearance.

- What are the exacerbating factors?
- Did you take your medications today?
- What can we do for you if one comes on?
- Is there someone we should contact if you have one?

Clinical Features

In some cases, the patient may have a brief warning or 'aura' that they are about to have a seizure. This may be in the form of a strange smell, visual or auditory hallucination, or other strange sensation. As a seizure begins the patient tremors, becomes rigid, and may give a cry, become cyanosed (*tonic phase*) and loses consciousness. The skeletal muscles contract and relax in waves and after a few seconds, there are jerking movements of the limbs; the tongue may be bitten (*clonic phase*). During this phase, these involuntary movements make the patient susceptible to injuries to the head, arms, or legs, and they may become incontinent of urine and stool. There may be frothing from the mouth. A seizure is followed by a period of drowsiness, confusion and extreme fatigue called the *postictal phase.* It is very important to evaluate the patient's injury during this phase.

Postictal Phase: Patient experiences lethargy, disorientation, apnea, obstructed airway, and cardiac arrhythmias.

Management

When observing a generalized motor seizure, knowing what not to do is as important as knowing what to do. Never attempt to place or force any object between the patient's teeth. Bite sticks are ineffective and may cause damage to oral structures. Do not attempt to restrain the patient's movements. Leave the patient in the chair in a supine position and do not attempt to move them. Do not attempt to ventilate the patient during a seizure. Do not restrain the patient during a seizure. The seizure typically lasts a few minutes. After a variable time the patient regains consciousness but may remain confused and disoriented and feel sleepy. Loosen any constrictive clothing and turn the patient on their side to protect their airway from vomiting and aspiration. Place padding beneath the patient's head to prevent injury and let the seizure run its course. After the seizure, place the patient in a recovery position and monitor the airway and vitals, and administer oxygen.

The *National Institute for Clinical Excellence* (NICE, UK) guidelines suggest that the indications for sending to hospital are:

- Status epilepticus
- High-risk of recurrence
- First episode
- Difficulty monitoring the individual's condition.

Medication should only be given if seizures are prolonged (convulsive movements lasting 5 minutes or longer) or recur in quick succession. In such cases, emergency services should be summoned immediately. According to the *American Red Cross*, emergency services should be called if:

- Seizures occur repeatedly
- A seizure lasts longer than five minutes
- The victim appears injured
- The victim has no history of a seizure
- The victim is pregnant
- The victim is diabetic
- The victim does not regain consciousness immediately after the seizure
- If the episode lasts longer than 10–15 minutes.

Pharmacological Management

If the emergency services have still not arrived and the seizure is lasting for more than 5 minutes, then dextrose 50 mL bolus of 50% glucose can be given in an adult patient. In children, 2 mL/kg 25% dextrose solution may be given. Benzodiazepines can also be given. Diazepam 5–10 mg IV/IM as an adult dose and pediatric dose is 0.2–0.5 mg/kg IV/IM may be given.

TRANSIENT ISCHEMIC ATTACK/CEREBROVASCULAR ACCIDENTS (STROKE)

A cerebrovascular accident (CVA or stroke) or a transient ischemic attack (TIA) is caused by an interruption of blood flow to the brain. This is a localized neurological disorder. This could be caused due to uncontrolled hypertension or any trauma to the head. These episodes are usually seen in older patients as a consequence of atherosclerosis. The interruption in flow may be due to a blood clot, spasm of the arteries, or even to rupture of a blood vessel in the brain. The different types are:

- Cerebral embolism—floating blood clot lodges in brain
- Cerebral infarction—decreased blood flow to the brain (atherosclerosis)
- Cerebral hemorrhage—rupture of a cerebral artery
- Cerebral thrombosis—obstruction of a cerebral artery due to clot formation.

Risk Factors for Stroke

- High blood pressure
- Smoking
- Diabetes: 5 times more likely to suffer stroke
- Heart disease

- Carotid artery disease
- High cholesterol
- Physical inactivity
- Obesity
- Heavy alcohol use.

Risk Factors You Cannot Change

- Aging—over 55
- Ethnicity
- A family history of stroke
- A prior stroke or heart attack
- Sickle cell disease.

Signs and Symptoms

Blood flow to the cerebral cortex is insufficient in these cases and the patient will exhibit symptoms within seconds. The signs and symptoms may be of short duration (TIA) which resolve spontaneously or persist for months or years. A transient ischemic attack is a forewarning of a major ischemic CVA; these patients must be evaluated by a physician to prevent such an occurrence.

- Headache, confusion and dizziness
- Unilateral weakness/paralysis (right or left side)
- Impaired speech
- Unequal pupils
- Difficulty breathing and swallowing
- Body veering to one side.

FAST: Signs can be used quickly to determine if a patient may be experiencing a CVA:

- Ask the person to smile (**F**ACE)
- Ask the person to raise both arms (**A**RM).
- Ask the person to speak a simple sentence (**S**PEECH)
- Call emergency services at any sign of stroke as time is crucial here (**T**IME).

Management

Terminate the procedure immediately as with any emergency. When faced with a TIA or CVA, emergency services should be called immediately. Place the patient on their side in a semi-supine position to maintain their airway, and suction oral secretions to prevent aspiration (as necessary). Monitor their vital signs. Oxygen may also be administered if the patient is having trouble breathing. Manage the patient symptomatically until help arrives.

Prevention

Try to make the patient comfortable and alleviate any anxiety/stress he/she may have about the dental visit. Do not treat for 6 months as there is a risk of restroke. Try to schedule their appointments in mid-afternoon as BP would be lower at that time. Consult with their physician if any precautions need to be taken.

HYPERVENTILATION

Anxiety, fear, overdose of medications, stimulants and pain in susceptible individuals can result in a conscious overdrive of ventilation called hyperventilation. This increased ventilation (breathing) in excess of what is required to maintain normal carbon dioxide levels can cause unpleasant symptoms which exacerbate the situation. Signs and symptoms include apprehension, air hunger (a sense that they "cannot catch their breath") coupled with numbness and tingling in the arms and legs, rapid shallow breathing, suffocating feeling, chest tightness and increased heart rate, all give the patient the sensation that something is seriously wrong. The hyperventilation may progress to the point where the patient may even lose consciousness.

Hyperventilation is the only emergency when oxygen administration is not administered. Terminate the procedure and reassure the patient. Make them realize that all of their symptoms are related to their fast respiratory rate. Coach the patient to take slow, regular breaths on a breath by breath basis (have the patient hold breadth for 10 sec interval). Monitor their vitals.

RESPIRATORY ARREST

The end result of bronchospasm, hypoxia, airway obstruction, aspiration, and laryngospasm may be respiratory arrest. Patients will become unresponsive and stop breathing. Call for help and emergency services immediately. Maintain the airway and ventilate with 100% oxygen (12/minute for adults and 20/minute for children). Repeat this step. Once the chest rises, stop the ventilation as over ventilation will distend the stomach with air and cause vomiting. Continue to monitor the vitals periodically until help arrives.

CONCLUSION

With the more frequent appearance in the dental office of individuals with underlying medical conditions, the possibility of problems/emergencies occurring will only increase. Obtaining a medical health and a drug history is the first step in identifying the patient likely to develop a medical emergency. With proper training, thorough preparation, and regular practice, the staff of the dental office will be able to provide appropriate medical care should the need arise.

BIBLIOGRAPHY

1. Advance cardiovascular life support (ACLS) provider manual, American Heart Association.
2. Alty CT. Coping with a Medical Crisis. RDH 2002 (Aug).
3. Anderson PE. Effectively handling medical emergencies. Dental Econ. 1989. pp.54-61.
4. Being prepared for office emergencies. The Dental Assistant Update. 1994;3(3): 3-8.
5. Bertold M. Florida mandates defibrillators in dental offices. *http://www.ada.org/prof/resources/pubs/adanews/adanewsarticle.asp?articlesid=1371.* Accessed 2/13.
6. Bird D, Robinson D. Modern Dental Assisting, 9th edn, Elsevier, St Louis, MO. 2009.
7. Curriculum guidelines for management of medical emergencies in dental education. J of Dental Educ. 1981;45(6):379-81.
8. Curriculum guidelines for management of medical emergencies in dental education. J of Dental Educ. 1990;54(6):337-8.
9. European Resuscitation Council 2005 European Resuscitation Council Guidelines Resuscitation.2005;67(1):181-9.
10. Grimes E. Medical Emergencies: Essentials for the Dental Professional. Pearson Education, Upper Saddle River, NJ, 2009.
11. Highlights of the 2010 American Heart Association CPR Guidelines. *http://www.heart.org/idc/groups/heart-public/@wcm/@ecc/documents/downloadable/ucm_317350.pdf.* Accessed 3/9/2011.
12. Malamed. Medical Emergencies, 5th edn, 2000.
13. Malamed SF. Managing medical emergencies. J of the Amer Dental Ass'n. 1993; 124(8):40-51.
14. Resuscitation Council (UK). Standards for Clinical Practice and Training for dental Practitioners and Dental care Professionals in General Dental Practice, July 2006. Revised Dec 2012.
15. Theisen FC, Feil PH, Schultz R. Self-perceptions of skill in office medical emergencies. J of Dental Educ. 1990;54(10):623-5.
16. Wahl MJ. Myths of dental-induced endocarditis. Compend. Cont Educ Dent. Vol.15(9):1100-1119.
17. Wall HK, Beagan BM, O'Neill HJ, Foell KM, Boddie-Willis CL. Addressing stroke signs and symptoms through public education: the Stroke Heroes Act FAST campaign. Prev Chronic Dis 2008;5(2). *http://www.cdc.gov/pcd/issues/2008/apr/07_0214.htm.* Accessed 2/13.

INDEX

Page numbers followed by *f* refer to figure and *t* refer to table

A

Abfraction 158
  causes of 158
  clinical features of 158
Abrasion 100, 156
  causes of 157*t*
  cervical 130
  clinical features of 158
Abrasive tooth surface 102*f*
Absorption 237
Acetaminophen 205, 209, 212, 230
Acid
  etch technique 136
  modified composite 133
Acyclovir 223
Adrenal insufficiency, acute 302
Adult
  and child choking algorithm 289
  basic life support algorithm 288
Agar-agar 141
Airway 294
  obstruction 295
    signs of 294
Alginate 141
Allergic reaction 293
Allergy 8, 16, 196, 298
Alloys, types of 143*t*
Aluminum
  chloride 58
  potassium sulfate 58
  sulfate 58
Alveolar
  crests, condition of 106
  inferior 12
Amalgam 122
  bonding systems 137
  restorations, safety of 125
  properties of 124
Amide 2, 247
  local anesthetics 248
Amlexanox 231
Amorphous calcium
  phosphate 193
Amoxicillin 221, 230, 266
Amphotericin 222
Ampicillin 266
Anaphylactic reaction 293
Anaphylaxis 299
Anemia 258, 268, 269, 309
  deficiency 268
  hemolytic 268
  mild 269
  moderate 269
Anesthesia
  failure of 6
  types of 11
Angina pectoris 293, 306
Angular bone loss 112
Anorexia nervosa 161*t*
Anti-anxiety drugs 47
Antibiotic 205, 215, 231, 267*t*
  associated colitis 216
  topical 220
Anticoagulants, oral 247
Antifungal therapy, topical 222*t*
Antiseptics, topical 226
Antiviral therapy 224*t*
Anxiety
  attack 310
  reduction 292
Aphthasol 231
Arrest, cardiac 293
Arrhythmias 274, 309
Articaine 2, 6, 9, 230
Aspirin 205–207, 212, 230, 243, 276

Asthma 296
  attack 208, 293
Attrited tooth surfaces 103*f*
Attrition 156
  clinical features of 156
Automatic external defibrillator 290
Azithromycin 230, 266

B

Bacterial
  endocarditis 265
  sialadenitis 204
Baseplate wax 149
Beclomethasone dipropionate 215
Benzocaine 230
Benzodiazepines 205, 224, 230, 252
Betamethasone
  sodium phosphate 215
Bisecting angle 80
Bleaching 193, 198
  extracoronal 199
  gels 196
  mechanism 194
Bleeding
  disorders 258, 270
  excessive 208
  internal 208
Blood
  picture, interpretation of 261*t*
  pressure, classification of 259*t*
Bone 108
  assessment tests 260
  loss
    extent of 108
    horizontal 113
    pattern of 108, 111
Breathing 294
Bronchial asthma 280
Bronchospasm 296
Brown fluorosis discolorations 196
Brushing 27
Bruxism 196
Buffering capacity 18
Bulimia nervosa 161
  clinical features of 161
Bupivacaine 2, 6, 9, 230
Burnout, cervical 104*f*

C

Calcium
  channel blockers 252
  hydroxide 126, 134
Calculus 106
Candida
  albicans 216, 222, 240
  associated
    angular cheilitis 222
    denture stomatitis 222
Candidiasis, oral 240
Carbamazepine 252
Carbamide peroxide 194
Carbohydrates 18
Cardiopulmonary resuscitation
  procedures 286, 288
Cardiovascular attack 273
Caries 164
  classification 93
  diagnosis of 26
  presence of 196, 197, 199
  radiographic diagnosis of 90
  types of 21
Cariogenic bacteria, properties of 20
Cast metal restorations 142
Casting gold alloys, types of 143
Cavity lining varnish 139
Cefazolin 266
Cellulitis 204
Cellulose wafers 49
Cementoenamel junction 105
Central nervous system 213, 249
Cephalexin 266
Cephalosporins 230
Cerebrovascular accidents 313
Chest pain 303
Chloral hydrate 250
Chlorhexidine 218, 226, 230
  mouth wash 28
Choline salicylate 206
Cimetidine 252, 252
Ciprofloxacin 221
Clamps 51*t*
Clarithromycin 266
Clavulanic acid 221
Clindamycin 218, 221, 230, 266
Clostridium difficile 216

Codeine 205, 212, 213, 230
Combination bleaching treatment 197
Community periodontal index 41, 42*t*
Complete blood count 260
Complex congenital heart disease 265
Composite resin 137, 138*t*
  restorations 201
Computed tomography 84, 85
Cone beam
  computed tomography 84, 85, 110
Congenital abnormalities 153
Congestive heart failure 275
Conscious sedation 12
Constipation 213
Conventional tomography 84
Coronary artery bypass grafts 275
Corticosteroids 205, 214
Cotton
  rolls 49
  wool appearance 88
Cracked tooth 204

D

Decay, diagnosis of 26*t*
Deciduous tooth restoration 130
Defective
  coronal restorations 196
  enamel formation 199
Denavir 232
Dental
  adhesives 120, 135, 135*t*
  amalgam 120, 123*t*
  anesthetic techniques 10
  caries 16
  cements 147, 148*t*
  considerations 255, 272
  floss 28
  hard tissue damage 198
  health education 38
  management 269, 270, 276, 280, 281, 283
  materials 119, 120*t*
    properties of 121*t*
  nerve block, inferior 11
  panoramic tomogram 82
  pit and fissure sealants 32
  porcelain 145
  procedures 266
  radiography 66
Dentin
  bonding systems 137
  caries 22
  desensitization 167
  discolorations 199
  hypersensitivity 171
    management of 178
Diabetes 306
  assessment tests 259
  blood tests for 262
  mellitus 276
Diabetic ketoacidosis 308
Diphenhydramine 291
Disclosing wax 150
Discolorations 185
  causes of 189*t*
  management of 190
Discolored teeth, treatment of 185
Disease 38
  arrest 38
  nature 268, 276
  suppression 37
Disorders, cardiac 258
Double cord technique 59, 62
Doxycycline 230, 241
Drug
  allergies 258
  in liver disorders 282*t*
  interactions 234
    types of 237
Dry mouth 18, 239
Dysgeusia 240

E

Elastic deformation 120
Electrical stimulation 176
Emergencies
  angina pectoris, cardiac 303
Emesis 213
Enamel
  bonding systems 136
  caries 21
    clinical manifestations of 21
    process 21
  hypoplasia 22, 188

Endemic fluorosis discolorations 197
Endocarditis
  infective 265
  prophylaxis 265–267
Endocrine disorders 258
Endodontic
  procedures 64
  therapy 167, 170
Enzymes 263
Epilepsy 279
Epinephrine 244, 247
  reaction 293
Erbium
  chromium yttrium selenium gallium garnet 60
  yttrium aluminum garnet 60
Erosion 159
  cavities 130
Erythematous hyperplastic candidiasis 222
Erythromycin 221, 230, 245, 252, 253
Esters 2
Ethoxy benzoic acid 134
Etidocaine 2
Ewing sarcoma 88
Extrinsic
  discolorations 189
  sugars 20

F

Facial nerve, blockage of 7
Fainting 309
Ferric sulfate 58
Fibrous dysplasia 88
Fissure
  sealant application 64
  sealing 130
Fits 258
Flora, oral 17
Flow rate 18
Fluconazole 230, 241
Fluocinonide 215
Fluoride
  absorption of 30
  application, topical 64
  delivery, methods of 31
  overdose, treatment of 35
  prenatal 231
  therapy 29
  toxicity 34
  varnish, application of 32
Fluorosis 34, 188
F-speed 79
Fungicide 3
Furcation exposure 112
  types of 113

G

Gardner syndrome 88
Gastrointestinal disorders 258
Gigantiform cementoma 88
Gingival
  abscess 116
  bleeding 106
  diseases 114, 117
  displacement 54
  enlargement 106
  hyperplasia 242
  inflammation 106
  protector 54
  recession 106
  redness 106
  retraction 54
    surgical methods of 59
Glass ionomer cement 129
  types of 130*t*
Glucagon 291
Gold casting alloy 142
Ground glass appearance 88
Gutta-percha points 147

H

Haugejorden and Slack 1975 classification 93
Heart
  attack 304
  failure 306
  transplants 275
Heat hardening treatment 122
Hematoma 7
Hemorrhage, intraoral 239
Heparin 276
Hepatitis 283*t*
High fusing porcelains 146

HIV/AIDS 284
assessment tests 261, 263
Hydrochloric acid 191
Hydrocodone 212
Hydrocortisone hemisuccinate 215
Hydrogen peroxide 193
Hygiene
instructions, oral 41
oral 15, 18
Hygoformic saliva ejectors 48
Hyperglycemia 308
Hyperparathyroidism 88
Hypersensitive teeth 196, 197
Hypersensitivity 204
classification 299
Hypertension 272
Hypertrophic cardiomyopathy 265
Hyperventilation 293, 310, 315
Hypo salivation 18
Hypoglycemia 293, 307, 309, 310
Hypotension, postural 293, 310
Hypothyroidism 278
Hypoxia 309

I

Ibuprofen 205, 209, 212, 230, 246
Idiopathic thrombocytopenic purpura 270
Infection, spread of 7
Infectious diseases 282
Inlay wax 149
In-office bleaching 196
technique 200
Interdental brushes 28
International normalized ratio 261*t*
Interproximal
caries 93
moderate 94
crater 112
Intraoral radiography, digital 110
Intraosseous hemangioma 88
Intrinsic discolorations, causes of 186*t*
Iontophoresis 182
Irrigation devices 32
Ischemic heart disease with angina 273
Isolation, methods of 46
Itraconazole 241

J

Jaundice 258

K

Ketoconazole 241
Kidney disease 258

L

Lamina dura 108
Langerhans cell disease 88
Laser 60, 182
activated bleaching 198
advantages of 61
Lateral periodontal abscess 204
Lidocaine 2, 6, 8, 230
transoral mucosal dental delivery system 232
Light enamel discolorations 197
Lignocaine 6
Lithium 246
Liver
assessment tests 260
disease 8, 258
disorders 281
function tests 264*t*
Local anesthesia 47
interactions 247
Local anesthetic
chemical structure of 5*f*
induced methemoglobinemia 249
molecule with
amide 5*f*
ester link 5*f*
solution 2, 10*t*
Low fusing
impression wax 150
porcelains 146

M

Macroabrasion 191, 192
Magnesium salicylate 206
Mandibular
anterior teeth 54
right quadrant 52
Marcaine 9

Maxillary
anterior teeth 53
left quadrant 53
right quadrant 53
Medium fusing porcelains 146
Mental nerve block 11, 12
Mepivacaine 2, 230
Mercury hygiene precautions 125
Metered dose inhaler 240
Methemoglobinemia 8
Methods of gingival tissue
displacement, classification of 46*t*
Metronidazole 218, 221, 230, 241
Miconazole 223
Microabrasion 191, 192
Mild yellow discolorations 196
Minocycline 241
Monitoring
radiation dose, methods of 70
Morphine 205, 214
Mucosal damage 199
Myocardial infarction 274, 293, 304, 306, 310

N

Nasopalatine 11
Nausea 213
Necrosis 243
Necrotizing
periodontal disease 114, 116, 117
ulcerative
gingivitis 116, 204
periodontitis 116
Needle
fracture 7
stick injury 7
Neutropenia, moderate 285
Nickel and cobalt-chromium alloys 143
Night guard bleaching 195
Nitroglycerin 292
Noncarious tooth surface loss 152
Noncervical carious lesions, clinical features of 164
Non-milk extrinsic sugars 20
Nonopioid analgesics 205, 206*t*
Nonsteroidal anti-inflammatory drugs 205, 246
Nonvital teeth, bleaching of 199
Nursing bottle caries 24
Nystatin 222, 230

O

Obstructive pulmonary disease, chronic 281, 296
Occlusal caries 97
Onion-skin appearance 88
Open interproximal contacts 106
Opioid analgesics 205, 210, 247
Osteitis deformans 88
Osteoma 88
Osteosarcoma 88

P

Pacemakers 275
Paget disease 88
Panoramic radiographs
advantages of 109
disadvantages of 109
Parallax
principles of 82
technique 82
Paralleling technique 80
Penciclovir 232
Penicillin 217, 230
Periapical
cemento-osseous dysplasia 88
periodontitis, acute 204
Pericoronal abscess 116
Pericoronitis 204
Periodontal
abscess 116
diagnosis 117*t*
disease 106, 113, 117
classification of 114*t*
types of 114
endodontic lesions 114
ligament space 108
therapy 167, 170
Periodontitis 114-117, 204
aggressive 114, 115, 117
radiographic diagnosis of 105

Periodontium,
  abscesses of 114, 116, 117
pH of saliva 18
Pit and fissure sealants 139
Plastic deformation 120
Polyether 142
Polysulphides 142
Polyvinyl siloxane,
  polymerization of 56
Porcelain, types of 145*t*
Preventive dentistry 15, 27
Prilocaine 2, 6, 9, 230
Procaine 2, 6
Proliferative periostitis 88
Prophylactic antibiotics 219
Prophylaxis 63
Propoxycaine 248
Prosthetic cardiac valves 265
Pseudomembranous 222
Pulmonary diseases 280
Pulp
  capping 134
  chamber, discolorations of 199
  horns, proximity of 197
Pulpal damage 164
Pulpitis, irreversible 204

R

Rampant caries 23, 24
Recurrent caries 23
Regional infection 8
Removable and fixed
  prosthesis 167, 169
Renal
  assessment tests 259
  disease 279
  failure, chronic 279
  function, blood tests for 262
Resin 137
  ionomer cement 132
  modified glass ionomer 133
Respiratory
  arrest 315
  depression 213
Restoration
  indirect 119
  wear 154
Restorative materials, indirect 144*t*
Retainers/clamps, types of 51
Retraction cords 56, 57*t*
  advantages of 57
  disadvantages of 57
Retraction
  paste 59
  strip 56
Reversible pulpitis 204
Reye's syndrome 208, 209
Rheumatic heart disease 265
Rifampicin 252
Root
  canal filling materials 147
  caries 23
  morphologies 106
  surface caries 130
Rubber dam 49, 56
  clamp 51
    forceps 51
  frame/holder 51
  holder, types of 51
  napkin 52
  punch 51
  set 50
  sheets 50, 50*t*
  template 51

S

Salicylates 205
Saliva 18
  ejectors 48
  ejectors, types of 48
  substitutes 205, 227
Salivary flow rate 18*t*
Seizures 293, 311
Septocaine 9
Severe
  caries 95, 269
  dark discolorations 197
  dentin loss 199
  enamel loss 196, 197
  neutropenia 285
  occlusal caries 97
Sialography 84, 85
Simple restorative procedures 64
Single retraction cord technique 63

Smooth surface caries 22
Sodium
  bicarbonate 193
  perborate 193
Staphylococcus aureus 218
Stephan's curve 19
Steroid
  crisis 310
  topical 215, 215*t*
Sticky wax 150
Stomatitis 242
Streptococcus
  mutans 16, 17, 21, 24
  salivarius 21
Stroke 273, 313
Strontium chloride 180
Subtraction radiography, digital 110
Sudden cardiac arrest 306
Sugars, classification of 20*t*
Sunburst radioopacities 88
Superficial enamel discolorations 196, 199
Syncope 293, 309
  types of 309*t*
Systemic fluoride methods 31

T

Temporomandibular
  imaging 84, 85
  joints 82
Tetracycline 219, 230, 241
  discolorations, mild 197
  staining classification 188*t*
Theophylline 246
Thermoluminescent dosimeters 73
Tongue 45
  depressors 47
  guards 47
Tooth
  discoloration 242
  mobility 106
  wear 155
    causes of 163*t*
    types of 155
Toothpastes, constituents of 29*t*
Total joint replacements 267
Traditional glass ionomer 126
Transient ischemic attack 313
Trendelenburg position 311
Triamcinolone
  acetonide 215
  mouthwash 215
Triazoles 223
Trismus 7
Tuberculosis 281

U

Ulceration, oral 243
Urinary retention 213
Use of local anesthetics 14
  during pregnancy 14
  in children 14

V

Vasoconstrictors 2, 57
Vasodepressor 309
Verbal rating scale 177*t*
Vertical bone
  defect 113
  loss 112
Viral hepatitis 283
Visual analogue scale 176, 177
Volume tomography, digital 111
Water fluoridation 33
Waxed dental floss 52
Wear, types of 153
White
  carious spot 22
  gold 143
  spot lesion 21

W

Wooden wedges 56

X

Xerostomia 18, 239
Xylitol 28

Z

Zinc
  oxide eugenol 126, 133
  phosphate cement 126
  polycarboxylate cement 126, 128